Clinical Medicine for Optometrists

Clinical Medicine for Optometrists

EDITORS

DAVID M. SHEIN, MD

Primary Care Physician, Wellesley Internal Medicine
Wellesley, Massachusetts
Physician, Department of Medicine, Mount Auburn Hospital
Cambridge, Massachusetts
Assistant Professor in Medicine, Harvard Medical School
Adjunct Associate Professor of Medicine,
New England College of Optometry
Boston, Massachusetts

RACHEL C. DRUCKENBROD, OD, FAAO

Attending Optometrist, VA Boston Healthcare System
Adjunct Assistant Professor of Optometry,
New England College of Optometry
Boston, Massachusetts

ASSOCIATE EDITOR

THOMAS F. FREDDO, OD, PHD, FAAO

Professor of Ophthalmology, Pathology, Anatomy and Neurobiology
(Emeritus)
Former Director of the Eye Pathology Laboratory, Boston University
School of Medicine
Boston, Massachusetts
Professor, MCP Health Sciences University
Worcester, Massachusetts

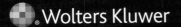 Wolters Kluwer

Philadelphia • Baltimore • New York • London
Buenos Aires • Hong Kong • Sydney • Tokyo

Acquisitions Editor: Chris Teja
Development Editor: Eric McDermott
Editorial Coordinator: Vinoth Ezhumalai
Marketing Manager: Kristin Ciotto
Production Project Manager: Sadie Buckallew
Manager, Graphic Arts & Design: Stephen Druding
Manufacturing Coordinator: Beth Welsh
Prepress Vendor: TNQ Technologies

9 8 7 6 5 4 3 2 1

Printed in China

Library of Congress Cataloging-in-Publication

ISBN-13: 978-1-975146-51-1

Cataloging in Publication data available on request from publisher.

shop.lww.com

This book honors the memory of my late father, Simra E. Shein, MD, a skilled surgeon, outstanding teacher, caring parent, and upstanding member of the community. My practice of medicine is influenced daily by his teaching of grace, humility, integrity, kindness, and skill.
—DMS

To those who have taught me the importance and fulfillment of optometric practice marked by compassion, collaboration, medical prowess, academic engagement, and sustained curiosity.
—RCD

Contributors

Jack L. Arbiser, MD, PhD
Thomas J. Lawley Professor of Dermatology
Department of Dermatology
Emory University School of Medicine
Winship Cancer Institute
Atlanta Veterans Administration Health Center
Atlanta, Georgia

Vanessa S. Cooper, MD
Clinical Fellow, Headache Medicine
Department of Neurology
Yale School of Medicine
New Haven, Connecticut

Jeffrey J. Dewey, MD
Assistant Professor
Department of Neurology
Yale School of Medicine
Yale New Haven Hospital
New Haven, Connecticut

Daniel T. Ginat, MD, MS
Associate Professor
Department of Radiology
University of Chicago
Chicago, Illinois

Emily R. Humphreys, OD, FAAO
Assistant Clinical Professor of Optometry
The New England College of Optometry
Boston, Massachusetts
Attending Optometrist, Lynn Community Health
    Center
Lynn, Massachusetts

Brianna M. Jones, MD
Resident Physician
Department of Radiation Oncology
Mount Sinai Health System
New York, New York

Gene Muise, RPh, MSc
Affiliate Assistant Professor
Bouvé College of Health Science School of Pharmacy
Northeastern University
Boston, Massachusetts

Emily E. Purcell, MD
Fellow Physician
Department of Rheumatology
University of Pennsylvania
Philadelphia, Pennsylvania

Kenneth E. Rosenzweig, MD
Chair and Professor
Department of Radiation Oncology
Icahn School of Medicine at Mount Sinai
System Chair
Department of Radiation Oncology
Mount Sinai Health System
New York, New York

Shiv T. Sehra, MBBS
Assistant Professor
Department of Medicine
Harvard Medical School
Boston, Massachusetts Chief
Division of Rheumatology
Program Director
Internal Medicine Residency
Mount Auburn Hospital
Cambridge, Massachusetts

Richard A. Serrao, MD
Clinical Associate Professor
Department of Medicine
Boston University School of Medicine
Lecturer on Medicine
Department of Medicine
Harvard Medical School
Attending Physician- Infectious Diseases
Department of Medicine
VA Boston Healthcare System
Boston, Massachusetts

Courtney E. Stull, MD
Fellow Physician
Department of Rheumatology
University of Pennsylvania
Hospital of the University of Pennsylvania
Philadelphia, Pennsylvania

Arti Tewari, MD
Resident
Department of Medicine
Mount Auburn Hospital
Cambridge, Massachusetts

Paola Andrea Olaya Urrea, MD
Department of Dermatology
Emory University School of Medicine
Atlanta, Georgia

Tanya G. Weinstock, MD
Instructor of Medicine
Harvard Medical School
Boston, Massachusetts
Medical Director
Division of Pulmonary and Critical Care Medicine
Mount Auburn Hospital
Cambridge, Massachusetts

Contents

CHAPTER 3: Lipid Disorders, Atherosclerosis, Cardiovascular Diseases, and Cardiac Testing   47

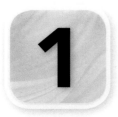

1

Evidence-Based Medicine and the Medical Literature
Principles of Laboratory Investigation

David M. Shein and Rachel C. Druckenbrod

LEARNING OBJECTIVES

We begin this first chapter by thinking about the power in the knowledge base that has enabled the fast pace of medical progress over the last century. From antibiotics isolated from mold that cure potentially fatal infections to the use of magnets for medical imaging, modern medicine has used observations as key building blocks. As clinicians, we rely on a vast, evolving reservoir of information to improve our clinical decisions. The effective clinician applies observation, from symptoms in history to findings on examination, to this growing knowledge base. Here, we present questions about how to include, interpret, and assess the relevancy of information in our daily practices. Section 1 provides an overview of medical literature analysis with practical examples. Section 2 covers principles of laboratory testing.

KEY CONCEPTS

Section 1: Analysis of Medical Literature
Part 1: Study design
   Study hypothesis
   Statistical significance
      Confidence interval and *P*-value
      Absolute and relative risk
      Number needed to treat
   Size of the effect
   Relevance to clinical practice

Part 2: Clinical examples
Section 2: Principles of Laboratory Testing
Reporting of laboratory values
   Sensitivity and specificity
   False positives and false negatives
Influential factors on laboratory test results
Primary and secondary prevention

SECTION 1: THE ANALYSIS OF MEDICAL LITERATURE
PART 1

When considering a research publication or a medical report, important factors to consider include:

- Study design
- Hypothesis
- Significance
- Size of the effect
- Relevance to clinical practice

STUDY DESIGN

Research publications encompass a range of trial types, and each brings its own strengths and limitations to the clinician in practice. Here we cover several commonly encountered study designs in the medical literature:

- Randomized controlled trial
- Cohort study
- Case-control study
- Meta-analysis
- Records review
- Case report

The following section brings important and representative studies of each type to simultaneously demonstrate the study type as well as to convey the important findings of the individual studies. The review of these studies also incorporates the statistical reporting of significance and determination of effect size covered above.

Randomized controlled trials (RCTs) are generally considered the gold standard of medical research, yet they are the most complex to perform and often costly as well. Despite their robust nature, in some situations, it may not be feasible or even ethical to conduct a RCT. When that is the case, researchers may develop a hypothesis that can be explored with data presently available for analysis, with an observational study.

In the prospective RCT, individuals are assigned randomly to one or more interventions or to a placebo group when present. Randomization creates balanced groups in each arm of the study, free of external influences that could drive different intervention groups to disproportionately experience certain effects. The groups are then monitored prospectively, typically with periodic contact from the researchers as the study progresses. Data may also be collected and monitored during the study.

In contrast to the prospective RCT, observational studies comprise individuals already engaged with the factors under study. External influences that relate to the factors being investigated may also influence the variables under study in unexpected ways. These external influences may actually be the cause of the observed outcome—and not the variable under study. An example could be a study comparing health impacts in cigarette smokers versus nonsmokers. Because it would be neither ethical nor practical to randomize individuals to smoke cigarettes versus placebo, the researchers would instead follow existing groups of smokers and nonsmokers over time. While any differences in outcomes that are observed could be due to smoking, it may also be that factors that influence the rate of tobacco smoking in a population (eg, overall less healthy lifestyle, socioeconomic status, educational attainment) and not the smoking itself that caused the results found in the study. Thus, one can see the benefit of the RCT, where the random assignment of the study groups avoids these pitfalls, termed bias and confounding, that might occur in an observational study.

The **cohort study** and **case-control study** are encountered commonly in the medical literature, often in situations when randomized trials are not possible. These include instances where data worthy of analysis presently exist, and the time frame required for a prospective trial would miss the chance to inform current practice. Cost may also be a factor as prospective randomized trials can be costly. Cohort and case-control studies can analyze data retrospectively by using currently available data in order to assess for relationships between disease and particular exposures. Cohort study design identifies a study group exposed to a particular factor and a control group not exposed to the factor and compares disease incidences between these two groups. Case-control studies are similar but use a slightly different sampling strategy: two groups—one with and one without the condition in question—are first identified and then prior exposures are compared between the groups. Both study types can indicate an association between disease and exposure, but are unable to conclusively determine cause-effect relationships.

Meta-analyses pool data from separate but similar research studies in order to summarize results and reach a consensus conclusion. By pooling data from several smaller studies (such as several RCTs), the meta-analysis achieves increased power for detection of statistically significant differences or associations between groups. Where small studies fail to detect statistical (or clinical) significance, meta-analyses can have success. Even studies that have variable research methods or different study populations may be acceptably subjected to meta-analysis, though these discrepancies can also contribute to conclusion bias. Pooled estimates determined by meta-analyses should be interpreted with caution and are criticized when biologic or statistical evidence suggests that the individual studies actually measured different factors.[1] Nonetheless, meta-analyses are powerful tools that utilize existing data and can lead to clear and guiding conclusions with impacts on clinical practice.

The **records review** can analyze trends and other patterns across an entire population. Due to the prevalence of electronic medical records and large insurance data sets (such as Medicare), it is now possible to analyze data on thousands or even millions of individuals to look for trends across one or multiple measures of healthcare delivery or outcomes. Unlike cohort or case-control studies, which compare outcomes by individuals, outcomes from record reviews are typically assessed across a population at different time points.

Case reports are straightforward and are frequently used in clinical practice, including settings such as bedside rounds and morbidity and mortality (M&M) rounds. These reports involve presenting a single or a few cases to inform the medical and scientific communities. Because they involve a limited number of cases and are not planned studies, case reports are the least robust of the study designs. Yet case reports are useful in several ways. For example, they can alert a public health authority when an increase in a communicable disease is reported, such as during influenza season or with a novel pathogen such as the 2019 coronavirus and COVID-19 illness. Hospitals use case reports of adverse outcomes to turn attention to necessary improvements in care delivery. Reports can educate the scientific community about a rare condition, and unexplained clinical findings may be the harbinger of a new disease. Rare adverse effects of newer drugs often come to light through case reports. Case reports also identify potentially important new areas of study that lead to further analysis via more robust trials.

STUDY HYPOTHESIS

Once the reader has considered the study design, the next step is to understand the *study hypothesis*. The hypothesis may be one of benefit (eg, a new medication), one of harm (eg, an environmental toxin), or the null hypothesis (when factors under study are expected not to have an impact). The hypothesis could be a novel concept, which is being newly explored in this trial; or prior work may have suggested the hypothesis, which is now being explored in a larger population or a subgroup to better understand the effect. It is important to ask the question, "Have the investigators addressed the original study hypothesis?" Robust study design involves one or more well-defined questions with associated predetermined hypotheses; additional questions and answers that arise during the course of the study or during analysis of the data should be regarded as secondary, and their validity is typically less robust.

SIGNIFICANCE

Turning next to the study results, any finding is either due to the effect of the factors under study or due to chance. The question of chance versus actual effect is addressed by determining statistical *significance*, which predicts the probability of an actual effect versus randomness or chance determining the outcome. Two of the more common methods for reporting statistical significance include the *P*-value and the confidence interval. The **P-value** describes the result of a statistical calculation that considers the likelihood that chance resulted in the outcome observed. A *P*-value of 0.05 or less (≤ 0.05) is considered significant, meaning it is so unlikely to be due to chance that the result is generally accepted as true in the scientific community (specifically, there is a 95% chance the result is true, and a 5% chance the result is due to random chance). Lower numbers (eg, $P = .01$) are even stronger from a statistical perspective. A *P*-value slightly higher than 0.05 may be described as showing a *trend*. A trend has a higher likelihood of being due to chance and is generally not considered significant, though it may serve as a hypothesis for further study.

The **confidence interval (CI)** describes a range for which an effect is likely based upon the data analyzed. It represents the range of values that are likely to occur if the same study is repeated by independent researchers on similar populations or data sets. The bounds of the interval (upper and lower numbers in the CI) typically describe with predefined confidence (usually 95% confidence) the **relative risk** (RR) of an outcome. The outcome may be more or less likely in the group under study. Mathematically, RR is a ratio calculated by dividing the probability of an outcome in an intervention group under study (eg, exposed to a certain risk or treated with an intervention) by that in a comparison group under study (eg, placebo, an alternate treatment, or unexposed). An RR below 1.0 indicates the outcome is less likely and subtracting the RR from 1.0 and then multiplying by 100 will yield a percentage reduction. For example, RR = 0.75 indicates an outcome 25% less likely ($1.0 - 0.75 \times 100\%$). An RR above 1.0 indicates the hypothesis is more likely and subtracting 1.0 from the RR and then multiplying by 100 will yield the percentage increase. For example, RR = 1.25 indicates an outcome 25% more likely ($1.25 - 1.0 \times 100\%$). An RR of 1.0 represents a null effect, since this indicates equal probabilities in outcomes between the groups (a ratio of 1.0). When the bounds of the CI associated with an RR value cross (contain) the number 1.0, the results are not considered significant, as this situation indicates that one end of the CI range (RR greater than 1.0) shows an increase in risk of the outcome, and on the other end (RR less than 1.0) there is a decrease in the outcome risk. Sometimes, a statistical analysis involves looking at *absolute differences* between groups rather than risk (for example, the difference in blood glucose level between groups prescribed different diabetes medications under study). CIs associated with a reported difference value are considered statistically significant only if the interval does not cross or contain zero, since an interval containing zero in this scenario indicates there is no difference in outcomes between the groups.

SIZE OF THE EFFECT

When considering reported risk values in the literature, it is important to distinguish between **relative risk** (or risk ratio) and **absolute risk**. Consider the data presented in **BOX 1.1**, reporting the impacts of statin therapy on various cardiovascular outcomes (Chapter 3). The study reported a risk ratio of

---

Box 1.1   Confidence Interval (CI), Relative Risk (RR), Absolute Risk, and Number Needed to Treat (NNT)

Consider statin treatment for cholesterol-lowering. The US Preventive Services Task Force reviewed published data to determine the benefits and risks for patients without known cardiovascular disease who consider taking a statin drug.

- Statin therapy decreased all-cause mortality:
  - Risk ratio, 0.86 (95% CI, 0.80-0.93)
  - Absolute risk difference −0.40% (95% CI, −0.64% to −0.17%)
- Statin use was not associated with an increased risk of serious adverse events:
  - RR, 0.99 (95% CI, 0.94-1.04)
- In one trial evaluating patients with multiple cardiovascular risk factors, NNT to prevent one cardiovascular event over ~2 years:
  - 94 in people younger than 70 years
  - 62 in people aged 70 years and older

Evidence Summary: Statins for Prevention of Cardiovascular Disease in Adults. Statin Use for the Primary Prevention of Cardiovascular Disease in Adults. Preventive Medication. U.S. Preventive Services Task Force; 2019. Available at https://www.uspreventiveservicestaskforce.org/Page/Document/evidence-summary-statins/statin-use-in-adults-preventive-medication1.

---

all-cause mortality of 0.86 among patients treated with statins, indicating a 14% (1.0−0.86 × 100%) lower risk in mortality when patients were treated with a statin versus when not treated with a statin. A reduction in RR of 14% seems impressive. However, consider the absolute risk difference. Absolute risk reflects the baseline risk of a given outcome and is calculated by subtracting the rate of an outcome among the treated group from the rate of an outcome among the control group. In the data presented in **BOX 1.1**, the absolute risk reduction in all-cause mortality was only 0.4%, a much smaller number than the 14% reported relative reduction in risk. This is because the actual number of people who have a heart attack or other cardiovascular event in the time frame under evaluation is relatively small at baseline, even without statin treatment. The relative reduction in risk benefits only the small fraction of the population estimated to actually have a cardiovascular event in this time frame. Thus, to interpret the magnitude of a study's conclusions regarding risk, one must know whether the authors report RR or absolute risk.

Number needed to treat (NNT) and number needed to harm (NNH) are useful ways to distill the complexity of relative and absolute risk into real numbers. NNT is defined as the number of patients needed to treat in order to prevent one adverse outcome. NNH reflects the number of people treated for one adverse event to manifest. In the study in **BOX 1.1**, patients with higher risk for a cardiovascular event due to an elevated C-reactive protein level were given statin treatment to prevent cardiovascular events[2] (Chapter 3). Over the nearly 2-year duration of the study, 94 people younger than 70 years had to take a statin to prevent one cardiovascular event (an NNT of 94). Thus, 93 of those patients who paid for their medication and remembered to take it every day experienced no benefit. One person benefited and did not have a cardiovascular event meeting the study's end point (heart attack, stroke, heart disease hospitalization, coronary artery procedure, or cardiac death). For patients aged 70 and over, the NNT was lower at 62. Thus, when counseling a patient with a high C-reactive protein level on the potential benefit from statin therapy, providers can more accurately predict the range of benefit for patients in different age groups while patients can better integrate this understanding into their preferences. A patient who is very fearful of having a cardiovascular event may want to take any relatively safe therapy. Others may prefer not to take medications unless a potential benefit is more likely than 1 in 94. In addition, patient baseline characteristics—in this case, age—can be used to provide a more accurate reference for patients to consider. It is important to understand that there is no universally acceptable NNT threshold; factors such as disease severity, treatment cost, risks, and individual patient perception of these factors play into the interpretation of NNT.

RELEVANCE TO CLINICAL PRACTICE

Relevance to clinical practice is important to consider both in terms of clinical significance and relevance to a population. Study conclusions may reach statistical significance, but not have meaningful clinical impacts. For example, consider a study comparing the impacts of two topical glaucoma medications on intraocular pressure, reporting that Drug A lowers eye pressure by 25% more than Drug B ($P = .001$). Before determining that Drug A is superior to Drug B for clinical practice, one important consideration is how much Drug A actually lowers eye pressure. There may be no clinically meaningful difference between the drugs for most glaucoma patients if Drug A achieves only 1 mmHg more pressure reduction than Drug B. However, for a patient with advanced glaucoma under strict intraocular pressure control, a clinician may find it worthwhile to choose Drug A over Drug B based on these study results (see below). Next, how does the population in the study compare to real-world populations, including patients in your practice? Can you apply the results of the study to your own population? Consider factors including gender, race, age, and socioeconomic status when extrapolating study results to patients for whom you provide care.[3] Consider the factors that your patient has in common with the study population that may predict similar outcomes for your patient. Also consider any differences that may drive a different outcome. Many existing studies of cardiovascular interventions were performed in middle-aged men. Later research focusing on women uncovered a different pattern of angina symptoms compared to men (Chapter 3). Individuals in other age groups may also respond differently, thus clinicians need to consider whether they can reach the same conclusions.

PART 2: CLINICAL EXAMPLES
THE WOMEN'S HEALTH INITIATIVE: A RANDOMIZED CONTROLLED TRIAL

In 1993, researchers began recruiting women to participate in the Women's Health Initiative,[4] an RCT of 16,608 women to evaluate multiple factors in the health of women after menopause. At that time, observational studies determined that after menopause, women who took estrogen and progestin had a lower risk of coronary heart disease (Chapter 3). Prior studies also indicated a reduced risk of bone density loss from taking estrogens, which could help protect against osteoporosis-related fracture risks (Chapter 6). However, observational data also suggested there was a small increase in the risk of breast cancer with estrogen supplementation. In aggregate, it was thought that postmenopausal therapy would prove beneficial and thus, prior to the Women's Health Initiative, physicians commonly recommend estrogen and progestin treatment for several years after menopause.[5]

The Women's Health Initiative, a large randomized, placebo-controlled trial to compare estrogen plus progestin versus placebo, presented results that fundamentally changed clinical practice. The trial was stopped early after 5.2 years of follow-up (8.5 years of follow-up was planned) due to a statistically significant increase in the risk of breast cancer in the estrogen plus progestin group as compared to placebo. In addition, women taking estrogen plus progestin had a higher risk of coronary heart disease (estrogen plus progestin was not protective), stroke, and pulmonary embolism. Compared with placebo, estrogen plus progestin was protective against colorectal cancer and hip fracture. There was no statistically significant impact on endometrial (uterine) cancer or death due to other causes.

To understand how the study results impacted clinical practice, begin by evaluating the *hypothesis*. The study goal was:

"To assess the major health benefits and risks of the most commonly used combined hormone preparation in the United States."

Two treatment arms were reported—estrogen plus progestin and placebo. Because less robust observational data suggested that estrogen plus progestin prescribed to women at the time of menopause would reduce the risk of coronary heart disease, this was evaluated as the primary benefit in the study with breast cancer risk as the primary adverse outcome. Secondary outcomes were also reported including risk of hip fracture, stroke, pulmonary embolism, endometrial cancer, colorectal cancer, and death due to other causes. Thus, the goal was to evaluate these health outcomes relative to placebo.

Results were reported as a hazard ratio (HR), similar to RR considering the timing of the events over the course of the study. The HR can reflect benefit (HR less than 1.00), harm (HR greater than 1.00), or null (HR = 1.00). Because study results can be influenced by chance, the HR is reported with a 95% CI indicating the range where the true result is likely to fall with 95% likelihood. As explained above, a CI that crosses 1.00 indicates that both benefit and harm are possible outcomes, and the results would therefore not be statistically significant. **TABLE 1.1** displays the HR for several outcomes from the Women's Health Initiative data with associated CIs.

The focus here will be on a subset of the results to highlight the statistical analysis and effect size. HR for coronary heart disease in **TABLE 1.1** is 1.29, indicating a 29% ($1.29 - 1.0 \times 100\%$) higher rate of heart disease in women taking estrogen plus progestin. The CI of 1.02 to 1.63 indicates that, with 95% confidence, the rate of coronary heart disease is higher in women taking this medication combination. Because the results at both ends of the range indicate an increase in risk, the HR result is statistically significant. Having determined a significant increase in risk, the next consideration is how this will impact a population taking this therapy, or the size of the effect. If coronary heart disease is a rare event, a 29% increase in the rate of the event may not affect that many individuals. On the other hand, if coronary heart disease occurs frequently, then a 29% increase may have a substantial effect on a population. The researchers made this task easy for readers here as they reported the *absolute excess risks* associated with estrogen plus progestin therapy per 10,000 person-years. For coronary heart disease, this risk was 7 more events.

Hip fracture rates were lower in the treatment group with an HR of 0.66, representing a 34% reduction in the rate of fractures. The CI indicates statistical significance with both upper and lower

TABLE 1.1   Key Outcomes of Statistical Significance From the Women's Health Initiative

Outcome	Hazard Ratio (HR)	Confidence Interval (CI)
Coronary heart disease	1.29	(1.02-1.63)
Breast cancer	1.26	(1.00-1.59)
Stroke	1.41	(1.07-1.85)
Pulmonary embolism	2.13	(1.39-3.25)
Colorectal cancer	0.63	(0.43-0.92)
Endometrial cancer	0.83	(0.47-1.47)
Hip fracture	0.66	(0.45-0.98)

bounds of the range (0.45-0.98) falling under 1.0. However, because the overall rate of hip fractures in the population under study was lower than the rate of coronary heart disease, this benefit of 34% reduction translated to 5 fewer hip fractures per 10,000 person-years for women taking estrogen plus progestin versus women not taking this treatment. Thus, in a similar population of women taking estrogen-progestin, more women would experience the harm of a cardiovascular event than protection from hip fracture.

HR for endometrial cancer is 0.83, or a 17% ($1.00 - 0.83 \times 100\%$) lower rate for this event, indicating that the effect of estrogen plus progestin may be protective. However, the CI of 0.47 to 1.47 indicates a range of statistically likely outcomes ranging from benefit (0.47) to harm (1.47) with 95% confidence. Thus, the result is not statistically significant, and the null hypothesis applies (no impact on endometrial cancer).

Physicians reading this study in 2002 needed to consider how the results would impact clinical practice. One important consideration is the population under study and how this translates to each individual patient in the practice. In this situation, as a study of postmenopausal treatments, the population under study and the population with clinical impact were female. Considerations including age, ethnicity, health status, comorbidities, and other risks are important. In the Women's Health Initiative, race/ethnicity was reported as follows: 84% of participants were white, 7.1% black, 5.1% Hispanic, 0.4% American Indian, and 2.1% Asian/Pacific Islander. For an individual patient in a racial or ethnic group not well represented by the study population, one could ask whether outcomes could be different due to factors not accounted for by the statistical analysis. Researchers addressed these questions with additional analysis to look at factors including race/ethnicity, diabetes, smoking status, and aspirin use. This did not reveal any interactions that would have impacted the outcomes for these subpopulations.

The Women's Health Initiative updated clinical knowledge on the impacts of estrogen plus progestin use in postmenopausal women. The findings resulted in substantial changes to medical practice, as oral estrogen-progestin prescriptions for postmenopausal women decreased dramatically after publication in 2002.[6] This was possible due to the randomized nature of the study and the large population that brought statistical power to the analysis.

Once-Daily Valacyclovir to Reduce the Risk of Transmission of Genital Herpes: A Randomized Controlled Trial

Herpes simplex virus causes a chronic infection (Chapter 9). The immune system typically suppresses the virus and prevents replication. A symptomatic outbreak occurs when the virus escapes immune control and actively replicates causing both symptoms and risk for transmission to uninfected people. When a person with herpes simplex is asymptomatic, there are two possible clinical scenarios: full viral suppression, in which case they are not infectious; or subclinical replication, during which time herpes simplex can be transmitted to close contacts despite the lack of symptoms. Herpes simplex type 2 (HSV-2) typically causes genital infections which are transmitted through sexual contact either during active outbreaks or with subclinical viral replication. HSV-2 is fairly prevalent in the United States with more than one-fifth of American adults aged 40 to 49[7] infected and over 700,000 new cases annually.[8]

In 2004, researchers published the results of a study using the antiviral valacyclovir to suppress viral replication and lower the risk of transmission.[9] This was an 8-month study of serologically discordant couples (one member had herpes antibodies indicative of infection and the other partner was susceptible). The antibody-positive member of the couple was given either valacyclovir or placebo for 8 months, and the status of the seronegative partner was evaluated during and after the trial. Results were reported as HRs with 95% CIs and P-values for statistical significance. Further evaluation was done to report the NNT.

Focusing on the results for acquiring an HSV-2 infection, the HR of time for the uninfected partner to acquire HSV-2 was 0.52, with a 95% CI of 0.27 to 0.99. The P-value was 0.04. Since the 95% CI was entirely less than 1.00 (indicating benefit) and the P-value was below 0.05, these results are statistically significant for decreasing the risk of HSV-2 acquisition over the 8-month study when the HSV-positive partner of an HSV-negative individual took daily valacyclovir. The reduction in risk was 48% ($1.00-0.52 \times 100\%$) when the partner with HSV-2 infection took valacyclovir. Further analysis revealed that the NNT is 38, indicating that 38 people with HSV-2 and a seronegative partner would need to be treated for 8 months to prevent one susceptible partner from acquiring HSV-2. Here again, NNT is a concept that is more easily communicated and better understood by patients who need to make a decision on whether they want to take this medication.

The randomized nature of the study as well as the concept of treating the asymptomatic seropositive partner has enabled clinicians to share this information with patients who often opt for long-term treatment. One limitation of this study is the relatively short time frame of 8 months. Although there was a reduction in transmission of close to 50% in the 8-month time frame, it is unknown how long this benefit would persist in a longer-term relationship between HSV-discordant partners.

A Population-Based Study of Measles, Mumps, and Rubella Vaccination and Autism: A Cohort Study

In 2002, researchers published the results of a retrospective analysis of MMR (measles, mumps, and rubella) vaccination to analyze the safety of the vaccine on long-term outcomes.[10] In this situation, randomization to vaccine versus placebo would not have been ethical. The length of time for a prospective study to gather these data would have been substantial and would have resulted in a long delay in the availability of information to inform doctors and patients. Data from the prior decade were available for retrospective analysis to inform current practice, however, making this an appropriate methodology.

Despite an excellent overall safety profile and marked decreases in the incidence of vaccine-preventable illnesses and their complications, there have been concerns about the safety of MMR. Given the close timing of MMR vaccination in children to the age when autism is often diagnosed, MMR has been investigated as a possible cause of autism. There are also biological associations of central nervous involvement with wild-type virus that triggered a concern for central nervous system involvement with the live virus vaccine. By taking advantage of comprehensive records available in Denmark, researchers cross-referenced the civil registry that tracked all live births with comprehensive health records for vaccination status and diagnoses of autism. This retrospective study looked at data recorded between January 1991 and December 1998 and followed up two groups or cohorts—children who were vaccinated for MMR and those who were not.

A total of 537,303 children were identified in this registry, 82% (440,655) of whom received the MMR vaccine. A total of 758 children in the cohort were diagnosed with autism or autistic spectrum disorders. Comparing the rate of autism and autistic spectrum disorders in the vaccinated versus unvaccinated groups, researchers found the following RR for autism:

$$0.92 \text{ (95\% CI 0.68-1.24)}$$

The upper and lower bounds of the CI cross 1.00 indicating that there is no statistical correlation. Thus, the hypothesized link between MMR vaccine and autism and autistic spectrum disorders is not realized statistically. Based upon this study in Danish children, readers can see solid evidence that there is no link between the MMR vaccine and autism.

A strength of this study is that it included a large and comprehensive cohort—all children born in Denmark. This eliminated possible bias from studying a subset of patients, for example, only those children followed in one or a limited number of geographic areas of a country. The comprehensive nature of the Danish healthcare system also limited possible bias that could occur because of missing data on autism and autistic spectrum disorders, diagnoses that one might not see in countries with multiple health systems, and limited access to all information. Researchers obtained 9 years of vaccine data and follow-up, resulting in a robust length of time for analysis. One potential limitation of this nonrandomized trial is whether an undetermined difference in the subset of children who were unvaccinated had an increased risk of autism and autistic spectrum disorders. This scenario is unlikely, and a robust retrospective study like this offers a high degree of reassurance about the safety of the MMR vaccine.

Meta-Analysis of Randomized Controlled Trials Comparing Latanoprost with Timolol in the Treatment of Patients with Open Angle Glaucoma or Ocular Hypertension

In 1978, the FDA approved Merck's Timoptic (timolol 0.5%), and the modern age of glaucoma pharmacotherapy began.[11] Topical ophthalmic beta-blockers provided excellent intraocular pressure (IOP)-lowering ability with only twice-daily dosing and avoided the undesirable side effects of pilocarpine (miosis/myopia) and epinephrine (conjunctival discoloration). For 20 years, timolol remained first-line therapy for medical glaucoma management, despite its risk for cardiac and pulmonary side effects in a minority of susceptible patients (eg, bradycardia, arrhythmia, and bronchoconstriction)[12] (Chapters 2 and 14). In the early 1990s, Pharmacia (later Pfizer) developed the first prostaglandin analogue, Xalatan (0.005% latanoprost). Xalatan offered no worrisome systemic side effects and seemed to have superior IOP-lowering action to Timoptic and to other modern glaucoma medications (eg, dorzolamide, a carbonic anhydrase inhibitor, and brimonidine, an alpha-adrenergic agonist). The replacement of timolol by latanoprost as a first-line glaucoma medication seemed promising.

In 2001, researchers performed a meta-analysis to formally compare the efficacy and side effect profiles of timolol and latanoprost among patients with primary open-angle glaucoma or ocular hypertension.[13] They performed an extensive search of electronic databases for reports of RCTs of latanoprost versus timolol published between 1966 and the end of July 2000. After filtering out RCTs that did not meet the specified inclusion criteria for the meta-analysis, they included 11 RCTs in the pool. Two researchers independently recorded study data such as trial design, length of study, number of subjects, patient age, type of glaucoma, baseline IOP, endpoint IOP, and medication side effects (including hyperemia, conjunctivitis, increased iris pigmentation, bradycardia, hypotension, and headache). Statistical analysis was performed to calculate mean IOP reduction and then differences in IOP reduction between treatment groups for each included RCT. RR and NNH with 95% CIs were determined for adverse effects.

A total of 1256 patients were included across the 11 RCTs. In all trials, patients received two bottles labeled morning or evening. For the timolol group, both bottles contained timolol, and for the latanoprost group, only one bottle contained the drug and the other a placebo. The difference in percent IOP reduction between timolol and latanoprost was analyzed for time periods 1 week, 1 month, 3 months, 6 months, and 12 months. Slightly different numbers of trials were available for pooled analysis at the various time points; for example, three trials were available for 1-week analysis, five trials were available for 3-month analysis, and only one trial was available for 12-month analysis (a study limitation). Both drugs significantly lowered IOP at all time points versus baseline. However, for all time points except 12 months, pooled analysis of the RCTs showed that percent IOP reduction was significantly greater for latanoprost than for timolol (range 4%-7% greater reduction). As an example, at 3 months timolol lowered IOP by $26.9 \pm 3.4\%$ while latanoprost lowered IOP by $31.2 \pm 2.3\%$. The difference in IOP reduction between timolol and latanoprost at 3 months was 5.0%

(95% CI 2.8-7.3, $P < .001$). The CI is significant here since the interval does not contain zero (indicating a non-zero difference between the groups), and the P-value is significant since it is less than 0.05 (**FIGURE 1.1**).

In terms of adverse effects, the data showed that patients taking latanoprost were at twice the risk for hyperemia compared with timolol (RR = 2.20, 95% CI 1.33-3.65). The NNH for hyperemia due to latanoprost was 21 (95% CI 14-42), indicating that (on average) treating 21 patients with latanoprost will lead to one additional patient developing symptomatic hyperemia. Additionally, no patients taking timolol developed iris pigmentation, while 4.39% of patients taking latanoprost had symptomatic darkening of the iris. Four of the 11 RCTs analyzed systemic adverse effects from timolol versus

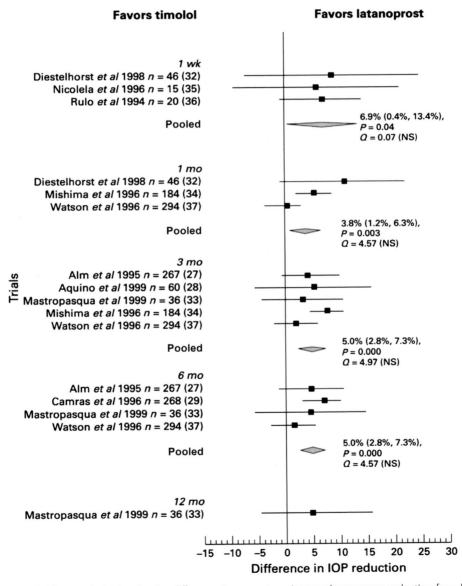

FIGURE 1.1 Meta-analysis data for the difference in percentage intraocular pressure reduction from baseline between latanoprost and timolol (mean difference and associated 95% CI). CI, confidence interval; IOP, intraocular pressure. (Zhang WY, Wan Po AL, Dua HS, Azuara-Blanco A. Meta-analysis of randomised controlled trials comparing latanoprost with timolol in the treatment of patient with open angle glaucoma or ocular hypertension. *Br J Ophthalmol.* 2001;85:983-990.)

latanoprost and two of them found statistically significant reductions in heart rate in the timolol group (for example, a reduction of 4 bpm (95% CI 2-6) for timolol and 1 bpm (95% CI −2-4) for latanoprost, $P < .01$). There were no differences in systolic or diastolic blood pressures between timolol and latanoprost groups.

These meta-analysis data suggest that latanoprost's IOP-lowering effect is superior to timolol's for ocular hypertension and open angle glaucoma, but also suggest that latanoprost has more ocular side effects than timolol. The analysis simultaneously demonstrated that timolol leads to a statistically significant reduction in heart rate while latanoprost does not. Beyond statistical significance, clinical relevance of data is critically important to consider before implementing study conclusions into clinical practice. The data showed that latanoprost reduces IOP by a maximum 7% more than timolol, which equates to a difference of 1.75 mm Hg for a patient with an untreated IOP of 25 mm Hg. While achieving an additional 1.75 mm Hg of IOP reduction may be critical for some patients (eg, those with end-stage glaucoma and strict IOP goals), for most patients this difference may be equivocal. The magnitude of slowing of the heart rate induced by timolol (4 bpm) was also quite small and may not be clinically relevant for most patients. The finding that latanoprost causes hyperemia at twice the rate of timolol may be clinically relevant; however, the overall incidence of hyperemia among patients taking latanoprost was also fairly low (8.7%, vs 4.0% of timolol patients).

While many clinicians choose latanoprost as a first-line agent in glaucoma management, data from this meta-analysis suggest that either drug is an acceptable first choice for effective IOP-lowering in open angle glaucoma and ocular hypertension. The decision to use one drug over the other should include risk analysis for ocular side effects and impacts on cardiovascular health for individual patients.

Use of Diagnostic Imaging Studies and Associated Radiation Exposure for Patients Enrolled in Large Integrated Healthcare Systems: A Records Review

Over the past few decades, there has been an increase in availability and use of costly diagnostic imaging with a concurrent increase in population-level radiation exposure. Aside from MRI and ultrasound, other imaging modalities expose patients to ionizing radiation (CT, PET, and nuclear imaging). The high cost of these tests has financial implications for both the individuals and the health systems who pay for them. The increase in imaging and concurrent radiation exposure had been demonstrated in the United States for patients with fee-for-service insurance that pays individually for each procedure or test. There is concern that fee-for-service systems generate more testing because there is no financial incentive for doctors and other providers to be economical when ordering imaging. On the other hand, integrated health systems typically work under a fixed budget, and doctors and other providers working in these systems often think more carefully about the costs of testing. In many cases, healthcare costs in integrated systems are lower. Thus, this study was undertaken to assess how the integrated health systems model impacted imaging rates over time.[14]

Six integrated health systems were analyzed with between one and two million members in each year of analysis. The outcomes of interest were imaging rates and cumulative annual radiation exposure in the population analyzed between the years of 1996 and 2010 (**TABLE 1.2**).

Results demonstrated substantial increases in the rates of advanced diagnostic imaging including CT scan, MRI, nuclear medicine, and PET scans. CT scans per 1000 nearly tripled, and for MRI that number almost quadrupled. Overall, radiation exposure increased from an average of 1.2 to 2.3 mSv per person during the course of this study.

Using the information readily available in electronic medical records, researchers were able to conduct an analysis of the overall trend in imaging use across populations of patients with a specific pattern of health system financing. Based upon the overall findings of increases in all advanced

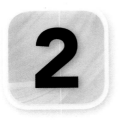

Hypertension

David M. Shein, Rachel C. Druckenbrod, and Thomas F. Freddo

LEARNING OBJECTIVES

Hypertension is the most prevalent chronic disease in the United States and is also a major cause of morbidity and mortality around the globe. Hypertension is a significant risk factor for serious cardiovascular conditions including heart failure and stroke and also impacts the eyes, kidneys, and other vital organs. Section 1 "Hypertension" reviews the epidemiology and pathophysiology of hypertension, the clinical impacts of elevated blood pressure (BP), how guidelines determine the blood pressure at which we diagnose hypertension, and the factors to consider for an individualized approach to treatment. Section 2 "Cardiovascular Drug Therapy" reviews important cardiovascular drug classes used to treat hypertension and their adverse effects, including ophthalmic considerations.

KEY CONCEPTS

Section 1: Hypertension
Epidemiology
Physiology
Diagnosis
    Essential/primary hypertension
    Secondary hypertension
    Hypertensive urgency
    Hypertensive emergency

Treatment
Clinical impacts
Section 2: Cardiovascular Drug Therapy
Angiotensin system agents
Adrenergic system antagonists
Calcium channel blockers
Diuretics

SECTION 1: HYPERTENSION

EPIDEMIOLOGY

As of 2008, the World Health Organization estimates that approximately 40% of the world's population older than 25 years has high blood pressure and that hypertension is uncontrolled in 1 billion of those people.[1] The US Centers for Disease Control and Prevention estimates that hypertension is present in 29% of Americans (approximately, 75 million people). Yet data show that only slightly more than 80% of Americans with high blood pressure are aware of their diagnosis. The percentage of these whose blood pressure is under control is just above 50%, suggesting inadequate therapy for many individuals who are on treatment. There are racial disparities in both the frequency of hypertension and the rate of control. Non-Hispanic black Americans have the highest prevalence of hypertension, yet data point to Caucasian populations as the group with the highest overall rate of blood pressure control.[2,3]

In 2003, the Seventh Report of the Joint National Committee on Prevention, Detection, Evaluation, and Treatment of High Blood Pressure[4] noted two statistics that are key in screening and managing hypertension:

1. Individuals with a blood pressure of 120/80 mm Hg at age 55 years have a 90% lifetime risk of developing hypertension
2. Most patients with hypertension will require two or more medications to control their blood pressure

These facts underscore two key points in the clinical management of hypertension. First, even with a seemingly "normal" blood pressure level at baseline, most Americans have a future risk of developing hypertension. Next, hypertension is not always a straightforward condition. Attention is needed for the proper diagnosis and management of this very common condition that is associated with significant morbidity and mortality.

Hypertension Pathophysiology

Factors that account for an individual's blood pressure include:

- Hydration status
- Sodium and potassium intake
- Sympathetic tone and arterial elasticity
- Cardiac contractility
- Renal function and hormonal factors
- Drugs (including Food and Drug Administration [FDA]-approved pharmaceuticals, dietary and herbal supplements, and illicit drugs)

The governing factors in determining blood pressure include mean arterial pressure (MAP), cardiac output, and peripheral resistance.

Mean arterial pressure is not simply the average of systolic blood pressure (SBP) and diastolic blood pressure (DBP); because the duration of diastole is longer than systole in each cardiac cycle, DBP is doubled, added to SBP and then averaged.

$$MAP = \frac{SBP + (2 \times DBP)}{3}$$

From a clinical and functional standpoint, cardiac output (CO) is the product of the heart rate (in beats per minute [BPM]) times stroke volume ejected with each beat, and MAP is the product of CO and peripheral vascular resistance (PR).

$$MAP = CO \text{ (cardia coutput)} \times PR \text{ (peripheral vascular resistance)}$$

These equations demonstrate that the factors most directly affecting blood pressure are cardiac output, vascular resistance, and plasma volume. Volume and pressure share a direct relationship: an increase in volume results in an increased pressure and the reverse is true as well.

The goal of the cardiovascular system is to maintain a constant flow of blood to vital organs. To do so, it is constantly adjusting pressure and volume to maintain homeostasis. In people with lower vascular volume—commonly seen with dehydration—the body employs various physiologic mechanisms to increase pressure (despite the reduced volume) to maintain a normal blood flow and avoid symptoms of hypoperfusion, including lightheadedness and syncope. These mechanisms normally disengage when blood volume is adequate to prevent an abnormally high blood pressure. In the setting of hypertension, many of the mechanisms that maintain normal blood pressure in volume depletion engage inappropriately despite a normal blood volume.

As noted above, the principal variables governing blood pressure include cardiac output, peripheral resistance, and blood volume. Thus, they represent the prime targets for therapeutic intervention as discussed later.

Cardiac Output

The heart receives substantial sympathetic innervation in the form of beta-1 adrenergic fibers that reach the sinoarterial (SA) node to accelerate heart rate and also reach the walls of the ventricles to increase the force of ventricular contraction (positive inotropic effect). The SA node also receives parasympathetic inputs from the vagus nerve (cranial nerve X) that modulate the sympathetic effects on heart rate. The electrically mediated release of calcium from stores in the sarcoplasmic reticulum of cardiac muscle cells leads directly to contraction.

Peripheral Resistance

Increases in blood pressure may result from changes in arterial tone due to increased alpha-adrenergic sympathetic stimulation and changes in vessel wall elasticity produced by vascular smooth muscle contraction. Atherosclerosis and arteriosclerosis also contribute to increased peripheral resistance. Sympathetic stimulation can occur with physiologic stressors such as exercise, psychological stress, and pharmacological triggers such as use of stimulants (which are often avoided in patients with hypertension), as well as excess catecholamine secretion such as from an adrenal tumor (Chapter 6). Increased tone is also a normal response to volume depletion to prevent organ hypoperfusion. In normal daily activities, the increased sympathetic stimulation that occurs during exercise causes transient blood pressure elevation. This transient blood pressure elevation is beneficial to maintain arterial elasticity and to meet the elevated demands for metabolites and oxygen during exertion. Sympathetic stimulation due to pain, fear, or anxiety causes tachycardia, tremulousness (psychomotor stimulation), and blood pressure increases. For example, "white coat syndrome" may occur where anxiety at medical visits triggers blood pressure increases in the examination room that may not be representative of the usual blood pressure. Patients experiencing pain also have an elevated blood pressure. Therefore, patients typically need outpatient follow-up in a nonacute setting before a diagnosis of hypertension can be made or antihypertensive medications adjusted after high blood pressure readings from emergency department visits from injury or other painful conditions. While episodic sympathetic stimulation can be beneficial, long-term, chronic sympathetic stimulation may be harmful. This can occur when people live in fear, such as in geographic regions of violent conflicts, or if they work in high-stress environments. The illicit use of stimulants, such as cocaine, may cause abrupt and sustained increases in blood pressure and vascular tone. These are especially harmful to the vascular system, potentially triggering acute cardiac and cerebrovascular events.

Humoral factors can also increase peripheral resistance by altering vessel diameter.

The most important hormonal factors that impact blood pressure are the components of the renin-angiotensin-aldosterone system (RAAS), which function to keep blood pressure in a normal range despite typical variations in sodium and water intake over the course of the day (**FIGURE 2.1**).

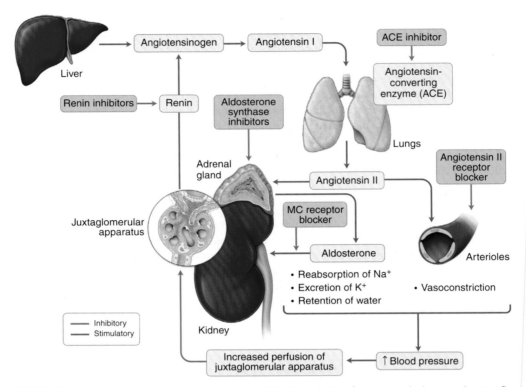

FIGURE 2.1 Renin-angiotensin-aldosterone system (RAAS) and sites for potential pharmacologic influence. The RAAS is a multisystem endocrine cascade that regulates electrolyte homeostasis, fluid balance, and blood pressure through action on the kidney and cardiovascular system. Decreased perfusion pressure in the kidney triggers the juxtaglomerular cells to release renin into the bloodstream and begin the cascade. Blue arrows indicate stimulatory action on the system; red arrows indicate inhibitory feedback and action of pharmaceutical agents. Examples of frequently used pharmaceutical agents that influence RAAS include mineralocorticoid (MC) receptor blockers (eg, spironolactone, eplerenone), angiotensin-converting enzyme (ACE) inhibitors (eg, captopril, enalapril), renin inhibitors (eg, aliskiren), and angiotensin II receptor blockers (eg, valsartan, losartan). Aldosterone synthase inhibitors are still in the experimental phase. (Reprinted with permission from Pawlina W, Ross M. *Histology: A Text and Atlas.* 8th ed. Philadelphia, PA: Wolters Kluwer; 2018.)

The kidneys, through the components of the juxtaglomerular apparatus (JGA), play a key role in the RAAS, monitoring systemic blood pressure and sodium concentration, then responding appropriately when blood pressure or the sodium level is out of range.

The Juxtaglomerular Apparatus

The JGA is a specialized structure formed by the distal convoluted tubule and the afferent arteriole leading to the glomerulus (**FIGURE 2.2**). Its main function is to regulate blood pressure and the filtration rate of the glomerulus. By doing so, this system also has a direct effect on plasma volume. A portion of the JGA is the macula densa, a collection of specialized epithelial cells in the distal convoluted tubule of the nephron that detect sodium concentration of the fluid in the tubule. In response to elevated sodium, the macula densa cells trigger contraction of the afferent arteriole, reducing blood flow to the glomerulus and the glomerular filtration rate. Derived from smooth muscle cells, the juxtaglomerular cells of the afferent arteriole secrete renin when blood pressure in the arteriole falls. Renin increases blood pressure via the RAAS.

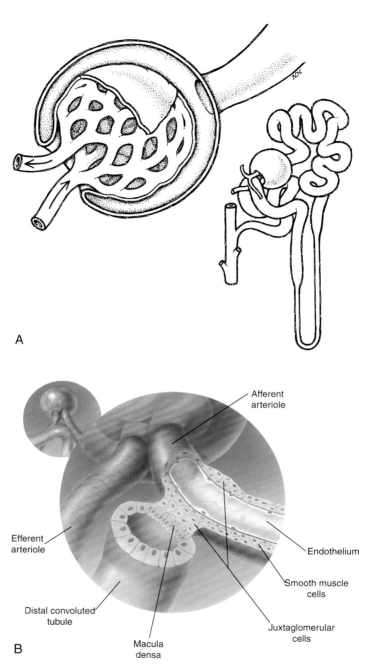

A

Afferent
arteriole

Efferent
arteriole

Endothelium

Smooth muscle
cells

Distal convoluted
tubule

Juxtaglomerular
cells

B

Macula
densa

FIGURE 2.2 A, Graphic glomerulus and juxtaglomerular apparatus (JGA). B, Histology of Juxtaglomerular apparatus labeled. (Asset provided by Anatomical Chart Co.)

When renin is released into the circulation, it cleaves a normally circulating protein produced by the liver called angiotensinogen, producing angiotensin I. Then, through the action of angiotensin-converting enzyme (ACE), produced primarily in the lungs, angiotensin I is converted to angiotensin II, a potent vasoconstrictor.

Arteriosclerotic changes in the afferent arteriole can stiffen its walls, prompting the JGA to misread its pressure as lower than it is. This misread will lead to inappropriate release of renin, elevating blood pressure in the mistaken belief that it was too low. As noted above, African Americans have a higher rate of hypertension, which is often less responsive to drugs that inhibit the RAAS. This clinical observation is supported by study of renal biopsies in hypertensive nephrosclerosis, revealing that that African Americans have more severe renal arteriosclerosis than whites.[5]

Plasma Volume

Normally, in response to low blood volume or low sodium intake, the nephron is triggered to augment its retention of sodium in order to sustain blood volume. As noted earlier, the macula densa senses both pressure and sodium concentration. When a low sodium concentration is detected, the adjacent juxtaglomerular cells secrete renin, which activates the RAAS system as noted earlier. When renin cleaves angiotensinogen, leading to production of angiotensin II, this hormone has activity beyond its vasopressor activity discussed earlier in relation to changes in peripheral resistance. This hormone also stimulates production of aldosterone by the zona glomerulosa of the adrenal cortex, causing an additional increase in sodium reabsorption by acting on sodium channels in the principal cells of the distal tubule of the nephron, thereby increasing blood volume and blood pressure. Locally produced prostaglandins are also important in the regulation of renal perfusion and sodium resorption via a paracrine effect. Inhibition with the use of nonsteroidal anti-inflammatories (NSAIDs) can adversely impact sodium management (see below).

Sodium is a key factor in regulating plasma volume and therefore blood pressure. In the euvolemic and normotensive individual, excess sodium intake is cleared by the kidneys to avoid fluid accumulation and blood pressure elevation. Many people with hypertension are unable to fully clear excess sodium, making their blood pressure so-called salt-sensitive. As sodium intake increases, even in the range of what we typically consider normal dietary amounts, higher blood pressure results. When salt-sensitive people with hypertension and prehypertension reduce sodium intake, blood pressure decreases. Data also support an opposite role for dietary potassium—abundant in many fruits and vegetables—such that *higher* potassium intake can *decrease* blood pressure. As the drop in blood pressure from sodium restriction and a high potassium intake reduces the risk for the health consequences of high blood pressure, diet is an important component of hypertension lifestyle management.

Pharmacologic Factors in Elevated Blood Pressure

Numerous pharmacologic agents used for noncardiovascular indications also impact blood pressure. Common examples include stimulants, nonselective NSAIDs, and cyclooxygenase-2 (COX-2) inhibitors. FDA-approved stimulants range from over-the-counter decongestants (such as pseudoephedrine) to medications for attention-deficit hyperactivity disorder (such as methylphenidate, sold under the common brand name Ritalin). In general, people with elevated blood pressure should be directed to alternative therapies that avoid stimulant use when possible. Both illicit use of prescription drugs (such as snorting FDA-approved stimulant medications) and illegal stimulants (such as methamphetamine and cocaine) trigger blood pressure elevations, sometimes to extremely dangerous levels with resulting cerebrovascular and cardiac complications. NSAIDs such as ibuprofen and naproxen are nonselective inhibitors of cyclooxygenase. By inhibiting prostaglandin synthesis, NSAIDs treat pain and inflammation, but the contributions of prostaglandins to the regulation of renal blood flow are also impacted, interfering with the ability of the kidneys to adjust to changes in blood volume and sodium concentration. The selective COX-2 inhibitor, celecoxib, has similar effects. By interfering with normal mechanisms of sodium and fluid balance, these drugs may further elevate blood pressure and contribute to fluid retention in people with high blood pressure. This can, in turn, exacerbate heart failure in people who are predisposed to this condition. While hypertension alone is usually not an absolute contraindication to NSAID use, it is good practice to limit both the frequency and total daily dose of NSAIDs in people with hypertension.

Definitions of Hypertension

Hypertension is defined according to its origin and also based on the degree of blood pressure elevation. Hypertension due to nonspecific causes (including interactions between genetic, environmental, and dietary factors) is known as primary hypertension or essential hypertension. The vast majority of patients with hypertension have essential hypertension. Secondary hypertension results from an identifiable medical condition or disease process, such as kidney disease or endocrine abnormalities.

Classification of hypertension by degree of blood pressure elevation is relevant since there are direct implications for hypertension management and prognosis. Perhaps surprisingly, the numeric cutoff for the diagnosis of hypertension is not consistent across all guidelines,[6,7] and recommendations may also vary with a patient's age, cardiovascular risk, and whether they have diabetes.[8] Different guidelines also vary in the naming conventions they apply to various stages of hypertension, and guidelines are often updated with new definitions over time. However, the framework of a continuum from small to medium, and ultimately larger risk as blood pressure measurements climb, is universal.

The continuum of blood pressure elevation begins at high normal, sometimes termed prehypertension, which represents an opportunity for patient education, lifestyle modification, cardiovascular risk factor evaluation, and closer monitoring. Depending upon the guideline, elevated blood pressure can be diagnosed as low as 120/<80 or at 130/85. Stage 1 hypertension is diagnosed when the blood pressure risk is judged to be high enough to warrant more directed intervention, typically including medication therapy. Classically, stage 1 hypertension was diagnosed at 140/90; however, newer guidelines make the diagnosis at 130/80. Stage 2 hypertension represents climbing risk of end-organ damage from increasing blood pressures, which typically warrants more intensive efforts to treat and often requires multiple pharmacologic agents to achieve a goal blood pressure. Classically diagnosed at 160/100, newer guidelines make the diagnosis at 140/90. Hypertensive urgency constitutes marked blood pressure elevation, often 180/120 or above, but without any complications of end-organ damage. Hypertensive emergency is defined by the same degree of blood pressure elevation and also includes detectable end-organ damage (which may include stroke, renal failure, coronary heart disease, or retinopathy). The distinction between hypertensive urgency and hypertensive emergency is critical since hypertensive emergency requires immediate hospitalization. Essential hypertension, secondary hypertension, and complications of severely elevated hypertension (including ophthalmic complications) are discussed in further detail later in the chapter.

DIAGNOSIS OF HYPERTENSION

As mentioned above, prehypertension has been defined to indicate a range at which there is enough increase in risk from blood pressure elevation that lifestyle measures (such as low sodium diet, increased exercise) should be undertaken. It is thus important to identify prehypertension, as it alerts patients and clinicians of a higher risk for progression to future hypertension. Prehypertension is asymptomatic and usually detected during routine blood pressure screening; it is an indication to

> **TABLE 2.1   Comprehensive Cardiovascular Risk Assessment for Prehypertension or New Diagnosis of Hypertension**
>
> - Lipid profile
> - Diabetes screening
> - Smoking status review and counseling as appropriate
> - Dietary review and counseling (emphasis on decreasing intake of sodium and processed food including "junk" food and fast food)
> - Physical exertion assessment
> - Family history (including cardiovascular disease, high blood pressure)

conduct a full cardiovascular risk assessment. When prehypertension is identified, it becomes even more important to address other cardiovascular risks, such as high cholesterol, smoking, and prediabetes or diabetes (**TABLE 2.1**).

The diagnosis of hypertension is made when the related increase in risk for the individual is high enough to warrant initiation of treatment. Current medical practice gives equal weight to the systolic and diastolic numbers, and the diagnosis of hypertension is confirmed when either number—or both—is elevated with a clinical picture consistent with the diagnosis. Because mild and moderate hypertension rarely cause symptoms, especially early in the disease when blood pressure elevations are mild, the diagnosis of hypertension is often made during routine blood pressure screening. As blood pressure climbs into the moderate to severe range, however, patients may experience and seek care for vague symptoms including headache, blurry vision, or dizziness. Severely elevated blood pressure can cause more dramatic symptoms due to acute, severe, and life-threatening complications of end-organ damage, such as papilledema, stroke, encephalopathy, acute kidney injury, and heart failure. Fortunately, severe and uncontrolled hypertension is uncommon in the industrialized world. When detected, this hypertensive emergency requires immediate care in an emergency medical setting (discussed further in the "Clinical Syndrome of Hypertension" section). The potential for life-threatening complications makes it important to diagnose and treat hypertension early in the course, before asymptomatic organ damage develops and certainly before symptoms occur.

The technique for blood pressure measurement is an important factor in the reliability of the reading.[9-11] Patients should be relaxed and comfortable, seated with the back supported and feet resting, uncrossed, on the ground. A patient who is running late for a medical visit, who is then whisked from a waiting room and placed in an uncomfortable position in the examination room for a quick blood pressure check, may well end up with an elevated reading—unsurprisingly! As discussed above, for patients in pain or in acute settings, clinicians should use caution in interpreting blood pressure results when making therapeutic decisions. Primary care follow-up should be considered. Also, when a single elevated reading is obtained in the medical setting, repeating the blood pressure after a few minutes when a patient is more comfortable and relaxed may result in a lower and more accurate reading. The cuff should be sized appropriately as indicated on the cuff; this is an especially important consideration for patients with either a high or low body mass index. A good-quality automated cuff for the upper arm is acceptably accurate for use in the clinical setting and may reduce the variation between observers conducting manual checks (**BOXES 2.1** and **2.2**).

Guidelines recommend repeating an initial elevated office blood pressure reading at a subsequent office visit before hypertension can be diagnosed. Increasingly, medical practice is recognizing the potential value of home readings, and the author (DS) often encourages patients to purchase a home sphygmomanometer and bring a log of home readings to future office visits (see **TABLE 2.2**).

integrity of intimal lining of the blood vessels. With sustained elevations in pressure, however, these compensatory influences are overwhelmed and damage the vascular lining results. This includes the development of atherosclerosis.

Cerebral effects of atherosclerosis result from carotid plaques that can occlude or embolize causing blindness from retinal infarction or ischemic stroke and disruption in the integrity of blood vessels in the brain that causes hemorrhagic stroke. The optometrist plays a vital role in stroke-risk mitigation when retinal cholesterol plaques (so-called Hollenhorst plaques) are discovered (Chapter 3). These small-caliber emboli, most commonly found at retinal vasculature branch points, are often nonocclusive due to their thin wafer shape. They may present in an asymptomatic patient, and thus be diagnosed incidentally, but occasionally lead to symptomatic transient or permanent vision loss from transient or fulminant retinal artery occlusion. Symptomatic Hollenhorst plaques share a well-known association with impending stroke and/or blindness,[16] and prompt evaluation is appropriate. Asymptomatic plaques found on routine examination represent a less acute risk, though they are often a marker for the presence of carotid artery disease. Outpatient carotid vascular evaluation as well as risk factor assessment and treatment should be pursued (Chapter 12).

Arterial plaque development leads to myocardial infarction when it occurs in the coronary arteries, and aortic involvement can result in aneurysm formation (especially with comorbid smoking as a risk factor), which can rupture with catastrophic results. This vascular effect also increases the risk to organs that are highly dependent on sensitive networks of arterial blood vessels. The negative effects on the vascular system are magnified when other risk factors for vascular damage are present including high levels of low-density lipoprotein (LDL) cholesterol and toxins from tobacco smoke, which also damage the arterial intima.

Cardiac effects from hypertension include concentric hypertrophy from chronic strain on the myocardium pumping against a higher arterial blood pressure. Hypertrophy is an adaptive mechanism to the increased wall stress resulting from increased pressure work. Recruitment and growth of the sarcomeres within the myocardial cells decreases the wall stress initially; over time, the response to wall stress is accompanied by fibrosis, which results in a stiff ventricle, and the negative effects of cardiac hypertrophy prevail. These include impaired diastolic filling in a stiff ventricle, which increases the risk of heart failure. Wall stress increases myocardial oxygen demand, and in concert with other risk factors that trigger coronary atherosclerosis, a mismatch between oxygen demand and delivery (through atherosclerotic vessels) results in cardiac ischemia, which can manifest as angina, arrhythmia, and myocardial infarction. Hypertrophy itself also increases the risk for arrhythmias and cardiovascular death.

Renal effects of hypertensive nephrosclerosis result from several mechanisms of kidney injury reflecting the impact of high pressures on the glomerulus and arterioles. As renal injury progresses, kidney function declines and the organ's ability to manage blood pressure further erodes. Comorbid diabetes, which is associated with a higher risk of hypertension, can itself impair renal function, and high blood pressure is an added risk factor which may ultimately lead to the need for renal replacement therapy—dialysis or renal transplant.

Similar to renal effects, ocular effects of elevated blood pressure are related to microvascular insult.[17-19] The presence of hypertension in the setting of diabetes independently increases the risk for development and progression of diabetic retinopathy.[6-8] Hypertension-related vasospasm and increased arteriolar tone create generalized and diffuse narrowing of the retinal arterioles. With continued blood pressure elevation, vessel sclerosis manifests as focal arteriolar narrowing, focal areas of venular compression by arterioles ("AV nicking"), and an increase in the arteriolar light reflex ("copper wiring") (**FIGURE 2.4**).

These changes are common among patients with chronic hypertension and may not improve even after normalization of blood pressure with intervention. Severe and acute blood pressure elevations disturb the blood-retinal barrier and lead to fluid exudation and retinal ischemia, with formation of hard exudates, macular edema, hemorrhaging (flame- and blot-shaped hemorrhages), microaneurysms, and cotton wool spots (focal infarctions of the retinal nerve fiber layer). Optic nerve head swelling and choroidal infarction result from the most severe blood pressure elevations. Interestingly,

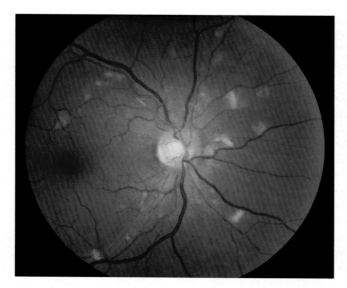

FIGURE 2.4 Hypertensive retinopathy demonstrating multiple cotton wool spots, arteriolar narrowing, and arteriovenous crossing changes. (Courtesy of Mayo Clinic, Jacksonville. Available at https://retinagallery.com/display-image.php?pid=6471.)

severe hypertensive retinopathy is more frequent among younger patients, perhaps because a greater proportion of this demographic suffers from secondary forms of hypertension (which can involve more acute and severe blood pressure elevation). There is also evidence that older patients with chronic primary blood pressure elevation may develop protective mechanisms against retinal vascular injury over time.[4,20]

Retinal vein occlusion (RVO) is an important, vision-threatening complication of hypertension that results from thrombus formation within the central retinal vein or its branches. The pathophysiology behind RVO is complex, and there are many distinct underlying etiologies, hypertension included.[21] The Blue Mountains Eye Study demonstrated an increased risk of RVO with increasing mean arterial blood pressure (OR 1.41 per 10-mm Hg increase) and atherosclerotic/hypertensive retinal vessels signs (OR 3.37 focal narrowing; 4.09 A/V nicking), as well as a significant association with older age (P = .03).[22] Additional risk factors for RVO include obesity, smoking, diabetes, carotid artery stenosis, and hypercoagulable states such as factor V Leiden mutation, protein C deficiency, hyperhomocysteinemia, antiphospholipid antibody syndrome, and monoclonal gammopathies.[11,23-25] Since a majority of RVO can be attributed to age-related systemic vascular disease, most patients do not require investigation beyond blood pressure measurement, serum lipid profile, and consideration for carotid artery evaluation for atherosclerosis on an individualized basis. However, it is generally recommended that a subset of patients undergo further evaluation for hypercoagulable states; these include patients younger than 50 years (especially in the absence of systemic cardiovascular risk factors), patients with a history of thrombosis, and patients with bilateral or rapidly sequential RVO. The prognosis for RVO depends on the distribution of the occlusion (ie, central vs branch vs hemiretinal vein occlusion [HRVO]) and the presence or absence of retinal ischemia and macular edema.[26] Ischemic central retinal vein occlusion (CRVO) and HRVO harbor the worst prognoses, and these patients require close monitoring for the onset of neovascularization, including at the iris and anterior chamber angle structures, with risk for neovascular glaucoma. Patients with RVO complicated by neovascularization and/or macular edema should be referred to a retinal specialist for treatment (**FIGURE 2.5**).

While the direct clinical implications of hypertensive eye disease are not entirely clear in terms of cardiovascular risk stratification, it is clear that hypertensive eye disease may herald further morbidity. The risk for cerebral infarction, congestive heart failure, renal impairment, and cardiovascular mortality is increased in the presence of hypertensive retinopathy.[6-8,27,28]

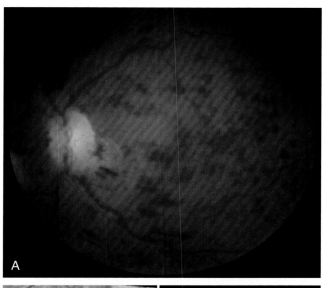

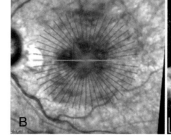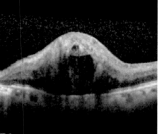

FIGURE 2.5 A, Central retinal vein occlusion (CRVO) of the left eye complicated by macular edema. B, Optical coherence tomography (OCT) imaging demonstrates significant, fovea-involving macular edema.

CLINICAL PEARLS

- Undiagnosed or poorly controlled hypertension may present to the optometrist in the form of hypertensive posterior segment disease.
- Workup of any patient presenting with cotton wool spots should include measurement of BP.
- Blood pressure measurement should be taken in office to determine severity of hypertension and thus urgency of management referral.
- Since hypertension is associated with increased risk for onset and progression of diabetic eye disease, patients with diabetes should be counseled on the importance of both blood glucose and blood pressure control.

When hypertensive retinopathy is observed on routine eye examination, blood pressure should be measured in the office to help determine the urgency of referral. Patients with severely elevated blood pressure and retinopathy should be directed to same-day emergency care for blood pressure management, since the retinal findings constitute a form of end-organ damage consistent with a hypertensive emergency. It is important to slowly reduce blood pressure in these cases as rapid lowering of elevated blood pressure can contribute to optic nerve infarction and permanent vision loss.[29] Patients with signs of mild hypertensive retinopathy and nonsevere elevation in blood pressure do not require emergent attention but should have a timely evaluation in a primary care setting to address blood pressure control. Serial eye examination is warranted to monitor for resolution of eye disease.

HYPERTENSION MANAGEMENT

Prehypertension

As mentioned previously, the management of hypertension may begin when prehypertension is identified. Prehypertension may be managed differently in patients depending on whether they have established cardiovascular or cerebrovascular disease (for example, prior myocardial infarction or ischemic stroke). Prehypertension in patients without cardiovascular disease is associated with a relatively small but definite increase in the risk of hypertension-related organ impacts and, as noted earlier, also predisposes to future increases in blood pressure and the eventual development of hypertension and its progression. While prehypertension is not generally treated with medications in patients without established cardiovascular disease, several actions are appropriate and can be considered treatment, albeit nonpharmacologic. First and foremost, the patient should be educated about the presence of prehypertension and the importance of this risk factor for developing further hypertension and related complications. Second, counseling should be provided on lifestyle interventions to lower blood pressure (see below for hypertension lifestyle management). Third, important cardiovascular comorbidities should be identified and addressed if present (**TABLE 2.3**) to reduce the risk of cardiac, cerebrovascular, and other complications. Lastly, the patient should be educated on the role of regular follow-up to monitor blood pressure for early identification and treatment of hypertension should it develop. Unfortunately, prehypertension is too often ignored, leading to missed opportunities for lifestyle interventions, which are effective and inexpensive.

In patients with established vascular disease (eg, cardiac, ocular, cerebral, renal), aggressive management of blood pressure may be pursued to reduce the risk of a recurrent event. The risk of future events is substantially higher in patients with established vascular conditions versus patients without established cardiovascular disease.

Hypertension: Blood Pressure Treatment Goal

For many years, blood pressure of 140/90 was generally accepted as the cutoff for the diagnosis of hypertension, and thus a treatment goal of <140/90 was established to minimize risk for hypertensive complications. More recent data demonstrated that in the setting of established cardiovascular disease or multiple cardiovascular risks (such as dyslipidemia, smoking, positive family history of

TABLE 2.3   Traditional Factors Considered for Cardiovascular Risk Assessment
Age and gender (male age > 45 y; female age > 55 y)
Family history of cardiovascular disease (first-degree relative male < 55 y, female < 65 y)
Cigarette smoking
Dyslipidemia (high LDL and/or low HDL)
Hypertension
Diabetes

HDL, high-density lipoprotein; LDL, low-density lipoprotein.

Adapted from Chobanian AV, Bakris GL, Black HR. The Seventh Report of the Joint National Committee on Prevention, Detection, Evaluation, and Treatment of High Blood Pressure (JNC 7). *Hypertension*. 2003;42:1206-1252.

may require emergency care to maintain breathing. While both ACE inhibitors and ARBs have been associated with this rare but life-threatening side effect, the rate of angioedema occurrence is higher with ACE inhibitors and is likely related to other substrates of angiotensin-converting enzyme (ACE) which do not occur with use of ARBs. Given the severity of angioedema, any patient on either of these drug classes should stop therapy immediately and initiate alternative treatment for blood pressure reduction. In situations where angiotensin antagonism is felt to be important enough, an ARB may be tried under close medical supervision when the angioedema occurred on an ACE inhibitor. Another ACE inhibitor should not be attempted, as the risk of recurrent angioedema is high.[39,40]

Monitoring on Therapy

In addition to routine monitoring of blood pressure, creatinine and potassium should also be checked after dose adjustments and during routine annual follow-up in patients on angiotensin-blocking drugs. Patients with chronic kidney disease or a history of high potassium may need to have these parameters monitored more frequently, especially if there are other medications or health conditions that could impact kidney function and potassium level.

BETA-BLOCKERS

Beta-blockers and related alpha-blockers are widely used medications with a broad range of indications. Both are sympathetic antagonists with clinical effects in many tissues, organs, and systems. Before considering the function of these antagonists, it is sensible to first consider the broad impacts of sympathetic agonists. There are both alpha- and beta-receptors for sympathetic stimulation, and different tissues respond either through alpha- or beta-receptors. Receptors are further classified into alpha and beta 1 and 2 subtypes.

In this section, an organ or tissue is identified, followed by its receptor type (alpha or beta) and the impact from receptor stimulation.

- Vascular smooth muscle (arteries): alpha stimulation results in contraction, increasing blood pressure
- Cardiac muscle: beta-1 stimulation is excitatory and increases both heart rate (chronotropy) and the force of cardiac contractions (inotropy)
- Bronchial (airways) smooth muscle: beta-2 stimulation results in relaxation of airways (improving airflow)
- Bladder neck (prostate region in men): alpha stimulation results in contraction and resistance to urine flow
- Metabolic effects: sympathetic stimulation results in increased availability of nutrients via glucose release from glycogenolysis in liver and muscle, as well as release of free fatty acids from adipose tissue
- Central nervous system: sympathetic stimulation results in excitatory action increasing wakefulness and psychomotor activity (sometimes termed the "fight or flight" reaction)
- Endocrine system: sympathetic stimulation increases renin which increases blood pressure through its effects on the RAAS
- Eye: sympathetic stimulation triggers mydriasis and also lowers intraocular pressure by suppressing aqueous production (eg, topical alpha-adrenergic agonists) and/or increasing outflow (eg, epinephrine[41]); sympathetic blockade with topical beta-adrenergic blockers also results in lower intraocular pressure, via decreased aqueous production

Clinical Effects and Indications

The most common uses of oral beta-adrenergic receptor blockers (beta-blockers) are for cardio-vascular indications. Beta-blockers lower blood pressure through several mechanisms of action. By blocking the effects of sympathetic stimulation on renin production by the kidney, vascular tone is reduced. The effects of sympathetic antagonism on heart rate and inotropy also reduce blood pressure by decreasing cardiac output.

Increases in blood pressure can be triggered by emotional stress, which causes an increase in sympathetic activity. Beta-blockers can be an especially effective antihypertensive treatment option in patients who experience blood pressure elevations in association with such stress. Other common clinical indications include use in tachyarrhythmias. By virtue of the above clinical effects, beta-blockers decrease myocardial oxygen demand and are an important component of care after myo-cardial infarction and in the medical management of cardiac ischemia and congestive heart failure.[42]

For years, beta-blockers were used as first-line antihypertensive agents. More recent guidelines have relegated beta-blockers to second-line use for treating uncomplicated essential hypertension as a single agent due to outcome data suggesting other medications may be more effective and because of their side effect profile.[13] When specific indications are present that require a beta-blocker (eg, tachyarrhythmia, myocardial ischemia), they can be used concurrently to address underlying hyper-tension. In addition, when multiple agents are necessary to control blood pressure, a beta-blocker may be used as an add-on to other medications.

CLINICAL PEARLS
- Use caution when prescribing topical (ocular) beta-blockers in patients on oral beta-blockers and those with baseline bradycardia, atrial fibrillation, or lung disease such as chronic obstructive pulmonary disorder (COPD) and asthma.
- Topical beta-blockers are available as nonselective (both beta 1 and beta 2) and cardioselective (only beta 1) for use in patients with respiratory disease.
- Patients should be educated on the potential adverse systemic side effects of beta-blockers including fatigue, shortness of breath, lightheadedness, and syncope.

Beta-blockers have a range of other uses. By inhibiting the effects of sympathetic stimulation, they can be used to prevent stage fright and other situations where the "fight or flight" reaction occurs resulting in symptoms such as tremor, tachycardia, or sweating. Another indication for use of beta-blockers in clinical practice is for migraine prophylaxis in patients with frequent migraines that are not otherwise well controlled.

In ocular use, topical beta-blockers decrease aqueous production and lower intraocular pressure.

Adverse Effects

General symptoms that can result from beta-blocker use include fatigue, dry eyes, and sexual dys-function, most often erectile dysfunction. Since beta-blockers lower blood pressure, hypotension can result especially at higher doses. The negative chronotropic qualities of beta-blockers can be helpful therapeutically in tachycardia but can also result in bradycardia in susceptible individuals. Thus, in patients with a low baseline heart rate or heart block, beta-blockers should be used cautiously if at all. All patients on beta-blockers need monitoring of blood pressure and heart rate.

Though systemic absorption of ocular beta-blockers is limited, in some patients, enough drug is absorbed to trigger beta-blockade side effects, including fatigue and bradycardia, in which case, an alternate agent should be used to manage intraocular pressure. Patients on oral beta-blockers and patients with baseline bradycardia, heart block, and/or with atrial fibrillation (especially those managed on cardioversion agents such as propafenone)[43,44] should be treated cautiously with topical ocular beta-blockers and the optometrist should discuss risks of initiating topical beta-blockers with the patient and the patient's medical team (primary care or cardiology) prior to initiation. Patients on topical beta-blockers should be educated on the adverse symptoms of beta-blockade and self-monitor for symptoms.

Specific clinical situations that have potential interactions with beta-blockers are the pulmonary conditions, asthma, and COPD (Chapter 14), as well as diabetes. As previously noted, beta-sympathetic stimulation results in airway relaxation to improve airflow. Inhaled medications available to manage acute asthma or COPD contain beta sympathetic agonists to reverse airway spasm. With beta-blocker use, the effect of these medications can be inhibited, decreasing the effectiveness of some inhaled pulmonary medications.

In diabetes, hypoglycemia is often the most common side effect that a patient will experience from insulin treatment. Hypoglycemia can also be seen with oral hypoglycemic agents. The physiologic responses to hypoglycemia that increase glucose production include the release of sympathetic agonist hormones to increase gluconeogenesis in the liver (Chapter 5). Along with gluconeogenesis, sympathetic agonists trigger the adrenergic symptoms of hypoglycemia including tremor, tachycardia, and sweating. These symptoms prompt the patient to take action, such as checking a blood sugar and eating glucose. With beta-blockade, the sympathetic response is blocked, and hypoglycemia unawareness may result. While this is an important clinical consideration, many patients with diabetes are treated with beta-blockers, as diabetes increases the risk for cardiovascular disease including ischemia, myocardial infarction, and congestive heart failure. The value of beta-blockers in these conditions often outweighs the risk of hypoglycemia unawareness. Similarly, hypertension is more prevalent in patients with diabetes, and when multiple medications are needed, or other first-line agents are not tolerated, beta-blockers are acceptable when used cautiously.

Monitoring on Therapy

The two most important parameters to monitor in patients treated for hypertension and ischemic heart disease are heart rate and blood pressure. While beta-blockers are beneficial in the management of heart failure for many patients, they must be started at a low dose and increased slowly, as too high a dose can also trigger worsening heart failure (Chapter 4). Thus, close monitoring in patients treated for congestive heart failure is also important.

ALPHA-BLOCKERS

Though not part of the A, B, C, D classes of cardiovascular drugs, alpha-blockers are important adrenergic drugs that have direct effects on the cardiovascular system.

Clinical Effects and Indications

Alpha-adrenergic antagonists, or alpha-blockers, are not a first-line treatment option for hypertension. Most often, they are prescribed for impaired urinary flow in benign prostate hyperplasia in older men. As noted, alpha stimulation results in contraction of smooth muscles in blood vessels and the bladder neck (**FIGURE 2.6**). Alpha blockade antagonizes the alpha stimulation of vascular smooth muscle, decreasing vascular resistance and lowering arterial blood pressure. Similarly, alpha-blockade in situations of poor urine flow and incomplete bladder emptying with prostate hyperplasia relaxes muscle tone at the bladder outlet, enabling more complete emptying of the bladder.

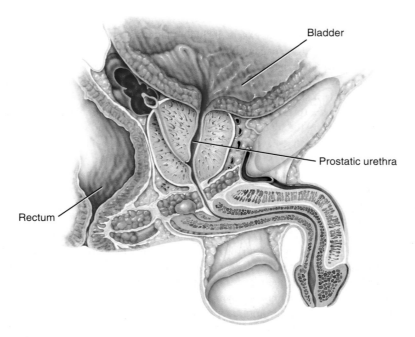

FIGURE 2.6 The prostate gland undergoes hyperplasia during normal aging. The enlarging prostate often compresses the prostatic urethra causing symptoms, including nocturia (awakening at night to void), hesitancy, slower stream, and postvoid dribbling. (Asset provided by Anatomical Chart Co.)

Topical alpha-adrenergic stimulation has several ocular effects as well, including alpha-1-mediated vasoconstriction of ocular blood vessels, (weak) pupillary dilation, and eyelid retraction and alpha-2-mediated intraocular pressure reduction. There is additionally a controversial role for alpha-2-mediated neuroprotection of the optic nerve fibers. The topical alpha-2 adrenergic agonists brimonidine and apraclonidine are commonly used in optometric practice for glaucoma management and (owing to some minor alpha-1 activity) to diagnostically blanch the superficial episcleral vessels when differentiating episcleritis from scleritis. Apraclonidine is also commonly used to diagnose Horner syndrome, which features upregulation of alpha-1 adrenergic receptors in the iris.

Adverse Effects

Arterial contraction under alpha stimulation is important for avoidance of postural or orthostatic hypotension. While supine, the feet and head are in line with the heart and the effect of gravity in these key areas is equal. Standing up adds gravity to the circulatory equation, and alpha stimulation of peripheral arteries in the lower extremities increases pressure and redirects blood against gravity to maintain brain perfusion. Alpha-blockade can inhibit this function and may cause symptoms of orthostatic hypotension, particularly with rapid standing.

When compared to thiazide diuretics, ACE inhibitors, and calcium channel blockers, a large randomized controlled hypertension study[35] demonstrated that alpha-blockers result in a slightly higher incidence of congestive heart failure. Thus, alpha-blockers are not frequently used as first-line agents in uncomplicated hypertension.

Muscle tone in the iris is maintained by alpha receptors, and blockade can decrease tone in the iris resulting in the intraoperative floppy iris syndrome. Though most eye surgeons will request discontinuation of alpha-blockers preoperatively, the effects on the iris may persist long term, requiring caution for many ocular surgeries for current or past alpha-blocker users.

Another pharmacologic consideration for the optometrist is the use of diagnostic mydriatic eye drops in the setting of elevated blood pressure. Topical phenylephrine 2% is a commonly used mydriatic eye drop with selective alpha-1 adrenergic activity that results in vasoconstriction and BP elevation. The small degree and transient nature of BP elevation from ophthalmic phenylephrine[8] is insufficient to warrant BP monitoring in all patients receiving topical phenylephrine during the eye examination, but consideration should be given if using higher concentrations of phenylephrine (eg, 10%), in the setting of baseline poorly controlled hypertension, those with arrhythmias, and among patients taking other drugs which can potentiate hypertensive crises (eg, monoamine oxidase inhibitors).

Finally, the use of the topical alpha-2 adrenergic agonists should be used with caution in infants and children due to potential risk for central nervous system depression, including severe hypotension, bradycardia, and apnea.[45]

CLINICAL PEARLS
- Alpha-adrenergic activity in the eye contributes to vasoconstriction, (weak) iris dilation, eyelid retraction, intraocular pressure reduction, and (controversial) neuroprotection.
- The use of topical phenylephrine (an alpha-1 agonist), particularly in the 10% rather than the 2.5% dose, carries systemic risk of hypertension and should be used with caution in patients with poorly controlled blood pressure, arrhythmias, or those taking MAOI (monoamine oxidase inhibitor) antidepressants.
- Infants and children may experience central nervous system depression with topical alpha-2 agonists such as brimonidine and apraclonidine.

Monitoring on Therapy

Blood pressure monitoring and assessment for symptoms of orthostatic hypotension are important. In addition, in men treated for prostate hyperplasia, inquiring about voiding symptoms including urine stream and nocturia can be used to assess the success of treatment.

CALCIUM CHANNEL BLOCKERS

Calcium channel blockers can be divided into two subclasses, dihydropyridines and nondihydropyridines, the latter of which there are only two currently used medications: verapamil (phenylalkylamine class) and diltiazem (benzothiazepine class). Each class has distinct clinical effects; verapamil and diltiazem have more cardiac effects, while the dihydropyridine class, which includes several different agents, is more selective for peripheral blood vessels.

Clinical Effects and Indications

Arterial smooth muscle contraction depends upon calcium movement across channels in the cell membrane (**FIGURE 2.7**). Calcium channel blockers inhibit arterial contraction and thereby lower arterial blood pressure. In addition, since verapamil and diltiazem are more selective for cardiac muscle, they also have negative chronotropic effects.

Hypertension is a common indication for calcium channel blockers. Due to the negative chronotropic effects of verapamil and diltiazem, they are also be used for tachyarrhythmias. The vascular effects can also be therapeutic in digital artery spasm (Raynaud disease) and for migraine prophylaxis.

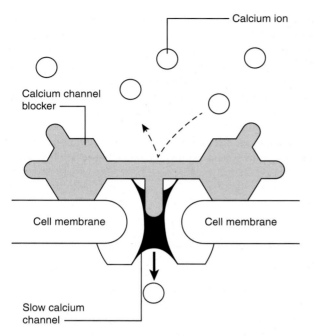

Calcium ion

Calcium channel blocker

Cell membrane

Cell membrane

Slow calcium channel

FIGURE 2.7 Calcium channel blockers work by inhibiting the movement of calcium ions across the cell membrane. (From Acosta RW. *Pharmacology for Health Professionals*. 2nd ed. Philadelphia, PA: Wolters Kluwer; 2012.)

Adverse Effects

As antihypertensives, calcium channel blockers can all cause hypotension. The negative chronotropic effects of verapamil and diltiazem can cause bradycardia in patients at risk. Peripheral edema is seen in drugs with more peripheral vascular action, typically developing in the lower legs and ankles. Headache is also a potential adverse effect. Inhibition of smooth muscle can also delay transit in the gastrointestinal tract resulting in constipation.

Monitoring on Therapy

Monitoring of both blood pressure and heart rate is necessary when patients take calcium channel blockers. Blood test monitoring is often considered optional for patients on no other drugs, as impacts on kidney and electrolytes are not typical with this drug class.

DIURETICS

Differing mechanisms of action are responsible for the effects of the various drugs in the diuretic class. The most commonly used diuretics for hypertension are the thiazides and thiazide-like diuretics. Loop diuretics are more potent than the thiazides, and while they can be used for hypertension, they cause substantial fluid clearance through the kidneys and are thus more useful in situations of fluid overload, such as congestive heart failure. The potassium-sparing diuretics may be combined with thiazides or used alone in specific clinical conditions, including heart failure and mineralocorticoid excess. They are also added in patients who have persistent hypertension despite multiple other agents (**TABLE 2.5**).

TABLE 2.5 Diuretics by Class			
Loop Diuretics	**Thiazide Class Diuretics**	**Aldosterone Antagonists**	**Potassium-Sparing Drugs**
Furosemide Bumetanide Torsemide Ethacrynic acid	Hydrochlorothiazide Chlorthalidone Indapamide	Spironolactone Eplerenone	Triamterene Amiloride

Clinical Effects and Indications

The thiazide drugs impact blood pressure through both diuresis and vascular mechanisms. Their ability to induce a mild diuresis occurs rapidly, and effects on vascular tone develop with longer term use. The diuretic effect of hydrochlorothiazide is achieved by inhibiting sodium reabsorption in the distal tubules (**FIGURE 2.8**). The result is loss of sodium, water, and potassium. For patients with mild edema, thiazides can clear excess fluid volume. When added to other antihypertensive drugs, thiazides augment the effects of angiotensin system antagonists and beta-blockers, providing significant additional blood pressure lowering. Thus, they are often included in multidrug regimens when more than one drug is needed for BP control. ACE inhibitors, ARBs, and beta-blockers are commonly combined with a thiazide diuretic in a single pill for convenience.

Loop diuretics reduce NaCl reabsorption in the thick ascending limb of the loop of Henle. They are rarely used for hypertension alone as they are more potent than the thiazides and most have shorter half-lives (which would require multiple doses per day). Fluid overload in conditions such as congestive heart failure typically responds to loop diuretics. If a patient with fluid overload also has hypertension, the loop diuretic may be effective for both.

Potassium-sparing diuretics include agents that directly result in sodium loss and others that are aldosterone antagonists. By inhibiting the sodium and water retention that results from aldosterone's effects, diuresis occurs. Sodium and potassium are exchanged at the cell membrane of the distal renal tubule, and the sodium chloride excretion that results in diuresis also results in potassium retention. These drugs may be used in patients with hypokalemia or combined with a thiazide to balance the

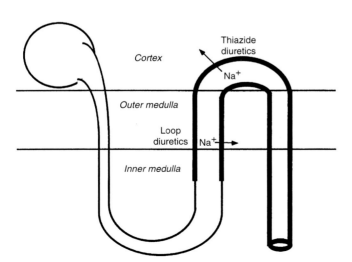

FIGURE 2.8 Site of action of loop and thiazide diuretics. Loop diuretics inhibit the Na-K-2Cl cotransporter in the medullary portion of the thick ascending limb of Henle, whereas thiazides block a simple NaCl carrier in the cortical portion of the distal tubule. These differences explain, in part, the susceptibility of individuals treated with thiazide-type diuretics to the development of hyponatremia. (Adapted from Iwasaki Y, Oiso Y , Yamauchi K, et al. Osmoregulation of plasma vasopressin in myxedema. *J Clin Endocrinol Metab.* 1990;70:534.)

thiazide kaliuretic effects. Resistant hypertension is often treated with the addition of a potassium-sparing diuretic to existing therapy with other drugs. While potassium-sparing diuretics can be used for hypertension, they are also indicated in congestive heart failure, while aldosterone antagonists are used in endocrine diseases that result in excess mineralocorticoid.

Adverse Effects

Hypotension and dehydration are among the most common adverse effects, and patients should be monitored for symptoms. Electrolyte management is altered to achieve diuresis, and lab monitoring is necessary. Diuretics can affect renal clearance of other plasma components and should be used cautiously in gout, where increased levels of uric acid from diuretic therapy (thiazides or loop diuretics) increase the risk for crystallization in joints causing acute inflammation short term, and accumulation in tophi long term.[46] Thiazides also carry a risk for glucose intolerance. This is a consideration in patients with prediabetes, diabetes, or significant risk factors for abnormal glucose metabolism (eg, obesity). While not fully contraindicated, thiazides may be reserved as second-line agents in these situations. The net benefit from well-controlled blood pressure exceeds the small risk of a mild increase in glucose levels, which itself can be managed with other approaches to lower risk. Some diuretics cause cutaneous photosensitivity, and patients should be advised to avoid prolonged sun exposure.

Monitoring on Therapy

Monitoring of blood pressure and fluid status is necessary in patients taking diuretics. Evidence of dehydration may require lowering the dose or even discontinuation. Fluid overload may require an increase in the dose, or for a patient on a thiazide, a change to a loop diuretic for increased potency of diuresis. Monitoring of serum electrolytes and kidney function is necessary. Patients on diuretic therapy who develop another cause of volume loss (eg, vomiting or intense sweating) may need especially close monitoring or temporary drug discontinuation.

REFERENCES

1. Mendis S, Puska P, Norrving B, eds. *Global Atlas on Cardiovascular Disease Prevention and Control.* Geneva, Switzerland: World Health Organization; 2011.

2. Yoon SS, Fryar CD, Carroll MD. *Hypertension Prevalence and Control Among Adults: United States, 2011–2014.* NCHS Data Brief, No 220. Hyattsville, MD: National Center for Health Statistics; 2015.

3. https://www.cdc.gov/bloodpressure/index.htm. Accessed June 2019.

4. Chobanian AV, Bakris GL, Black HR. The Seventh Report of the Joint National Committee on Prevention, Detection, Evaluation, and Treatment of High Blood Pressure (JNC 7). *Hypertension.* 2003;42:1206-1252.

5. Marcantoni C, Ma LJ, Federspiel C, et al. Hypertensive nephrosclerosis in African Americans versus Caucasians. *Kidney Int.* 2002;62:172-180.

6. Welton PK. 2017 ACC/AHA/AAPA/ABC/ACPM/AGS/APhA/ASH/ASPC/NMA/PCNA guideline for the prevention, detection, evaluation, and management of high blood pressure in adults: a report of the American College of Cardiology/American Heart Association Task Force on Clinical Practice Guidelines. *Hypertension.* 2018;71(6):e13-e115.

7. Williams B, Mancia G, Spiering W, et al. 2018 ESC/ESH guidelines for the management of arterial hypertension. *Eur Heart J.* 2018;39(33):3021-3104.

8. American Diabetes Association. Standards of medical care in diabetes – 2019 abridged for primary care providers. *Clin Diabetes.* 2019;37(1):11-34.

9. Handler J. The importance of accurate blood pressure measurement. *Perm J.* 2009;13(3):51-54.

10. Muntner P, Shimbo D, Carey RM, et al. Measurement of blood pressure in humans: a scientific statement from the American Heart Association. *Hypertension.* 2019;73(5):e35-e66.

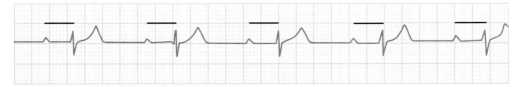

FIGURE 3.6 Note consistent PR intervals greater than one large block (>0.20 seconds). (Reprinted with permission from *Yao and Artusio's Anesthesiology: Problem-Oriented Patient Management. 7th ed. Philadelphia, PA. Lippincott Williams & Wilkins; 2011.)*

duration to severe delays and beats that do not get conducted from the atria to the ventricles. These conditions are termed AV block, classified as first, second, or third degree.

- First-degree heart block is seen as a consistent prolongation in the PR interval (>0.20 seconds or one large box on the ECG). This condition is asymptomatic (**FIGURE 3.6**).
- Second-degree heart block is subdivided into two types: Mobitz I (also called Wenckebach) and Mobitz II
  - Mobitz I is characterized by an increasing PR interval from beat to beat until one P wave is not conducted or "dropped" (P without following QRS); the PR then shortens and the cycle begins again (**FIGURE 3.7**).
  - Mobitz II is characterized by a periodic pattern of nonconducted P waves (eg, every third or fourth) without the interval prolongation seen in Mobitz I. Patients with Mobitz I or II are usually asymptomatic, but may sense the dropped beats or occasionally feel lightheaded (**FIGURE 3.8**).
- In third-degree or complete heart block, the electrical activity from the atria does not pass through the AV node due to conduction system disease. The ventricles thus beat independently which is termed an escape rhythm, typically at a slow rate. On the ECG, there are both P waves and QRS complexes, but their progression across the tracing shows no relationship as each chamber beats independently. Third-degree heart block is usually accompanied by significant bradycardia, which leads to fatigue, pre-syncope or syncope and triggers ischemia in patients at risk.

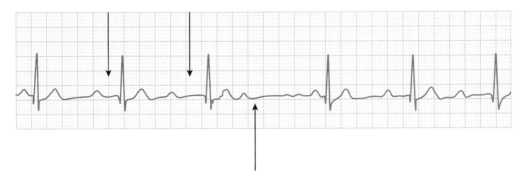

FIGURE 3.7 Mobitz I (Wenckebach); note prolonging PR intervals (downward arrows) followed by a nonconducted P wave (without QRS) (upward arrow). (Reprinted with permission from *Yao and Artusio's Anesthesiology: Problem-Oriented Patient Management. 7th ed. Philadelphia, PA. Lippincott Williams & Wilkins; 2011.)*

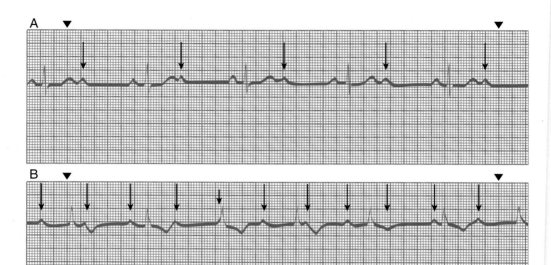

FIGURE 3.8 Heart block rhythms. A, Second-degree heart block: Mobitz type II. Arrows denote P wave not followed by QRS complex. B, Third-degree heart block (complete atrioventricular block). Arrows denote P waves. Note the lack of relationship between the atria (P wave) and ventricles (QRS). (A and B, From Huff J. *ECG Workout.* 4th ed. Philadelphia, PA: Lippincott, Williams & Wilkins; 2002:150-156.)

In the setting of PR prolongation with AV block, an assessment for triggers considers:

- Ischemia
- Intrinsic disease in the cardiac conduction system
- Infectious causes (including endocarditis [Chapter 4] and Lyme disease [Chapter 9])
- Medications, including ocular beta-blockers (Chapter 2)

The use of beta-blockers (including topical) should be avoided in any second-degree heart block because of their negative chronotropic effects, which increase the risk of progression to symptomatic third-degree block.

The patient history assesses risk factors, including symptoms of atherosclerosis, concurrent infections, and medications, to address the factors that impact conduction. Treatable causes should be addressed. Significant conduction system disease and symptomatic AV block require treatment, such as pacemaker implantation.

CLINICAL PEARLS

Topical beta-blockers for the treatment of glaucoma are contraindicated in patients with greater than first-degree heart block. Given the other classes of efficacious medications available to treat glaucoma (eg, prostaglandins), it is prudent to avoid topical beta-blockers in patients with any degree of heart block.

BUNDLE BRANCH BLOCK

Following the path of electrical activity, after the AV node, the His bundle splits into right and left bundle branches, leading to the respective ventricles.

While diseases that slow conduction can impact both the right and left bundle branches, the causes often differ. In general, a right bundle branch block (RBBB) is considered benign when it occurs in isolation and without other cardiac symptoms. In these cases, extensive evaluation may not be necessary. In contrast, when a left bundle branch block (LBBB) develops, ischemic cardiac disease is a more likely cause. An evaluation of cardiac blood flow is typically a part of the evaluation of a new onset LBBB. Bundle branch blocks are identified because of the slowed conduction in the affected ventricle, with ventricles thus depolarizing at different times. Normally, the ventricles depolarize simultaneously, and the large QRS spike occurs. When the ventricles depolarize separately due to a bundle branch block, a second peak called R′ appears when the delayed ventricle depolarizes after the R wave from the ventricle with normal conduction. This is colloquially termed the rabbit ear pattern, which is a hallmark of the RBBB (**FIGURES 3.9** and **3.10**).

ARRHYTHMIAS

The normal heart rate or pulse rate is typically between 60 and 80 beats per minute (BPM). Some people, such as fit athletes, can have a resting pulse in the 50s or even 40s. Under ordinary physiologic stresses that trigger catecholamine release, such as with exercise or acute fright, the heart rate will transiently increase. Pathological states of tachycardia and bradycardia may be accompanied by symptoms. Palpitations or heart fluttering can occur with fast rates. Presyncope or syncope can occur with either fast or slow heart rates. Arrhythmias can occur due to disease states that are external to the heart (eg, excess catecholamine release) or due to intrinsic disease in the atria, ventricles, or both.

Conditions affecting the SA node can result in fast, irregular, or slow heart rates. Atrial tachycardia is called sinus tachycardia when originating in the normal pathway of SA or sinus node activation. It can be due to external causes or intrinsic cardiac triggers. Triggers of atrial or sinus tachycardia include exercise, a normal physiologic response. Thyrotoxicosis (Chapter 6) is a pathologic noncardiac cause of atrial tachycardia. Stimulants, whether in clinical use (eg, for treatment of attention deficit hyperactivity disorder or inhaled beta-adrenergic agonists for asthma—Chapter 14), social use (eg, caffeine), or illicit use (eg, cocaine, methamphetamine), can also increase the heart rate. In these situations, the heart is responding normally to an external trigger.

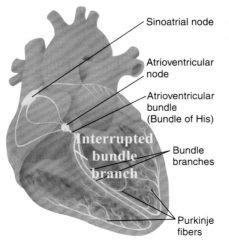

FIGURE 3.9 Diagram of bundle branch block. (Reprinted with permission from Jensen S. *Nursing Health Assessment.* 3rd ed. Wolters Kluwer; 2018.)

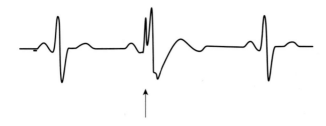

FIGURE 3.10 Doubled QRS (arrow; rabbit ear pattern; right bundle branch block).

Tachycardia also occurs due to disease in the cardiac conduction system. Atrial fibrillation is an atrial arrhythmia that is not a sinus rhythm and usually presents with tachycardia. In atrial fibrillation, the normal process for initiating the heartbeat in the SA node is replaced by erratic beating from many sites in the cardiac atria, resulting in a disorganized pattern that does not effectively pump blood. The rate is always irregular. There is no organized atrial contraction, and P waves are not present. The hallmarks of atrial fibrillation on an ECG are thus:

- An irregular rhythm
- No P waves present

Atrial fibrillation deserves special attention due to important clinical considerations including the association with risk of embolic stroke and retinal artery embolism (Chapters 4 and 12) (**FIGURE 3.11**).

Sinus bradycardia due to SA node activation at a low rate can be normal (or physiologic). In individuals who are physically fit and in overall good health, the normal heart rate will often slow below 60 BPM during sleep. Drugs such as beta-blockers will slow the heart rate, and in susceptible individuals, trigger bradycardia—even when used topically such as ocular applications, as noted above (also Chapter 2). Disease of the SA node can also slow its activation resulting in bradycardia, which may cause symptoms.

While the ventricles normally beat in response to conduction initiated in the SA node and conducted across the AV node, there are conditions in which the ventricles will beat on their own. The

A
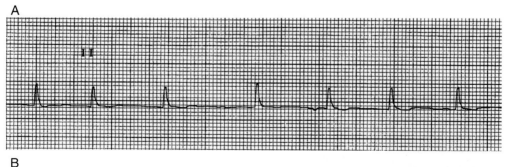

B
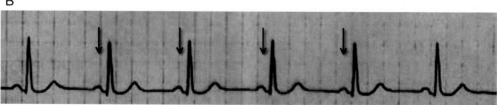

FIGURE 3.11 A, Atrial fibrillation: Note the absence of P waves and irregular of QRS complexes. B, Normal sinus rhythm: P waves (arrows) precede each QRS complex with regular spacing.

key ventricular tachyarrhythmias are ventricular tachycardia and ventricular fibrillation. Ventricular tachycardia, in which the rapid ventricular rate does not allow ample time in diastole to fill normally, results in poor systemic perfusion and usually causes symptoms (presyncope, syncope, cardiac ischemia) or death if circulation is severely impaired. In addition, ventricular activation outside of the normal conduction pathways is highly abnormal, and the presence of ventricular arrhythmias is usually indicative of severe underlying cardiac disease or life-threatening extracardiac conditions such as drug toxicity or electrolyte disturbances. Conditions in which the ventricles do not contract at all, such as ventricular fibrillation, are seen as cardiac arrest and a cause of sudden cardiac death. Ventricular arrhythmias are life-threatening and require immediate treatment. If there is no circulation, CPR must be administered in the short term. Ultimately, a shock delivered via a defibrillator is required to restore a perfusing rhythm. The underlying condition triggering the ventricular arrhythmia also needs immediate treatment. Clinicians should be aware of the location of emergency kits and automated external defibrillators in their clinical settings, as well as in recreation centers, airports, and other public places.

HYPERTROPHY

Other key findings on the ECG include hypertrophy and infarction, with both reflecting abnormalities in the cardiac muscle. Cardiac muscle hypertrophy of the left ventricular wall is most commonly associated with hypertension, although other conditions such as inherited cardiomyopathies and cardiac valvular diseases can also result in hypertrophy (Chapters 2 and 4). Left-sided hypertrophy can be seen as abnormally large QRS waves accompanied by abnormalities in repolarization. When hypertrophy is present on the ECG, an echocardiogram can be used to confirm the finding and explore the underlying cause, such as valvular disease or an asymmetric pattern of hypertrophy in an inherited cardiomyopathy. The left ventricular hypertrophy of hypertension affects all areas of the ventricle and is often called concentric hypertrophy. The underlying cause for hypertrophy should be determined and treated as appropriate when present (**FIGURE 3.12**).

ISCHEMIA AND INFARCTION

Cardiac muscle receives its blood supply from the coronary arteries, or the epicardial circulation. When these arteries are narrowed or occluded due to atherosclerosis (Section 3), or suffer spasm, impaired myocardial blood flow is seen clinically as ischemia, often experienced as angina. Angina may manifest with chest pressure, left arm pain, and/or jaw pain, often accompanied by nausea and

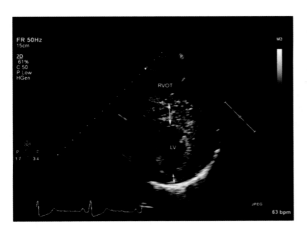

FIGURE 3.12 Echocardiographic image with thickened left ventricular muscle (myocardial hypertrophy) indicated by the large arrow; normal myocardial thickness is indicated by the small arrow. LV, left ventricle; RVOT, right ventricular outflow tract. (Reprinted with permission from Armstrong WF, *Feigenbaum's Echocardiography*. 8th ed. Wolters Kluwer; 2018.)

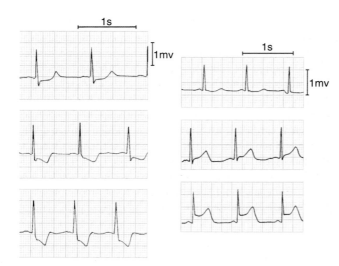

FIGURE 3.13 Myocardial ischemia. Shown are ECG tracings depicting ST segment depression (left) and ST elevation (right). (Reprinted with permission from Gravlee GP. *Hensley's Practical Approach to Cardiothoracic Anesthesia.* 6th ed. Wolters Kluwer; 2018.)

shortness of breath. When angina is untreated and cardiac muscle ischemia persists, myocardial infarction results. When a patient presents with symptoms that could reflect angina, especially when risk factors for cardiac ischemia are present, assessment is necessary to rule out ischemia. The initial assessment includes the ECG. If the ECG displays a pattern suggesting cardiac ischemia or infarction, then symptomatic cardiovascular disease can be diagnosed, and focus on cardiac treatment can be pursued. It is important to note that since the sensitivity of the ECG is not 100%,[2] even if it does not clearly indicate the presence of ischemia or infarction, when suspicion for epicardial arterial disease is high enough, further testing is necessary to assess function or to visualize flow through the arteries.

Cardiac ischemia such as with angina and acute infarction can be reflected in abnormalities in the ST segment and T waves. A depressed ST segment and inverted T wave is often an indicator of ischemia. On a stress test, it would indicate an abnormal test (see below), leading to a diagnosis of cardiovascular disease and subsequent therapeutic interventions. ST segment elevation is indicative of acute infarction (**FIGURE 3.13**). In an emergency setting, these findings require prompt medical treatment, which often includes cardiac catheterization and stent placement (see below). After a significant myocardial infarction (MI), the presence of the infarcted myocardium can be seen on the ECG as Q waves, thus the term *Q wave MI.*

The cardiac stress test is used to evaluate for cardiac ischemia in a patient with possible symptoms such as chest pressure, left arm or jaw pain, or exertional shortness of breath. (The pain along the left side of the neck and jaw, plus the pain radiating down the left arm, is referred pain into the dermatomes of C3, 4, and 5 from irritation of the left phrenic nerve.)

CARDIAC TESTING

For some patients, blood flow through a narrowed epicardial blood vessel is adequate to deliver oxygen at rest, yet with exertion such as exercise, the increased oxygen demand outstrips the ability of the narrowed artery to deliver. Thus, to trigger symptoms during the medical evaluation, a functional test that increases myocardial oxygen demand is necessary. The standard exercise stress test or exercise tolerance test entails walking on a treadmill that progressively speeds up and increases in incline. In patients who cannot exercise, a drug such as persantine that mimics the vascular effect of exercise on the heart is injected under observation. Myocardial oxygen demand is increased and exertional ischemia can be triggered and thus diagnosed. The ECG tracing is monitored during exercise to diagnose ischemia when provoked by the stress test. When the baseline ECG is abnormal, including prior infarction or bundle branch block, or when medication is used in lieu of exercise, the ECG cannot reliably detect ischemia, and a test to image the heart during exercise to compare function or blood flow before and after exercise is necessary. Perfusion images with a radioisotope (thallium) that is taken up by normal heart muscle but not by ischemic or infarcted muscle can be used to differentiate these states. If there is perfusion at rest, but not with exercise, this suggests ischemia, and treatment can be initiated. Complete perfusion with both exercise and rest is a normal result. Nonperfusion at rest and the same region of nonperfusion with exercise are indicative of infarcted myocardium.

CARDIAC CATHETERIZATION

When patients present with ischemic angina symptoms that represent very high risk (such as angina at rest), or with evidence of acute infarction, the epicardial circulation is assessed. Usually done with a cardiac arteriogram or catheterization (commonly called *cardiac cath*), an incision into the femoral artery in the groin or an artery in the arm (brachial or radial) enables the catheter to be thread to the openings of the coronary vessels just above the aortic valve to introduce contrast dye. Fluoroscopic images are followed to determine the arterial anatomy and state of the blood vessels. Narrowed or occluded epicardial arteries that are triggering cardiac ischemia or active infarction can be opened with a balloon and secured with a stent to hold open the blood vessel (**FIGURES 3.14** and **3.15**).

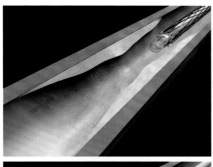
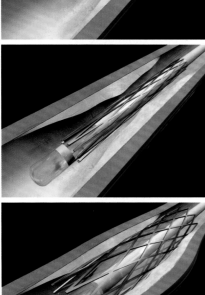

FIGURE 3.14 Cardiac stent procedure: A catheter containing a collapsed stent over a balloon is inserted into the symptomatic atheromatous lesion via catheter. Once the stent is positioned within the lesion, the balloon is inflated to expand the artery and deploy the stent. The balloon is then deflated and the catheter is removed, leaving the expanded arterial stent in place.

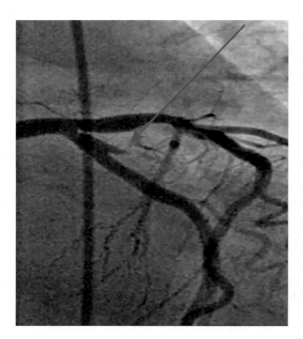

FIGURE 3.15 Coronary arteriogram showing total occlusion of the anterior marginal branch of the circumflex artery (red arrow). (Reprinted with permission from Clements SD. *The Digital Echo Atlas.* Wolters Kluwer; 2018.)

CARDIAC BLOOD TESTS

When myocardial infarction or severe ischemia is present, blood tests detect the enzymes leaking from damaged heart muscle. The ubiquitous muscle enzyme **creatine phosphokinase** (CK or CPK) was used for many years to assess for acute myocardial infarction by evaluating the myocardial band (MB) fraction, an isoform of the enzyme found only in cardiac muscle. An elevated MB fraction in the presence of suspected myocardial infarction (often based upon symptoms and ECG) confirmed the diagnosis of myocardial infarction. While some medical facilities continue to use CK and MB fraction to look for infarction, more sensitive testing for the muscle protein **troponin** is used more often. Troponin, the component of thin filaments (actin) in the sarcomere to which calcium binds to initiate contraction, is released from infarcted myocardial cells into the circulation. Elevation of troponin levels in the setting of high clinical suspicion for ischemia is useful in determining prognosis and guiding therapy.

C-reactive protein (CRP) is a serum marker for systemic inflammation. Inflammation from any source can contribute to plaque formation, rupture, and vascular occlusion. Very high levels of CRP (>10 mg/L) indicate systemic inflammation such as with infection or other inflammatory conditions (eg, rheumatoid arthritis). However, even within the range of normal, more subtle increases in CRP can be used to predict cardiovascular risk.[3] A high-sensitivity C-reactive protein (hsCRP) level can thus provide added predictive value to select patients. As with any other risk factor, results should be considered with the aggregate of risks; the hsCRP result alone should not drive treatment decisions. The value of the test is highest when traditional risk factor analysis (see below) does not provide clarity to decisions regarding medical management. High-risk patients with multiple cardiovascular risk factors that warrant treatment will generally have no benefit from an hsCRP level as it will not alter their treatment recommendations. The corollary, in patients with no other cardiovascular risk factors, an elevated hsCRP alone cannot justify medication therapy. The hsCRP should thus be reserved for situations when the risk/benefit assessment for lipid-lowering medications is uncertain, such as for patients with borderline risk profiles. The CRP level can decrease in response to statin therapy[4] and other interventions that improve the quality of

Diet and related management of weight are also important considerations. Meaningful and long-term change will often best result from sensible and incremental changes. Thus, rather than suggest that patients change everything they eat, reviewing dietary patterns for the key pitfalls enables the clinician to make specific recommendations for areas to improve. Published outcomes correlate high carbohydrate intake to both diabetes (such as rice[23]) and slower metabolic rates after weight loss (making it harder to sustain weight loss).[24] Thus, recommending alternatives to rice (such as chopped vegetables, eg, riced cauliflower), white bread (such as whole wheat bread—or eliminating the bread calories entirely), and other processed carbohydrates colloquially termed *carbs* can help with weight management and lower lipid levels, blood pressure, and overall cardiovascular risk.

The Mediterranean diet has been advocated as a healthy approach to eating, and studies have reinforced its value for lowering the risk of developing diabetes, cardiovascular disease, and stroke.[25] Key components of the diet include:

- Daily consumption of nuts (one serving), fruits, and vegetables
- Daily consumption of whole grains (as opposed to highly processed carbohydrates)
- Weekly consumption of fish and poultry, eggs, beans
- Moderate consumption of dairy
- Limited consumption of red meat and sweets

In terms of items to reduce or eliminate, there is much guidance for clinicians to provide. Sugared beverages, including soft drinks and sports drinks, have known health risks and have been correlated with increased weight in children and adults.[26] Often called empty calories, they are a product of the modern food industry, serve no beneficial purpose, and should be eliminated. Observational data on beverages with sugar substitutes (such as diet soft drinks) have not correlated their consumption with any better weight outcomes. High-calorie *junk foods* (including candy bars, ice cream, chips) should also be consumed only on occasion. Replacing these snack foods with fresh vegetables and fruit can improve overall health. Portion size should be managed for home food preparation and restaurant eating.

COMORBID RISK FACTORS

While hypertension and smoking also contribute to cardiovascular disease, they are not directly tied to development of dyslipidemia. When present, both hypertension and smoking should be considered together with dyslipidemia as part of an overall risk-reduction strategy. Prescribing a cholesterol-lowering medication to a smoker should be accompanied by the equally important counseling on smoking cessation. Similarly, initiating cholesterol medication in a patient with hypertension should also be accompanied by measures to manage hypertension to more powerfully impact cardiovascular risk. While considering comorbid conditions may take more time and effort, when doctors and other health providers deliver comprehensive counseling patients are given opportunities for the best health outcomes through increased personal health awareness and participation in their care. Eyecare providers are in a key position to have such discussions with patients, including counseling and referral for management of comorbid cardiovascular risks when evaluating patients who have ocular findings of dyslipidemia or hypertension, such as Hollenhorst plaques or hypertensive retinal changes.

Drug Therapy for Dyslipidemia

Several drugs are available to treat lipid disorders. The most commonly prescribed drugs primarily lower the LDL level and may have a small beneficial impact on triglycerides and HDL. There are also drugs that target triglycerides and increase HDL a small amount. There are no drugs currently available that substantially increase the HDL level with proven cardiovascular risk reduction.

Current lipid treatment guidelines focus recommendations based upon two factors in the evaluation of the patient.[27] The first is an overall cardiovascular risk assessment, and the second is the LDL cholesterol level. Factors that contribute to the highest level of risk include established cardiovascular diseases and diabetes. Established cardiovascular disease includes:

- Patients who have had an *acute cardiovascular or other vascular event* including myocardial infarction, ischemic stroke, RAO, amputation due to peripheral vascular disease
- *Symptoms or findings of chronic cardiovascular disease* including angina, aortic aneurysm, carotid artery stenosis, OIS, transient ischemic event including amaurosis fugax
- *Cardiovascular procedures* including arterial stent (coronary artery, carotid artery, aorta), cardiac bypass surgery

In patients with established cardiovascular disease as above, lipid-lowering therapy is considered secondary prevention to prevent disease progression and recurrent events.

Patients with diabetes are also identified as similarly high risk, as diabetes carries a two to four fold higher rate of cardiovascular events including myocardial infarction and stroke.

Once these highest risk states are identified, aggressive management of LDL cholesterol with pharmacotherapy, along with attention to all other cardiovascular risk factors, is important to lower that risk.

In primary prevention for patients without diabetes, LDL level should be considered.

- Very low levels (70 mg/dL and below) are typically associated with low risk in the absence of other competing risk factors.
- Very high levels (over 190 mg/dL) warrant consideration of pharmacotherapy to reduce the LDL level due to this very high lipid-related risk.
- For patients whose risk falls in the middle, based upon age (45+ for men, 55+ for women) and LDL level (between 70 and 190 mg/dL), cardiovascular risk can be estimated with the ASCVD Risk Estimator.

The Risk Estimator is a calculator that considers several key risk factors and provides an estimate of the percentage risk for an event in the next 10 years.[28] Ten-year risk above 7.5% warrants consideration for statin therapy according to these guidelines that first advocated the use of the calculator. Notably, not all clinicians agree with that cutoff. At 10% 10-year risk, there is a greater consensus on the benefit of initiating statin therapy[29] (see **TABLE 3.2**) (http://tools.acc.org/ASCVD-Risk-Estimator-Plus/#!/calculate/estimate/).

TABLE 3.2   Traditional Risk Factors in ASCVD Risk Assessment[17]
Age
Gender (M/F)
Race (Caucasian, African American, other)
Systolic BP
Diastolic BP
Total cholesterol
HDL cholesterol
Diabetes (Y/N)
Smoker (current, former, never)
On therapy for hypertension (Y/N)

BP, blood pressure; HDL, high-density lipoprotein.

STATINS

The medications in this drug class are used most commonly for lipid treatment and are referred to as statins due to this common suffix in their generic names. These medications all inhibit the 3-hydroxy-3-methylglutaryl-CoA reductase or HMG-CoA enzyme and are thus also known as HMG-CoA reductase inhibitors. HMG CoA reductase is the rate-limiting enzyme in cholesterol biosynthesis. Thus, by inhibiting this enzyme, these drugs slow the process of hepatic cholesterol production. The different drugs in this class vary primarily in their potency and metabolism. Potency impacts the degree to which they lower the LDL level, and metabolism can impact the risk of drug-drug interactions. The more potent statin drugs can lower LDL by 50% or more when given at higher doses (**FIGURE 3.21**). High-potency statin doses also lower triglycerides a small amount and increase HDL by about 10%.

Statins are also associated with additional vascular benefits beyond their lipid-lowering abilities, often referred to as pleiotropic effects. Contributing to vascular endothelial stability, statins additionally decrease the risk for the plaque rupture that leads to acute vascular events. These benefits are seen both long term and short term; statin therapy is thus initiated in the acute setting of a cardiovascular event for patients not previously on treatment.[30]

Multiple studies have investigated statin use in cardiovascular disease. Statins have been found to decrease the risk of cardiovascular events, including myocardial infarction, the need for cardiovascular interventions, cardiovascular death, and strokes, both in secondary prevention and for primary prevention in patients with multiple cardiovascular risk factors when compared to placebo. Researchers subsequently demonstrated that there is incremental benefit from a high-dose versus a low-dose statin,[31] an important consideration in current treatment guidelines.[27]

Statins are generally well tolerated; however, there are a number of important clinical considerations, and monitoring for adverse effects is necessary. Because this drug class is used so widely, even infrequent events will occur in a relatively large absolute number of people. Most statins have extensive hepatic metabolism, and other drugs that are metabolized through these pathways can either speed up or slow down statin metabolism. The former situation could lead to reduced drug levels and lower efficacy of therapy, and in the latter situation higher drug levels can result, increasing the risk of statin toxicity. Conversely, statins can have these effects on co-administered therapy for other

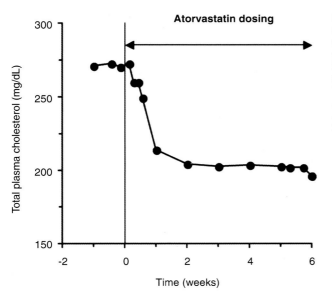

FIGURE 3.21 Within about 2 weeks of initiating therapy with a low dose of atorvastatin (5 mg), this patient's plasma total cholesterol has decreased by about 25%. (Reprinted with permission from Derendorf H. *Rowland and Tozer's Clinical Pharmacokinetics and Pharmacodynamics: Concepts and Applications.* 5th ed. Wolters Kluwer; 2019.)

conditions, especially anti-infectives, where more rapid breakdown could compromise the effectiveness of therapy. Thus, careful consideration of drug-drug interactions is important when starting statins or initiating other drugs in the setting of long-term statin use.

Statins are known to cause two syndromes involving muscles. The most severe condition, myositis, occurs very rarely with statin monotherapy at approved doses and in the absence of interacting drugs. In myositis, muscle inflammation occurs resulting in muscle pain and elevated blood levels of the muscle enzymes creatine phosphokinase (CK or CPK) from skeletal muscle breakdown. Myositis can be severe, and the drug should be stopped if myositis is suspected or confirmed. Statins can also cause a less serious syndrome of myalgias or muscle soreness without an elevated CPK level. Because muscle soreness is a nonspecific complaint (many people not taking statins have myalgias), it is not always possible to definitively determine the cause. While there are abundant reports of myalgias associated with statin use, in a placebo-controlled clinical trial, the rate of myalgia has been shown to be similar in the placebo group as compared to the group taking statin therapy.[32] For patients with significant myalgias while on statin therapy, a trial off the drug for a few weeks can be used to assess whether the statin is a trigger. If the myalgias resolve, yet statin therapy is important due to underlying cardiovascular risk, a different statin can be initiated and monitored. Studies and broad clinical experience with this drug class support tolerance of other agents in the class when myalgias develop with one drug. For patients who cannot tolerate any statin, other lipid management approaches may be necessary, such as the use of a second-line lipid-lowering agent.

Due to the hepatic metabolism of statins, significant liver dysfunction is generally considered a contraindication to statin therapy. Before statins are initiated, liver function should be checked. Once on a statin, patients should be monitored for liver toxicity clinically, with assessment for symptoms of liver disease on history (such as nausea, jaundice, abdominal pain), and assessing for jaundice, hepatomegaly, or right upper quadrant tenderness during the physical examination. Routine monitoring of liver enzyme blood tests is not considered necessary in patients with no underlying liver disease who are not taking other drugs that could interfere with liver function[33] (**TABLE 3.3**).

PCSK-9 INHIBITORS

The newest drug class for lipid treatment inhibits the enzyme proprotein convertase subtilisin–kexin type 9, thus PCSK-9 inhibitors. PCSK-9 binds the LDL receptor resulting in its degradation, lowering the number of LDL receptors. When present, the LDL receptor removes LDL from the serum, thus lowering serum LDL levels and reducing cardiovascular risk. Inhibiting PSCK-9 prevents the enzyme from degrading the LDL receptor, resulting in longer lifespan for LDL receptors, more LDL uptake from serum, and a lower serum LDL level. LDL reductions are often dramatic, dropping well beyond 50% from pretreatment levels. PCSK-9 drugs are monoclonal antibodies delivered by injection.

The PSCK-9 inhibitors have been shown to lower the risk of recurrent cardiovascular events when used in secondary prevention as add-on therapy in patients already taking maximally tolerated doses of a statin.[34] The benefits of cardiovascular risk reduction accrue the most in patients with higher

TABLE 3.3   Prescription Stains Available in the United States
Atorvastatin
Fluvastatin
Lovastatin
Pitavastatin
Pravastatin
Rosuvastatin
Simvastatin

pretreatment LDL levels. Due to their cost and the barrier of parenteral administration, these drugs are generally reserved for patients who are at very high risk for cardiovascular events and either have inadequate LDL level reductions from statin therapy or cannot tolerate statin therapy.

PCSK-9 therapy is usually tolerated well, with side effect rates generally similar to those of placebo. Local reactions at the injection site are usually mild and are the most common adverse effects. The liver and muscle risks with statin use have not been found to be a concern with this drug class. There are no known drug-drug interactions. Monitoring on therapy consists of periodic lipid profiles and checking the drug injection sites.

EZETIMIBE

This oral medication inhibits cholesterol absorption at the intestinal brush border and has a small impact on lipid levels. Used alone, its impact on LDL levels and cardiovascular outcomes is not robust, but when combined with a statin drug, it has been shown to reduce cardiovascular event rates.[35] It is thus used most commonly in patients at high cardiovascular risk with an inadequate LDL reduction on a statin, either the highest available dose or the maximum tolerated dose. With the availability of the potent PCSK-9 inhibitors for LDL lowering with statin failure, ezetimibe is used most often when the additional LDL reduction goal is relatively small or with barriers to PCSK-9 use, such as when cost or self-injection is an issue for the patient.

Ezetimibe is generally well tolerated with few side effects. Periodic measurement of the lipid profile is usually the only necessary monitoring.

FIBRATES

This drug class is most effective at lowering triglyceride levels and increasing serum HDL. Several mechanisms are responsible for these favorable clinical effects on triglycerides and HDL. Fibrates activate peroxisome proliferator-activated receptors, which are nuclear transcription factors. The result is an increase in HDL synthesis, while also increasing triglyceride uptake into cells and increasing the catabolism of VLDL.[36] Studies have not consistently shown a reduction in cardiovascular events from fibrate therapy.[37,38] In practice, fibrates are used most often for patients with very high triglycerides who are at risk for pancreatitis or to treat complex lipid disorders along with statins or other drugs.

While usually tolerated well, there are a number of drug-drug interactions, and a review of current therapies is indicated before a fibrate is initiated or before a new prescription is added to current fibrate therapy. There are also potential important interactions with statin drug metabolism, and when used together for patients with severe dyslipidemias, monitoring of liver tests is often necessary and some physicians monitor CPK enzyme levels as well.

NIACIN

Niacin or nicotinic acid is the common name for vitamin B3. In very high doses, it can lower triglycerides and increase HDL. The mechanism of action is not completely understood, but is hypothesized to be multifactorial, including inhibiting free fatty acid release from muscle and increasing the breakdown of chylomicron particles. Despite these positive impacts on the lipid profile, studies have not conclusively demonstrated reductions in cardiovascular events from niacin use. In addition, the high doses required for clinical effectiveness cause significant adverse effects that limit tolerability and can exacerbate other conditions. Flushing is an adverse effect that typically accompanies the high doses necessary for effectiveness. While taking the dose with aspirin can help minimize this effect, many patients still cannot tolerate the necessary dose. Other side effects include glucose intolerance, exacerbation of gout, peptic ulcers, and liver test elevations. There are also a number of important drug-drug interactions for which prescribing doctors need to be alert. Thus, niacin is not commonly prescribed in clinical practice.

FISH OIL

Fish oils include eicosapentaenoic acid and docosahexaenoic acid. Ingestion of high levels—often substantially higher intakes than from merely eating fish—have been shown to decrease triglyceride levels and possibly slow the progression of atherosclerosis and the occurrence of arrhythmias and cardiac death. While many fish oil supplements are marketed directly to consumers and available without a prescription, there is a specific prescription formulation available for hypertriglyceridemia. Potential cardiovascular benefits have been evaluated in numerous studies with mixed results—some positive, while others showed no benefit. A particularly large trial that received attention showed no benefit for lowering cardiovascular events including myocardial infarction, cardiac death, or arrhythmias.[39] Since fish oil has not been found to pose any harms, eating fish at least once or twice a week remains a commonly recommended component of a healthy diet (including the Mediterranean diet). The prescription fish oil preparations remain an option for managing hypertriglyceridemia.

ASPIRIN THERAPY

Acetylsalicylic acid or aspirin has many clinical effects, some of which offer benefit in specific situations. Yet due to the complex actions of aspirin, benefits are accompanied by significant potential for adverse effects. Its role in inhibiting the cyclooxygenase enzyme blocks prostaglandin synthesis. By inhibiting the prostaglandins that cause inflammation, aspirin can be helpful in treating fevers and inflammatory pain such as joint injuries and inflammatory arthritis. On the other hand, other prostaglandins are necessary to maintain renal blood flow and mucosal integrity. These prostaglandins are also inhibited by aspirin, which can impair renal blood flow and trigger gastric ulcers and bleeding. Aspirin also inhibits thromboxanes, which contribute to platelet aggregation. In the setting of atherosclerotic vascular disease, where platelet aggregation and clot formation in arterial plaques leads to acute ischemia, platelet inhibition has been shown to be beneficial; aspirin therapy is standard emergency treatment for patients suffering an acute myocardial infarction. However, this reduction in platelet function that can help in atherosclerotic vascular disease can lead to serious adverse effects elsewhere, including the gastrointestinal (GI) tract, where compromised gastric mucosal integrity can lead to ulcer formation and bleeding. In situations where the risk of hemorrhagic stroke is elevated, such as in chronic hypertension or acute blood pressure elevation, aspirin will increase the bleeding risk. Clinicians must understand and balance the potential benefits and known risks in recommending aspirin.

Many studies of aspirin have been published since the randomized Physicians' Health Study reported a reduction in myocardial infarction in men treated with aspirin for primary prevention (325 mg every other day)[40] in 1989. However, this highly publicized reduction in myocardial infarction incidence was limited to men older than 50 years and was not accompanied by a decrease in cardiovascular disease death compared to placebo. While bleeding complications including GI bleeding and intracranial hemorrhage occurred infrequently, they were more common occurrences in the aspirin treatment group. The aspirin treatment group was also more likely to receive blood transfusions due to bleeding. Lower doses of aspirin have since been advocated to maintain the protective antiplatelet benefit while lowering the risks of GI toxicity. However, studies of lower aspirin doses have also found an increase in the risk of bleeding, confirming that the antiplatelet effect is a double-edged sword.[41]

More recent studies reflect the additional knowledge and therapeutics available in the decades since the Physicians' Health Study was completed. A meta-analysis that evaluated more recent aspirin prevention trials and also considered outcomes in women reached a different conclusion with respect to primary prevention.[42] There remained a reduction in the incidence of myocardial infarction as well as a small decrease in ischemic stroke, yet similar to the Physicians' Health Study, there was no reduction in cardiovascular mortality. GI bleeding and intracranial hemorrhage occurred at about the same rate as the cardiac benefits. Similarly, when a low dose (100 mg) of aspirin was compared to placebo for primary prevention in patients with diabetes, the cardiovascular benefit of 1 fewer event per 100 patients treated for 7.5 years was offset by one additional major bleeding event.[43] Thus, aspirin therapy for primary prevention has fallen out of favor, particularly for older patients and those otherwise at a higher risk of GI bleeding. However, it remains important to be sure that in a situation of equipoise with respect to the trade-off of risks, patients understand the information and have the opportunity to voice their preference. Some individuals may want to prevent a heart attack at higher cost, as gastric bleeding can usually be treated and cured, versus the permanence of a myocardial infarction.

Two footnotes on aspirin therapy: In the setting of established cardiovascular disease, the studies on aspirin use in primary prevention no longer hold. Established cardiovascular disease is a substantial risk for a future event and will alter the risk-benefit balance. In particular, patients with cardiac stents, which are more prone to developing occlusive clots, often require antiplatelet therapies that may include aspirin. While aspirin has been shown to reduce the risk of precancerous colon polyps,[44] in most evaluations, it does not offer net benefit to people at average risk, and reductions in colon cancer are not proven. As with myocardial infarction prevention, for patients at especially high risk of colon cancer, an overall consideration of risk-benefit may look different than it does for the average-risk patient.

ATHEROSCLEROSIS

The process of atherosclerosis contributes to arteriosclerosis or hardening of the arteries. Arteriosclerosis is a progressive disease that involves inflammation and degeneration of the inner lining, or intima, of medium and large arteries. Since arteries are key conduits for delivering oxygen and nutrients to the body cells and organs, compromise of arterial function leads to disease in many systems. There are many well-known risk factors for the development of atherosclerosis and the resulting arteriosclerosis; an individualized assessment enables each patient's vascular disease risk to be determined. When done in concert with approaches to modify these risks, treatment can effect reductions in the complications of atherosclerosis.

The process of atherosclerosis was not well understood for many years and common thinking about this disease has not consistently caught up with modern scientific understanding. Atherosclerosis is not a diffuse but a focal process, characterized by individual lesions, marked by inflammation and immune dysregulation. The process of atherosclerosis leads to arteriosclerosis in vessels of a size, type, and caliber that deal with pulsatile flow of blood (ie, larger than arterioles). Precursor lesions evolve, grow, and coalesce, resulting in larger areas causing more diffuse vascular damage. Circulatory impairment often occurs from the acute rupture of relatively small, but unstable plaques that trigger accumulation of platelets and clot formation, rather than from a progressive deposition of lipid.

Atherosclerosis begins with damage to the tunica intima of medium and large vessels, leading to deposition of LDL within the vessel wall. Oxidation of LDL in the arterial intima is an important early event in the early lesions of atherosclerosis. The oxidized LDL particles attract monocytes and macrophages which ingest the oxidized LDL and become foam cells. Accumulation of large numbers of foam cells corresponds to the early stage of arteriosclerosis known as the fatty streak.

The foam cells in turn elaborate factors that trigger inflammation and propagation of the plaque including interleukins, chemotactic hormones, and growth factors that cause the arterial smooth muscle cells to proliferate and invade the tunica intima, while also attracting inflammatory cells and platelets. The smooth muscle cells attempt to cap these areas of arterial damage, resulting in the formation of a fibrous cap.

The fibrous cap and its interaction with the local environment play a pivotal role in the direction that the arterial intima lesion takes. A thin fibrous cap is at higher risk of rupture in a harmful local environment of scouring high blood pressure, toxic chemicals from cigarette smoke, and local inflammation from oxidized LDL. On the other hand, a stable fibrous cap is more likely to result when exposed to a normal blood pressure and low levels of inflammation such as with LDL cholesterol management on statin therapy. The stable cap in a low risk environment is less likely to rupture.

Rupture of the fibrous cap is the critical event that moves an atherosclerotic lesion from an observer to bad actor. When the protective cap ruptures, the core of the atherosclerotic lesion is exposed. The lesion, which is filled with foam cells and necrotic material from the death of leukocytes, is an inflammatory milieu that has resulted from the atherosclerotic process. This mix combined with turbulent blood flow over the irregular surface is thrombogenic, attracting and activating platelets, which adhere and form a clot. As this clot propagates, it grows out of the lesion and can occlude the artery causing acute ischemia and ultimately infarction[45] (**FIGURE 3.22**). Portions of such lesions can also be dislodged, producing emboli that can occlude smaller vessels downstream.

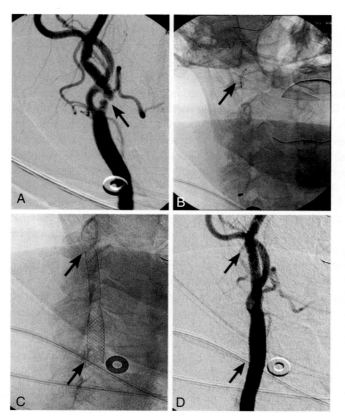

FIGURE 3.22 An 82-year-old, right-handed woman with hypertension, hyperlipidemia, coronary artery disease, and progressive right internal carotid artery stenosis despite aggressive medical therapy with anti-platelet and statin medications. A, Right common carotid arteriography demonstrates severe (greater than 90%) stenosis of the proximal right internal carotid artery (arrow). B, Fluororadiograph demonstrates placement of a vascular filtration device across the site of stenosis prior to stent-angioplasty (arrow). C and D, Fluororadiograph and right common carotid arteriogram demonstrate placement of the endovascular stent with restoration of normal blood flow in the right carotid artery (arrows). The patient tolerated the procedure very well and was discharged the following morning. (Reprinted from Rowland LP. *Merritt's Neurology.* 11th ed. Philadelphia, PA: Wolters Kluwer; 2005.)

in the skin integrity, whether from a pebble, splinter, or ungroomed toenail, can result in a limb-threatening infection. Avoidance of barefoot walking and treatment of cracked skin and tinea pedis along with fastidious toe-nail grooming help avoid skin breaks and maintain the integrity of the epidermal barrier.

Overview of Risk Determination and Prevention

The clinical manifestations of cerebrovascular, peripheral vascular, and coronary artery disease such as stroke, amputation, and myocardial infarction all result in significant morbidity and represent major causes of mortality in the Western world. This underscores the role of risk factor identification and modification for the health and longevity of individuals and populations. In addition, the efficient use of healthcare resources is important to consider. Prevention is much more effective than late-stage interventions which are always more resource-intensive and initiated at a later stage when organ dysfunction and associated impairment in quality of life is already present.

Observational data over many years have shown a clear correlation between higher LDL levels and cardiovascular events.[27] Inflammation also plays a key role in the formation of fatty streaks and their progression to occlusive arterial lesions. Inflammation can be triggered by infection, smoking, and chronic inflammatory diseases. Pneumonia,[70] influenza infection,[71] and other infectious conditions have been correlated with a higher risk of acute coronary artery events. The inflammation from chronic inflammatory conditions such as rheumatoid arthritis[72] has also been found to correlate with a higher risk of cardiovascular events.

LDL-lowering with statin therapy and PCSK-9 inhibitor treatment provides net benefit when elevated cardiovascular risk warrants therapy.[22] Regular exercise, healthy eating, and maintaining a healthy weight are also factors that can decrease inflammation and reverse other risk triggers; they correlate with lower risks for cardiovascular events. Smoking cessation can lower cardiovascular risk by as much as 50% in the first year after quitting. Influenza and pneumococcal vaccination, by preventing their respective infections, will lower the risk for acute cardiovascular events and is sensible for overall health.

Arterial damage from hypertension has been strongly linked to risks for cardiovascular disease as well. Hypertension treatment has been shown repeatedly to offer cardiovascular risk reduction across ages and in patients with other cardiovascular comorbidities, especially diabetes.[73]

Diabetes (Chapter 5) deserves special mention, as it has been shown to increase the risk for cardiovascular disease including myocardial infarction and stroke (macrovascular disease) by two to four times compared to people without diabetes. This risk relationship was identified as far back as the 1970s.[74] Several theories exist to support this observation, and it is likely that multiple mechanisms explain the reasons for this increase in risk. Management of glucose is also an important component of health management for patients with diabetes and can reduce cardiovascular events. A growing body of data indicates that various oral and noninsulin injected drugs have differential effects on cardiovascular risk, and attention to specific medical therapy can also favorably impact cardiovascular risk.[75-77] In addition, smoking has added hazards for patients with diabetes since it also increases the risk for microvascular complications, highlighting the need for intensive efforts at education and cessation support for smokers who have diabetes.

Family history of cardiovascular disease is also an important consideration. Occurrence of a cardiac or other vascular event in a first-degree relative before the age of 55 in males and 65 in females is considered a risk factor. Indeed, asking a single question about the presence of cardiovascular disease in any first-degree relative performed similarly as a risk predictor to taking a more complex family history.[78]

Many approaches are available for risk assessment and treatment to reduce cardiovascular complications associated with atherosclerosis. Since no one approach will be an exact predictor of risk, interpreting results and providing sensible explanations and recommendations to our patients is also an important role for the clinician. Once risk is assessed, the clinician should make recommendations that are concordant with guidelines, while also considering each patient's preferences and expectations to maximize patient engagement in any prevention strategy.

REFERENCES

1. Dubin D.. *Rapid Interpretation of EKG's*. 6th ed.. Tampa, FL: Cover Publishing; 2000.

2. Herring N, Paterson DJ. ECG diagnosis of acute ischaemia and infarction: past, present and future. *QJM: An International Journal of Medicine*. 2006;99(4):219-230. doi:10.1093/qjmed/hcl025.

3. Markanday A. Acute phase reactants in infections: evidence-based review and a guide for clinicians. *Open Forum Infect Dis*. 2015;2(3), ofv098. doi:10.1093/ofid/ofv098.

4. Albert MA, Danielson A, Rifai N. Effect of statin therapy on C-reactive protein levels. *J Am Med Assoc*. 2001;286(1):64-70.

5. Elias-Smale SE, Proença RV, Koller MT, et al. Coronary calcium score improves classification of coronary heart disease risk in the elderly: the Rotterdam Study. *J Am Coll Cardiol*. 2010;56:1407-1414.

6. Schuetz GM, Zacharopoulou NM, Schlattmann P, Dewey M. Meta-analysis: noninvasive coronary angiography using computed tomography versus magnetic resonance imaging. *Ann Intern Med*. 2010;152:167-177.

7. Hollander JE, Chang AM, Shofer FS, McCusker CM, Baxt WG, Litt HI. Coronary computed tomographic angiography for rapid discharge of low-risk patients with potential acute coronary syndromes. *Ann Emerg Med*. 2009;53:295-304.

8. Friedewald WT, Levy RI, Fredrickson DS. Estimation of the concentration of low-density lipoprotein cholesterol in plasma, without use of the preparative ultracentrifuge. *Clin Chem*. 1972;18:499-502.

9. Grundy SM, Cleeman JI, Merz CN, et al. Implications of recent clinical trials for the national cholesterol education program adult treatment panel III guidelines. *Circulation*. 2004;110(2):227-239. doi:10.1161/01.CIR.0000133317.49796.0E.

10. The Emerging Risk Factors Collaboration; Di Angelantonio E, Sarwar N, Perry P, et al. Major lipids, apolipoproteins, and risk of vascular disease. *J Am Med Assoc*. 2009;302:1993-2000.

11. Zech LA Jr, Hoeg JM. Correlating corneal arcus with atherosclerosis in familial hypercholesterolemia. *Lipids Health Dis*. 2008;7:7. PMCID: PMC2279133 PMID: 18331643.

12. Diekman T, Lansberg PJ, Kastelein JJP, Wiersinga WM. Prevalence and correction of hypothyroidism in a large cohort of patients referred for dyslipidemia. *Arch Intern Med*. 1995;155(14):1490-1495. doi:10.1001/archinte.1995.00430140052004.

13. Mora S. Nonfasting for routine lipid testing: from evidence to action. *JAMA Intern Med*. 2016;176(7):1005-1006. doi:10.1001/jamainternmed.2016.1979.

14. Cogan DG. The corneal arcus. *N Engl J Med*. 1974;291:1356.

15. Rosenman RH, Brand RJ, Sholtz RI, et al. Relation of corneal arcus to cardiovascular risk factors and the incidence of coronary disease. *N Engl J Med*. 1974;291:1322-1324.

16. Fernández A, Sorokin A, Thompson PD. Corneal arcus as cardiovascular disease risk factor. *Atherosclerosis*. 2007;193(2):235-240.

17. Olsen TW, Pulido JS, Folk JC, Hyman L, Flaxel CJ, Adelman RA. Retinal and ophthalmic artery occlusions Preferred Practice Pattern®. *Ophthalmology*. 2017;124(2):120-143. doi:10.1016/j.ophtha.2016.09.024.

18. Ghosh C, Ghosh T. Eyelid lesions. In: Trobe J, Givens J, eds. UpToDate. Accessed June 4, 2019. www.uptodate.com/contents/eyelid-lesions.

19. Bowling B. Chapter 1: eyelids. In: Bowling B, ed. *Kanski's Clinical Ophthalmology: A Systematic Approach*. 8th ed. Elsevier; 2016:1-62. Available at https://www.elsevier.com/books/kanskis-clinical-ophthalmology/kanski/978-0-7020-5572-0.

20. Stearns S, Friedman E, Lugitch M, Hoffman SH. Lipemia retinalis: report of a case. *N Engl J Med*. 1948;238:16-17.

21. Zahavi A, Snir M, Kela YR. Lipemia retinalis: case report and review of the literature. *J AAPOS*. 2013;17(1):10-11.

22. Maki KC, Bays HE, Dicklin MR. Treatment options for the management of hypertriglyceridemia: strategies based on the best-available evidence. *J Clin Lipidol*. 2012;6(5):413-426.

23. Hu EA, Pan A, Malik V, Sun Q. White rice consumption and risk of type 2 diabetes: meta-analysis and systematic review. *Br Med J*. 2012;344:e1454.

24. Ebbeling CB, Feldman HA, Klein GL, et al. Effects of a low carbohydrate diet on energy expenditure during weight loss maintenance: randomized trial. *Br Med J*. 2018;363:k4583.

25. Martínez-González MA, Gea A, Ruiz-Canela M. The mediterranean diet and cardiovascular health: a critical review. *Circ Res.* 2019;124:779-798.

26. Vartanian LR, Schwartz MB, Brownell KD. Effects of soft drink consumption on nutrition and health: a systematic review and meta-analysis. *Am J Public Health.* 2007;97:667-675.

27. Grundy SM, Stone NJ, Bailey AL, et al. 2018 AHA/ACC/AACVPR/AAPA/ABC/ACPM/ADA/AGS/APhA/ASPC/NLA/PCNA guideline on the management of blood cholesterol. *J Am Coll Cardiol.* 2019;73(24):e285-e350. doi:10.1016/j.jacc.2018.11.003.

28. http://tools.acc.org/ASCVD-Risk-Estimator-Plus/#!/calculate/estimate/Visited June 2019.

29. US Preventive Services Task Force. Statin use for the primary prevention of cardiovascular disease in adults: US preventive services task force recommendation statement. *J Am Med Assoc.* 2016;316(19):1997-2007. doi:10.1001/jama.2016.15450.

30. Whayne TF Jr. A viewpoint on statin effects – benefits and problems. *Int J Angiol.* 2008;17(4):178-180. doi:10.1055/s-0031-1278305.

31. LaRosa JC, Grundy SM, Waters DD, et al. Intensive lipid lowering with atorvastatin in patients with stable coronary disease. *N Engl J Med.* 2005;352:1425-1435.

32. Gupta A, Thompson D, Whitehouse A, et al. Adverse events associated with unblinded, but not with blinded, statin therapy in the Anglo-Scandinavian Cardiac Outcomes Trial – Lipid-Lowering Arm (ASCOT-LLA): a randomised double-blind placebo-controlled trial and its non-randomised non-blind extension phase. *Lancet.* 2017;389:2473-2481. doi:10.1016/S0140-6736(17)31075-9.

33. Jose J. Statins and its hepatic effects: newer data, implications, and changing recommendations. *J Pharm Bioallied Sci.* 2016;8(1):23-28. doi:10.4103/0975-7406.171699.

34. Schwartz GG, Steg PG, Szarek M, et al. Alirocumab and cardiovascular outcomes after acute coronary syndrome. *N Engl J Med.* 2018;379:2097-2107.

35. Cannon CP, Blazing MA, Giugliano RP, et al. Ezetimibe added to statin therapy after acute coronary syndromes. *N Engl J Med.* 2015;372:2387-2397.

36. Staels B, Dallongeville J, Auwerx J, Schoonjans K, Leitersdorf E, Fruchart JC. Mechanism of action of fibrates on lipid and lipoprotein metabolism. *Circulation.* 1998;98(19):2088-2093.

37. Jun M, Foote C, Lv J, et al. Effects of fibrates on cardiovascular outcomes: a systematic review and meta-analysis. *Lancet.* 2010;375:1875-1884.

38. Elam MB, Ginsberg HN, Lovato LC, et al. Association of fenofibrate therapy with long-term cardiovascular risk in statin-treated patients with type 2 diabetes. *JAMA Cardiol.* 2017;2(4):370-380. doi:10.1001/jamacardio.2016.4828.

39. Rizos EC, Ntzani EE, Bika E, Kostapanos MS, Elisaf MS. Association between omega-3 fatty acid supplementation and risk of major cardiovascular disease events: a systematic review and meta-analysis. *J Am Med Assoc.* 2012;308(10):1024-1033.

40. Steering Committee of the Physicians' Health Study Research Group. Final report on the aspirin component of the ongoing physicians' health study. *N Engl J Med.* 1989;321:129-135.

41. De Berardis G, Lucisano G, D'Ettorre A, et al. Association of aspirin use with major bleeding in patients with and without diabetes. *J Am Med Assoc.* 2012;307:2286-2294. doi:10.1001/jama.2012.5034.

42. Abdelaziz HK, Saad M, Pothineni NV, et al. Aspirin for primary prevention of cardiovascular events. *J Am Coll Cardiol.* 2019;73:2915-2929.

43. The ASCEND Study Collaborative Group; Bowman L, Mafham M, Wallendszus K, et al. Effects of aspirin for primary prevention in persons with diabetes mellitus. *N Engl J Med.* 2018;379:1529-1539. doi:10.1056/NEJMoa1804988.

44. Grau MV, Sandler RS, McKeown-Eyssen G, et al. Nonsteroidal anti-inflammatory drug use after 3 years of aspirin use and colorectal adenoma risk: observational follow-up of a randomized study. *J Natl Cancer Inst.* 2009;101:267-276.

45. Ross R. Atherosclerosis – An inflammatory disease. *N Engl J Med.* 1999;340:115-126.

46. Berenson G. S., Srinivasan SR, Bao W, Newman WP III, Tracy RE, Wattigney WA. Association between multiple cardiovascular risk factors and atherosclerosis in children and young adults. *N Engl J Med.* 1998;338:1650-1656.

47. Yoon PW, Bastian B, Anderson RN, et al. Potentially preventable deaths from the five leading causes of death – United States, 2008-2010. *MMWR Morb Mortal Wkly Rep.* 2014;63(17):369-374.

48. Go AS, Mozaffarian D, Roger VL, et al. American Heart Association statistics committee and stroke statistics subcommittee heart disease and stroke statistics – 2013 update: a report from the American Heart Association. *Circulation.* 2013;127:e6-e245.

49. Hemingway H, McCallum A, Shipley M, Manderbacka K, Martikainen P, Keskimäki I. Incidence and prognostic implications of stable angina pectoris among women and men. *J Am Med Assoc.* 2006;295:1404-1411.

50. Zaacks SM, Liebson PR, Liebson PR, Calvin JE, Parrillo JE, Klein LW. Unstable angina and non-Q wave myocardial infarction: does the clinical diagnosis have therapeutic implications? *J Am Assoc Cardiol.* 1999;33(1):107-118.

51. BARI Investigators. Seven-year outcome in the bypass angioplasty revascularization investigation (BARI) by treatment and diabetic status. *J Am Coll Cardiol.* 2000;35:1122-1129.

52. Lamas GA, Hochman JS. Where does the occluded artery trial leave the late open artery hypothesis? *Heart.* 2007;93(11):1319-1321. doi:10.1136/hrt.2007.123489.

53. Lee J, Inoue M, Mlynash M, et al. MR perfusion lesions after TIA or minor stroke are associated with new infarction at 7 days. *Neurology* 2017;88:2254-2259. doi:10.1212/WNL.0000000000004039.

54. Furie KL. Pathophysiology of symptoms from carotid atherosclerosis. In: Dashe JF ed. UpToDate. Waltham, Mass: UpToDate; 2019. Accessed August 22, 2019. www.uptodate.com.

55. Jashari F, Ibrahimi P, Nicoll R, et al. Coronary and carotid atherosclerosis: similarities and differences. *Atherosclerosis.* 2013;227(2):193-200.

56. Lefevre M. Screening for asymptomatic carotid artery stenosis: U.S. Preventative services task force recommendations statement. *Ann Intern Med.* 2014;161:356-362.

57. Furie KL. Evaluation of carotid artery stenosis. In: Dashe JF, ed. *UpToDate.* Waltham, Mass: UpToDate; 2019. Accessed August 23, 2019. www.uptodate.com.

58. Fairman RM. Management of symptomatic carotid atherosclerotic disease. In: Dashe JF, Collins KA, eds. *UpToDate.* Waltham, Mass: UpToDate; 2019. Accessed August 23, 2019. www.uptodate.com.

59. Barnett HJM, Taylor DW, Eliasziw M, et al; North American Symptomatic Carotid Endarterectomy Trial Collaborators. Beneficial effect of carotid endarterectomy in symptomatic patients with high-grade carotid stenosis. *N Engl J Med.* 1991;325:445.

60. European Carotid Surgery Trialists' Collaborative Group. MRC European Carotid Surgery Trial: interim results for symptomatic patients with severe (70-99%) or with mild (0-29%) carotid stenosis. *Lancet.* 1991;337:1235.

61. Randomised trial of endarterectomy for recently symptomatic carotid stenosis: final results of the MRC European Carotid Surgery Trial (ECST). *Lancet.* 1998;351:1379-1387.

62. Brott TG, Hobson RW II, Howard G, et al; CREST Investigators. Stenting versus endarterectomy for treatment of carotid-artery stenosis. *N Engl J Med.* 2010;363(1):11-23. doi:10.1056/NEJMoa0912321.

63. Hayreh SS, Podhajsky PA, Zimmerman MB. Retinal artery occlusion: associated systemic and ophthalmic abnormalities. *Ophthalmology.* 2009;116(10):1928-1936.

64. Callizo J, Feltgen N, Pantenburg S, Wolf A, et al. Cardiovascular risk factors in central retinal artery occlusion: results of a prospective and standardized medical examination. *Ophthalmology.* 2015;122(9):1881-1888.

65. Benavente O, Eliasziw M, Streifler J, Fox AJ, Barnett HJ, Meldrum H; North American Symptomatic Carotid Endarterectomy Trial Collaborators. Prognosis after transient monocular blindness associated with carotid artery stenosis. *N Eng J Med.* 2001;345:1084-1090.

66. Streifler JY, Eliasziw M, Benavente OR, et al. The risk of stroke in patients with first-ever retinal vs hemispheric transient ischemic attacks and high-grade carotid stenosis. North American Symptomatic Carotid Endarterectomy Trial. *Arch Neurol.* 1995;52:246.

67. Bakri SJ, Luqman A, Pathik B, Chandrasekaran K. Is carotid ultrasound necessary in the evaluation of the asymptomatic Hollenhorst plaque? *Ophthalmology.* 2013;120(12):2747-2748.E1.

68. Guirguis-Blake JM, Beil TL, Senger CA, Whitlock EP. Ultrasonography screening for abdominal aortic aneurysms: a systematic evidence review for the US preventive services task force. *Ann Intern Med.* 2014;160:321-329.

69. Karthikesalingam A, Vidal-Diez A, Holt PJ, Loftus Ian M. Thresholds for abdominal aortic aneurysm repair in england and the United States. *N Engl J Med.* 2016;375:2051-2059.

70. Musher DM, Rueda AM, Kaka AS, Mapara SM. The association between pneumococcal pneumonia and acute cardiac events. *Clin Infect Dis.* 2007;45:158-165.

71. Kwong JC, Schwartz KL, Campitelli MA. Acute myocardial infarction after laboratory-confirmed influenza infection. *N Engl J Med.* 2018;378:2538-2541.

72. Solomon DH, Karlson EW, Rimm EB, et al. Cardiovascular morbidity and mortality in women diagnosed with rheumatoid arthritis. *Circulation.* 2003;107:1303-1307.

73. 2017 ACC/AHA/AAPA/ABC/ACPM/AGS/APhA/ASH/ASPC/NMA/PCNA guideline for the prevention, detection, evaluation, and management of high blood pressure in adults: a report of the American College of Cardiology/American Heart Association Task Force on Clinical Practice Guidelines. *J Am Coll Cardiol.* 2018;71:e127-e248.

74. Kannel W, McGee DL. Diabetes and cardiovascular disease: the framingham heart study. *J Am Med Assoc.* 1979;241(19):2035-2038.

75. Imprialos K, Faselis C, Boutari C, et al. SGLT-2 inhibitors and cardiovascular risk in diabetes mellitus: a comprehensive and critical review of the literature. *Curr Pharm Des.* 2017;23:1510. doi: 10.2174/13816128236661701241 23927.

76. Roumie CL, Chipman J, Min JY, et al. Association of treatment with metformin vs sulfonylurea with major adverse cardiovascular events among patients with diabetes and reduced kidney function. *J Am Med Assoc.* 2019;322(12):1167-1177. doi:10.1001/jama.2019.13206.

77. Bethel MA, Patel RA, Merrill P, et al. Cardiovascular outcomes with glucagon-like peptide-1 receptor agonists in patients with type 2 diabetes: a meta-analysis. *Lancet Diabetes Endocrinol.* 2018;6:105-113.

78. Patel J, Al Rifai M, Scheuner MT, et al. Basic vs more complex definitions of family history in the prediction of coronary heart disease: the multi-ethnic study of atherosclerosis. *Mayo Clin Proc.* 2018;93(9):1213.

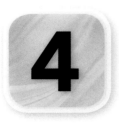

4 Intrinsic Cardiovascular Disorders

David M. Shein and Rachel C. Druckenbrod

LEARNING OBJECTIVES

While coronary artery disease (Chapter 3) represents the single most common cardiovascular condition in the developed world, other important conditions also affect the heart. Many have manifestations in other systems including ocular findings and symptoms. This chapter will cover a diverse set of conditions, including cardiac valvular disease, acute infections, long-term infectious complications, genetic disorders, and rhythm abnormalities due to disease of the conduction system. Atrial fibrillation, an arrhythmia affecting about 1% of the American population, is a substantial cause of embolic stroke and is also covered in this chapter.

KEY CONCEPTS

Section 1: Valvular Heart Disease
Aortic stenosis
Aortic insufficiency
Mitral stenosis
Mitral insufficiency
Marfan syndrome
Section 2: Cardiac Complications of Infectious Diseases
Rheumatic fever

Endocarditis
Section 3: Cardiomyopathy and Congestive Heart Failure
Cardiomyopathy
Congestive heart failure
   Cardiac physiology review
Section 4: Cardiac Arrhythmia
Atrial fibrillation

SECTION 1: CARDIAC VALVULAR DISEASE

The four cardiac valves are delicate structures that allow unidirectional blood flow through the heart, separating each atrium and ventricle, and controlling outflow through the aorta and pulmonary artery. The aortic valve is normally a triple-cusp valve that floats freely, responding to pressure from blood flow to trigger opening and closing.

The mitral valve is a complex valve with attachments to papillary muscles in the ventricle via chordae tendineae (**FIGURE 4.1**). The pulmonic valve is similar to the aortic valve in structure, while the tricuspid valve (between the right atrium and right ventricle) is more similar to the mitral valve. The left-sided valves play a large role in the integrity of the systemic circulation and, when diseased, generally cause more symptoms than right-sided valve disease. Heart valve failure occurs chiefly through two mechanisms: stenosis (narrowing) or insufficiency (regurgitation) (**FIGURE 4.2**).

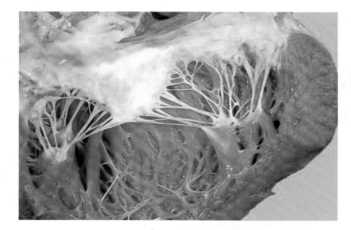

FIGURE 4.1 A normal mitral valve with chordae tendineae inserting into the papillary muscles. (From Mills SE. *Histology for Pathologists.* 5th ed. Philadelphia, PA: Wolters Kluwer; 2019.)

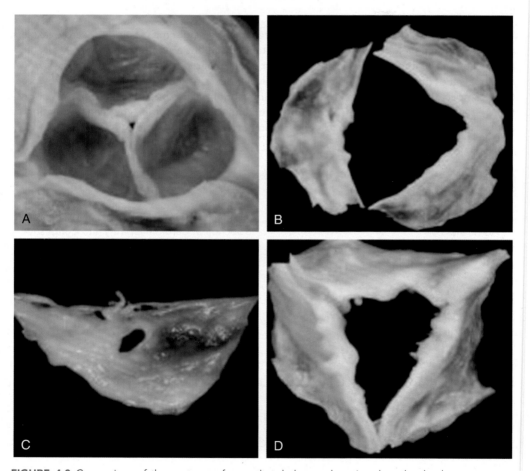

FIGURE 4.2 Comparison of the anatomy of normal and abnormal aortic valves that lead to severe aortic regurgitation. A, Normal aortic valve. A cephalad view of a normal aortic valve from a young adult is shown. The size of the cusps and the distance between each of the commissures are roughly equal. B, Regurgitation secondary to dilated aortic root and bicuspid aortic valve. The excised valve shows a bicuspid aortic valve with the larger conjoint cusp shown on the right side. There is mild thickening of the free edge without calcification. C, Regurgitation secondary to healed endocarditis. A semilunar valve cusp shows a large central perforation as a sequela of infective endocarditis. D, Trileaflet aortic valve with regurgitation. A trileaflet aortic valve shows marked thickening and retraction of cusps. The cusp retraction by fibrous tissue results in failure of coaptation at the center of the valve. The fusion in two of the three commissures also results in valve stenosis. (Courtesy of Drs. E. Rene Rodriguez and Carmela D. Tan. Availabe at www.e-heart.org.)

Ventricular fibrillation is a fatal arrhythmia unless treated with circulatory support (cardiopulmonary resuscitation or CPR) and timely defibrillation. Defibrillation can be administered by healthcare professionals in a hospital setting, in the field by trained field personnel (such as emergency medical technicians), and by bystanders with automatic external defibrillators (AEDs) in public places. AEDs are straightforward to use, as the device provides instructions to administer CPR and allow the machine to administer defibrillating shocks using internal algorithms based upon a machine reading of the electrocardiogram (ECG).

Atrial fibrillation affects about 2.5 million people in the United States,[21] with increasing age as a significant risk factor such that by the age of 80 years, about 10% of the population has atrial fibrillation.[22] Atrial fibrillation is also seen more commonly in males.[23] Additional risk factors for atrial fibrillation include atrial enlargement (such as with valvular disease, as above), congestive heart failure, hypertension (Chapter 2), hyperthyroidism (Chapter 6), pulmonary disease (Chapter 14), and acute alcohol intoxication. Atrial fibrillation is commonly seen after cardiac surgery, although in this setting it is often temporary.

Without organized atrial electrical activity, no organized atrial contractions occur. The arrhythmia will always result in an irregular heart rate with only the ventricle contracting during systole. The irregular rate can be detected on cardiac examination and with examination of the pulse; on ECG, the irregular ventricular rate is seen without P waves (Chapter 3). For most patients with untreated atrial fibrillation, the rate is also rapid.

Symptoms can result from the rapid rate itself (eg, feeling palpitations, racing heart) along with circulatory symptoms from impaired ventricular filling during the shorter time spent in diastole. Loss of the atrial kick plus impaired ventricular filling from a rapid heart rate can lower cardiac output and trigger symptoms of poor perfusion, including presyncope, syncope, and heart failure.

Stroke risk is an additional important consideration in atrial fibrillation. Without organized contraction, blood pools in the region of the atrial appendage and clot may form. When thrombotic material from an atrial clot breaks away and enters the systemic circulation, embolic consequences such as stroke or retinal artery embolism may result (Chapter 12). Thus, an assessment of stroke risk and appropriate therapy are critically important in managing atrial fibrillation. Since valvular disease is a significant risk factor for clot formation and stroke risk, patients with so-called valvular atrial fibrillation should be prescribed long-term anticoagulation in the absence of a contraindication. For nonvalvular atrial fibrillation, consideration of the known risk factors such as advancing age, underlying hypertension, and the presence of diabetes can be assessed and a risk score determined[24,25] with a tool such as CHA_2DS_2VASc (see **BOX 4.1**). The score informs clinical decision-making that considers the risks and benefits of long-term treatment with oral anticoagulant therapy to reduce stroke risk.

Anticoagulation in high-risk atrial fibrillation requires either warfarin (vitamin K antagonist) or a direct oral anticoagulant (DOAC), which includes the factor Xa inhibitors rivaroxaban, apixaban, and edoxaban. Aspirin is not as effective in preventing stroke when high-risk features are identified.[26] For patients with substantial risk of bleeding such as a high risk of falls, or those with difficulty adhering to medications, a discussion of the risks and benefits of anticoagulation is appropriate, and community outreach for social supports to help with home safety and medication adherence warrants consideration. An additional option for patients with high-risk atrial fibrillation and contraindications to long-term oral anticoagulation is a mechanical device that ties off the clot-prone left atrial appendage.[27] For patients with transient high-risk for bleeding, such as pending surgery or active medical risk (eg, gastric ulcer), temporary discontinuation of anticoagulation may be needed until the acute risk resolves. For elective cataract surgery, the bleeding risk is low enough that many surgeons do not require perioperative discontinuation of anticoagulation.[28]

Box 4.1   The CHAD2 DS2 VASc Scoring System to Assess for Stroke Risk in Nonvalvular Atrial Fibrillation

CHA_2DS_2-VASc	Score If Positive
Congestive heart failure	1
Hypertension	1
Age ≥ 75 y	2
Diabetes mellitus	1
Stroke/TIA	2
Vascular disease[a]	1
Age 65-74 y	1
Sex category (female)	1

MI, myocardial infarction; TIA, transient ischemic attack.

Score ≥ 2—oral anticoagulants recommended.[17]

[a]prior MI, peripheral arterial disease, or aortic plaque.

Atrial fibrillation in a low-risk individual, also called lone atrial fibrillation, carries a low risk for embolic events, and anticoagulation is not recommended as the risks likely outweigh the benefits. In this setting, many physicians do recommend daily aspirin.

Since atrial fibrillation carries risks including embolic stroke, difficulty with rate control, and loss of atrial kick, newly diagnosed atrial fibrillation is often treated with cardioversion to convert the arrhythmia back to normal sinus rhythm. Some patients spontaneously return to sinus rhythm without treatment; a subset of these patients will fluctuate between sinus rhythm and atrial fibrillation, known as paroxysmal atrial fibrillation. Cardioversion to restore sinus rhythm can be done medically or electrically. Electrical cardioversion employs a lower energy shock as compared to defibrillation for ventricular fibrillation. Before attempted cardioversion, patients should either be assessed for clot in the atria or treated for several weeks with an anticoagulant to assure that the organized atrial contraction from a successful cardioversion will not propel an established clot into the circulation, triggering an acute embolic event. Risk factors for failure to remain in sinus rhythm after cardioversion include atrial enlargement and longer duration spent in atrial fibrillation. When attempts to restore sinus rhythm are unsuccessful in patients who remain asymptomatic with atrial fibrillation, there are two treatment approaches: restore sinus rhythm with addition of antiarrhythmic medications and repeated attempts at cardioversion; or control heart rate and stroke risk while allowing atrial fibrillation to persist. Several studies have addressed these options,[29,30] and the general consensus is that quality of life and medical outcomes are similar, making patient preference and individualized medical considerations the determining factors in whether *rate control* in atrial fibrillation or *rhythm control* to sinus rhythm should be pursued.

Heart rate control in atrial fibrillation is usually accomplished with a beta blocker or calcium channel blocker with negative chronotropic effects such as diltiazem. There are also a number of antiarrhythmic agents that can be used. When medications fail, or in the more unusual situation of a very slow heart rate with atrial fibrillation, an implanted pacemaker may be necessary.

REFERENCES

1. Tzemos N, Therrien J, Yip J, et al. Outcomes in adults with bicuspid aortic valves. *J Am Med Assoc*. 2008;300:1317-1325.
2. Cowell SJ, Newby DE, Prescott RJ, et al. A randomized trial of intensive lipid-lowering therapy in calcific aortic stenosis. *N Engl J Med*. 2005;352:2389-2397.

3. Mack MJ, Leon MB, Thourani VH, et al. Transcatheter aortic-valve replacement with a balloon-expandable valve in low-risk patients. *N Engl J Med*. 2019;380(18):1695-1705. doi:10.1056/NEJMoa1814052.

4. Popma JJ, Deeb GM, Yakubov SJ, et al. Transcatheter aortic-valve replacement with a self-expanding valve in low-risk patients. *N Engl J Med*. 2019;380(18):1706-1715. doi:10.1056/NEJMoa1816885.

5. Freed LA, Levy D, Levine RA, et al. Prevalence and clinical outcome of mitral-valve prolapse. *N Engl J Med*. 1999;341(1):1-7.

6. Esfandiari H, Ansari S, Mohammad-Rabei H, Mets MB. Management strategies of ocular abnormalities in patients with Marfan syndrome: current perspective. *J Ophthalmic Vis Res*. 2019;14(1):71-77.

7. Carapetis JR, Steer AC, Mulholland EK, Weber M. The global burden of group A streptococcal diseases. *Lancet Infect Dis*. 2005;5(11):685-694.

8. Gewitz M, Baltimore R, Tani L, et al. Revision of the Jones criteria for the diagnosis of acute rheumatic fever in the era of Doppler echocardiography: a scientific statement from the American Heart Association. *Circulation*. 2015;131:1806-1818.

9. Remenyi B, Carapetis J, Wyber R, Taubert K, Mayosi BM; World Heart Federation. Position statement of the World Heart Federation on the prevention and control of rheumatic heart disease. *Nat Rev Cardiol*. 2013;10:284-292.

10. Loughrey PB, Armstrong D, Lockhart CJ. Classical eye signs in infective endocarditis. *QJM*. 2015;108(11):909-910.

11. Thuny F, Disalvo G, Belliard O, et al. Risk of embolism and death in infective endocarditis: prognostic value of echocardiography. A prospective multicenter study. *Circulation*. 2005;112:69-75.

12. Okada AA1, Johnson RP, Liles WC, D'Amico DJ, Baker AS. Endogenous bacterial endophthalmitis. Report of a ten-year retrospective study. *Ophthalmology*. 1994;101(5):832-838.

13. Nishimura RA, Otto CM, Bonow RO, et al. 2017 AHA/ACC focused update of the 2014 AHA/ACC guideline for the management of patients with valvular heart disease: a report of the American College of Cardiology/American Heart Association Task Force on clinical practice guidelines. *J Am Coll Cardiol*. 2017;135(25):e1159-e1195.

14. Salmon J. *Kanski's Clinical Ophthalmology*. 9th ed. China: Elsevier; 2019.

15. Kimizuka Y, Kiyosawa M, Tamai M, Takase S. Retinal changes in myotonic dystrophy. Clinical and follow-up evaluation. *Retina*. 1993;13(2):129-135.

16. Yusuf S, Hawken S, Ounpuu S, et al; INTERHEART Study Investigators. Effect of potentially modifiable risk factors associated with myocardial infarction in 52 countries (the INTERHEART study): case-control study. *Lancet*. 2004;364:937-952.

17. Kushwaha SS, Fallon JT, Fuster V. Restrictive cardiomyopathy. *N Engl J Med*. 1997;336(4):267-276.

18. Mozzafarian D, Benjamin EJ, Go AS, et al; on behalf of the American Heart Association Statistics Committee and Stroke Statistics Subcommittee. Heart disease and stroke statistics – 2016 update: a report from the American Heart Association. *Circulation*. 2016;133:e38-e360.

19. Akintoye E, Briasoulis A, Egbe A, et al. National trends in admission and in-hospital mortality of patients with heart failure in the United States (2001-2014). *J Am Heart Assoc*. 2017;6:e006955. doi:10.1161/JAHA.117.006955

20. McAlister FA, Wiebe N, Ezekowitz JA, Leung AA, Armstrong PW. Meta-analysis: β-blocker dose, heart rate reduction, and death in patients with heart failure. *Ann Intern Med*. 2009;150:784-794.

21. Feinberg WM, Blackshear JL, Laupacis A, Kronmal R, Hart RG. Prevalence, age distribution, and gender of patients with atrial fibrillation: analysis and implications. *Arch Intern Med*.1995;155:469-473.

22. Singer DE. A 60-year-old woman with atrial fibrillation. *J Am Med Assoc*. 2003;290(16):2182-2189. doi:10.1001/jama.290.16.2182.

23. Go AS, Hylek EM, Phillips KA, et al. Prevalence of diagnosed atrial fibrillation in adults. National implications for rhythm management and stroke prevention: the AnTicoagulation and Risk Factors in Atrial Fibrillation (ATRIA) study. *J Am Med Assoc*. 2001;285(18):2370-2375. doi:10.1001/jama.285.18.2370.

24. Lip GY, Nieuwlaat R, Pisters R, Lane DA, Crijns HJ. Refining clinical risk stratification for predicting stroke and thromboembolism in atrial fibrillation using a novel risk factor-based approach: the euro heart survey on atrial fibrillation. *Chest*. 2010;137(2):263-272. doi:10.1378/chest.09-1584.

25. January CT, Wann LS, Alpert JS, et al. 2014 AHA/ACC/HRS guideline for the management of patients with atrial fibrillation: a report of the American College of Cardiology/American Heart Association Task Force on practice guidelines and the Heart Rhythm Society. *J Am Coll Cardiol*. 2014;64:e1-e76.

26. Hsu JC, Maddox TM, Kennedy K, et al. Aspirin instead of oral anticoagulant prescription in atrial fibrillation patients at risk for stroke. *J Am Coll Cardiol*. 2016;67(25):2913-2923.

27. Majule DN, Jing C, Rutahoile WM, Shonyela FS. The efficacy and safety of the WATCHMAN device in LAA occlusion in patients with non-valvular atrial fibrillation contraindicated to oral anticoagulation: a focused review. *Ann Thorac Cardiovasc Surg*. 2018;24(6):271-278. doi:10.5761/atcs.ra.18-00014.

28. McMahan LB. Anticoagulants and cataract surgery. *J Cataract Refract Surg.* 1988;14:569-571.

29. Carlsson J, Miketic S, Windeler J, et al; STAF Investigators. Randomized trial of rate-control versus rhythm-control in persistent atrial fibrillation: the Strategies of Treatment of Atrial Fibrillation (STAF) study. *J Am Coll Cardiol.* 2003;41(10):1690-1696.

30. Hagens VE, Ranchor AV, Van Sonderen E, et al; RACE Study Group. Effect of rate or rhythm control on quality of life in persistent atrial fibrillation. Results from the Rate Control Versus Electrical Cardioversion (RACE) Study. *J Am Coll Cardiol.* 2004;43(2):241-247.

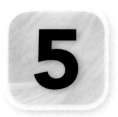

Diabetes Mellitus

David M. Shein and Rachel C. Druckenbrod

LEARNING OBJECTIVES

Diabetes is a chronic disease with an increasing prevalence worldwide. The costs of the grow-ing disease burden are reflected in several ways, including direct medical costs and costs of diabetic complications, as well as related disability and lost productivity. Many factors are contributing to the rising worldwide burden of diabetes and all healthcare providers play an important role in diabetes prevention, disease management, and risk reduction for short-term and long-term complications.

Because diabetes is a leading cause of preventable blindness around the world, the optome-trist's disease knowledge should include screening, diagnosis, and monitoring of ocular disease along with an understanding of pathophysiology, systemic manifestations, therapies, and the fac-tors that patients employ for self-care. This includes diet and lifestyle management, glucose self-monitoring, clinical laboratory testing, insulin, and other treatments.

KEY CONCEPTS

Classification of diabetes and prediabetes	Complications of diabetes
Epidemiology	Ocular
Glucose homeostasis and insulin	Systemic
Diagnostic criteria and diabetes-related tests	Hypoglycemia and its management
	Treatment of diabetes

DIABETES CLASSIFICATION

Based upon prevalence, there are two major types of diabetes mellitus: type 1 and type 2. Although less common, other subtypes are also clinically important, including gestational diabetes, monogenic causes of diabetes, and diabetes associated with other systemic diseases such as pancreatic failure. This chapter covers diabetes mellitus, which, untreated, results in an increased urine volume due to excess glucose. Diabetes mellitus is differentiated from diabetes insipidus, where increased urine volume is caused by abnormalities in the level of antidiuretic hormone or renal clearance of filtered serum (Chapter 6).

Type 1 diabetes develops due to autoimmune destruction of pancreatic beta cells, the sole source of endogenous insulin. Insulin is thus required for type 1 diabetes treatment. While often seen in children, type 1 diabetes can develop at any age. Important racial and geographic associations are seen with diabetes type 1, which is more common in non-Hispanic whites and also occurs at a higher rate in geographic regions as distance from the equator increases.[1] An interaction between genetic risk and environmental triggers factors into the development of type 1 diabetes.

Type 2 diabetes develops due to the combination of insulin resistance and relative insulin deficiency, and the degree to which each factor contributes varies by patient. Even in an individual patient, these factors vary over time. There are strong genetic risks associated with type 2 diabetes, although often the environment (including lifestyle factors) plays a significant role in disease expression. Insulin resistance is typically present in patients who are overweight or obese and can improve with weight loss. As noted above, insulin resistance is often coupled with some degree of insulin deficiency. Unlike type 1 diabetes, the defects that lead to type 2 diabetes develop slowly over years, leading to an intermediate state of impaired glucose tolerance which does not meet the criteria for diabetes, and is commonly known as prediabetes. Over time, insulin production typically decreases; medications and ultimately exogenous insulin may be necessary for treatment of type 2 diabetes. The importance of healthy eating (such as a Mediterranean diet, see below), weight management, and physical activity cannot be overemphasized, even in the setting of medication use.

Latent autoimmune diabetes in adults (LADA) is an uncommon form of diabetes with adult-onset similar to type 2 diabetes, but like type 1 diabetes, patients demonstrate circulating autoantibodies to pancreatic islet cells. It may be considered on a spectrum of insulin resistance between type 1 and type 2 diabetes and has a variable association with obesity. Patients do not initially require insulin, but many progress to insulin dependence over time (months to years).

Gestational diabetes occurs during pregnancy and is associated with insulin resistance, which increases during pregnancy. Untreated, there are both short- and long-term risks to the mother and the fetus. Women who develop gestational diabetes are at risk for developing diabetes type 2 in the future. Access to prenatal care is an important factor in helping both mother and fetus; screening for gestational diabetes and treating affected women is a component of that care.

Less often, diabetes can be caused by other specific factors. Because pancreatic beta cells produce insulin, significant pancreatic injury can trigger diabetes. A range of causes, including systemic illness (eg, marked hypertriglyceridemia—Chapter 3), toxin exposure (such as alcohol abuse), and genetic diseases (eg, hemochromatosis, cystic fibrosis—Chapters 8 and 14, respectively) cause general pancreatic injury without sparing the beta cells. When pancreatic injury affects insulin production, a nonautoimmune type of diabetes that resembles type 1 (insulin-requiring) occurs due to the impact on insulin production. Medications, including certain HIV treatments (Chapter 10) and glucocorticoid therapy, can result in glucose intolerance and diabetes. Health conditions such as adrenal glucocorticoid excess in Cushing syndrome (Chapter 6) can result in hyperglycemia, often termed secondary diabetes. Unlike the complex interaction of multiple genes and the environment that is seen in the more common type 1 and 2 diabetes, the rare monogenic diabetes results from single-gene mutations that dramatically increase the risk for diabetes.

EPIDEMIOLOGY OF DIABETES

Currently, the worldwide estimated prevalence of diabetes is between 8% and 9%[2]; in the United States, the prevalence is greater than 9% of the population, amounting to about 30 million Americans.[3] However, the prevalence of diabetes is not evenly distributed in the population, with substantial racial and ethnic variation[2] with highest rates occurring among American

Indians and Alaskan Native populations; non-Hispanic black populations have the second highest rates, followed by Hispanics, Asian Americans, and non-Hispanic whites, who have the lowest incidence.[4]

Prediabetes, which reflects impairment in glucose homeostasis without the full criteria to meet the diagnosis of diabetes, is both a risk factor for developing diabetes, and itself can contribute to vascular, renal and other complications seen with abnormally high blood glucose levels. More than 25% of adults in the United States have prediabetes.

Lack of awareness is also an important consideration. In the United States, about 25% of people with diabetes are unaware of this diagnosis. The International Diabetes Federation estimates that about 50% of diabetes worldwide is undiagnosed, with the highest rate of undiagnosed diabetes in Africa.[2]

Most people with diabetes have type 2 diabetes, with both the incidence and prevalence increasing across the globe. The United States has seen a dramatic increase in diabetes over the past few decades.[4] Regions such as Africa and the Middle East are predicted to see rates more than double within the next 30 years.

The increase in type 2 diabetes is correlated with both environmental risks and advances in treating communicable diseases. Environmental factors contributing to a rise in diabetes include a move toward living and working situations that entail less physical activity (urbanization), leisure time activities that are increasingly sedentary and focused around video screens versus outdoor activities and exercise, and a shift in eating habits toward diets with more processed, calorie-dense foods (often called a Western diet). At the same time, lower death rates from infectious diseases enable people to live longer, which can lead to the development of chronic diseases like diabetes that are associated with advancing age (**FIGURE 5.1**).

In the United States, diabetes is listed as the seventh most common cause of death[5,6]; however, this is often considered an underestimate because of the risk that diabetes adds to the occurrence of cardiovascular diseases and stroke.

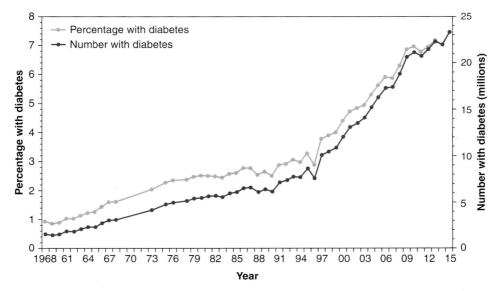

FIGURE 5.1 Number and Percentage of US Population with Diagnosed Diabetes, 1958-2015. CDC's Division of Diabetes Translation. United States Diabetes Surveillance System available at http://www.cdc.gov/diabetes/data. (https://www.cdc.gov/diabetes/statistics/slides/long_term_trends.pdf.)

PATHOPHYSIOLOGY: HORMONES AND GLUCOSE HOMEOSTASIS

Insulin is the hormone that is affected in all types of diabetes mellitus. Receptors for insulin are present on many cells, most abundant in muscle, fat, and liver. Circulating insulin binds and activates the insulin receptor, resulting in the uptake of glucose and potassium into cells. Activation of the receptor results in intracellular signals that trigger anabolic activities, such as increasing glycogen storage and shutting down the body's own glucose production. Insulin levels are normally high after carbohydrate intake and typically very low during fasting states. Symptoms can occur from insulin deficiency, receptor downregulation, abnormal receptor intracellular signaling, and hypoglycemia.

Insulin Deficiency and Ketone Production

In the absence of insulin, such as with autoimmune diabetes, the insulin receptor cannot move glucose into cells, resulting in an elevated serum glucose and cellular starvation. The functions that the insulin receptor plays in cellular signaling in the presence of a climbing serum glucose are also lost. In response, ketones are produced as an alternate energy source from fat and muscle breakdown. Ketones are normally produced in response to the need for energy at the cellular level when carbohydrate consumption is inadequate to meet the body's demands for glucose. Examples of inadequate carbohydrate intake that result in ketone production include intentional fasting, starvation, and very-low-carbohydrate diets (often for weight loss). For similar reasons (cellular hypoglycemia), ketone production also occurs in states of severe insulin deficiency. Thus, in the setting of hyperglycemia, the presence of ketones in urine or serum is indicative of insulin deficiency, usually due to type 1 diabetes.

Insulin Resistance

A complex response to an abnormal metabolic state that is often triggered by obesity, insulin resistance includes downregulation of the insulin receptors on the cell surface, in addition to abnormalities in the receptor's intracellular signaling which impair glucose control. In insulin resistance, more insulin is needed to affect a normal response to a climbing serum glucose level.

In obesity, the levels of free fatty acids (FFAs) rise and there is an inverse correlation between FFA levels and insulin sensitivity. Excess nutrients such as FFAs and glucose are proinflammatory. This inflammatory component is not mediated by an autoimmune process as in type 1 diabetes, but rather by proinflammatory cytokines that are secreted in response to the excess nutrients. This results in both insulin resistance and β-cell dysfunction, which impair insulin production. Excess FFAs within macrophages and β-cells lead to secretion of the cytokine interleukin (IL)-1β, which in turn mediates the secretion of additional proinflammatory cytokines from macrophages, islet cells, and other cells. Cytokines are released into the circulation and act on the major sites of insulin, triggering insulin resistance. Thus, excess FFAs can impede insulin signaling directly within peripheral tissues, as well as indirectly through the release of proinflammatory cytokines.

Because insulin resistance often occurs in conjunction with a degree of impaired insulin production, it results in serum hyperglycemia. Unless steps are taken to reverse these processes, this dual physiologic insult will typically worsen over time and the degree of hyperglycemia will progress.

Hypoglycemia

When blood glucose levels are low—for example, with fasting, during ongoing energy expenditure such as exercise, or when an excessive amount of insulin is administered—endogenous energy sources (within the body) are utilized. The counter-regulatory hormones (glucagon, cortisol, and

increases the risk for genital yeast infections, seen more often in females and in young children in diapers. Vision is also impacted by sustained hyperglycemia (see below).

In response to insulin deficiency, as explained earlier, ketone production occurs. The presence of diabetic ketosis is accompanied by acidosis because the major ketone, beta-hydroxybutyrate, is acidic. Because carbon dioxide is also acidic, patients with diabetic ketoacidosis (a metabolic acid) will have an increased rate of respiration as the body compensates to clear acid by exhaling more carbon dioxide (respiratory compensation for the metabolic acidosis). This increase in respiration commonly takes the form of deep, labored breathing (also known as *Kussmaul breathing*). Thus, the common name diabetic ketoacidosis (DKA) reflects the range of laboratory abnormalities present in the setting of insulin deficiency.

The acidosis, hyperglycemia, and resulting dehydration result in alterations in mental status ranging from lethargy to coma, when severe. Decreased appetite and vomiting can also occur, sometimes leading to a misdiagnosis of a gastrointestinal illness when patients present with new onset of type 1 diabetes.

Treatment for diabetic ketoacidosis requires administration of intravenous fluid, insulin, glucose, and potassium. With insulin, blood glucose levels will fall as glucose enters cells, ketone production will cease, and volume status will return to normal with fluid replacement and resolution of glycosuria. Another key factor in the emergency management of diabetic ketoacidosis is potassium monitoring. With insulin, potassium moves intracellularly along with glucose. With insulin deficiency, cellular potassium levels drop, the serum potassium level increases, and excess potassium in the serum is lost in the urine. Once insulin is administered, potassium rapidly returns intracellularly, and the serum potassium level can rapidly drop to dangerous levels. Thus, even though the serum potassium level is often elevated in patients presenting with diabetic ketoacidosis, total body potassium is often depleted, and the serum level must be closely monitored to prevent hypokalemia. Risks from hypokalemia include muscle weakness or paralysis, muscle cramping, and abnormal heart rhythms, which can be fatal if untreated.

While diabetic ketoacidosis can be a presenting symptom of diabetes, it is also seen in the setting of poor diabetes control that can occur with acute infection and with insulin nonadherence.

For all patients with newly diagnosed type 1 diabetes, insulin treatment is required. Managing insulin and meals, understanding hypoglycemia (see below) and its treatment, as well as the psychosocial aspects of the diagnosis and changes it requires, always takes a team. For children and adolescents, as well as for older adults, management often requires the assistance of others, including family members. Even for independent adults, a partner or spouse, close friends, roommates, and others may be members of the informal team that assists, advises, and supports the individual with type 1 diabetes.

Type 2 Diabetes

Type 2 diabetes typically has a slower onset, developing over many years. The diagnosis may be detected anywhere along a continuum from early asymptomatic to later-onset with symptoms of hyperglycemia, secondary complications, or an acute hyperosmolar state. Because of this slow and progressive process, in addition to the high prevalence of the disease, screening for type 2 diabetes, as discussed above, results in earlier detection and the opportunity for earlier intervention, both in the prediabetes state as well as with early diabetes.

Ketoacidosis occurs infrequently in type 2 diabetes, although it may occur in certain circumstances, including a rare complication with SGLT-2 medication use (see treatment below).

Depending upon the individual and the risks for the development of diabetes, two and sometimes three simultaneous pathological situations are typically at play to varied degrees. Insulin resistance is described above, resulting in higher insulin requirements to achieve the desired response of glucose transport into cells. The pancreas is often unable to keep up with this demand and a relative insulin deficiency develops; without the insulin resistance, glucose levels could stay normal. When hyperglycemia is present, a third situation called glucose toxicity develops, and the pancreatic beta cell function further declines, with less insulin production. Over time, progressive loss of pancreatic endocrine function occurs and insulin production continues to decrease. While lifestyle factors such as exercise, weight loss (for overweight and obese patients), and medications can improve both insulin sensitivity and insulin output, the insulin deficiency typically progresses and diabetes appears to worsen over time, requiring more medication or the addition of insulin.

When type 2 diabetes is poorly controlled, hyperglycemia will progress. As with type 1 diabetes, hyperglycemia results in glycosuria and volume depletion. However, unlike type 1 diabetes, there is typically enough insulin circulating in type 2 diabetes that ketones are not formed, and acidosis does not develop. Without the acute symptoms related to ketoacidosis, hyperglycemia will often progress to markedly elevated levels, along with ongoing glycosuria causing dehydration, until enough water is lost that the serum concentration of solutes increases to the point of hyperosmolarity. The result is a hyperglycemic, hyperosmolar state (sometimes also termed hyperosmolar, nonketotic state). Lethargy, confusion, and, when severe, coma can result. Fluids and insulin are necessary to reverse this state. Triggers can include infection and poor medication adherence.

There are a range of treatment options available for type 2 diabetes including oral medications, insulin, and injected noninsulin drugs; all are reviewed below. Lifestyle management is also critical, especially for patients who are overweight or obese.

Gestational Diabetes

Pregnancy may be accompanied by some degree of insulin resistance, and in women at risk, this can result in the development of glucose intolerance and gestational diabetes. For an individual woman, risk factors for developing gestational diabetes include older age, a family history of diabetes, obesity, delivering a previous baby over nine pounds, and a history of chronic anovulation. There is also a difference in risk among ethnic groups; in the United States, African American, Hispanic, Pacific Islander, and South or East Asian women are at higher risk than white women.[10] Gestational diabetes increases the risk for a number of adverse perinatal outcomes including maternal high blood pressure, large baby for gestational age, macrosomia (large head), birth trauma, cesarean delivery, and hypoglycemia in the newborn. Routine prenatal care involves screening for gestational diabetes, typically with the OGTT (as described above).[11]

COMPLICATIONS OF DIABETES

Diabetes is a complex disease with significant impacts from both metabolic effects of acute and chronic hyperglycemia as well as impacts on other organs and systems. Risks for acute and chronic complications vary by individual, comorbidities, and type of diabetes.

Acute complications are mostly related to issues of glycemic control, including development of hyper- and hypoglycemia. As discussed above, hyperglycemia can cause a range of symptoms. With very poor diabetes control (including new onset of type 1, acute infection, and poor treatment adherence), diabetic ketoacidosis or the hyperosmolar state can develop depending upon the underlying defect(s) that lead to the development of diabetes. Vision may be transiently impacted by hyperglycemia-induced refractive changes of the lens, either in a myopic or hyperopic direction, which resolves with improved glucose control.[12] Vision is also impacted in diabetics by more rapid cataract development as compared to nondiabetics, and by posterior segment complications like macular edema, macular ischemia, vitreous hemorrhage, or retinal detachment from proliferative diabetic retinopathy. Ophthalmic complications in diabetes are discussed further below.

Hypoglycemia can occur with both very tight blood glucose management or erratic diabetes control, most often in a situation where a patient is taking insulin or an insulin secretagogue (oral pill to increase pancreatic insulin production used in type 2 diabetes—see below). Studies show a close correlation with tighter glucose control and higher risks for hypoglycemia[13] (see **FIGURE 5.3**).

Symptoms of hypoglycemia occur due to two key processes. The first, neuroglycopenia, reflects inadequate delivery of glucose to the brain. The brain requires glucose as its energy source, and in the setting of a low glucose level, symptoms from mild confusion to coma occur along a continuum as blood glucose levels drop. Other symptoms can include headache, blurred vision, and weakness. The other category of hypoglycemic symptoms reflects sympathetic activation as a result of counter-regulatory hormone release. Catecholamine secretion occurs as part of the normal process to counter hypoglycemia, and the sympathetic effects of catecholamines, including tremulousness, tachycardia, mydriasis, sweating, and hunger, are important signals that hypoglycemia may be developing. Hypoglycemia unawareness occurs when the sympathetic symptoms do not occur. This is seen in several situations, including frequent hypoglycemic episodes; sympathetic antagonist (eg, beta blocker) use; and advanced neuropathy. When patients with frequent hypoglycemia develop hypoglycemia unawareness, new glucose management goals are typically set. For patients aiming to have tight control, a period of looser control with tolerance for higher glucose levels will return the awareness of hypoglycemia and lower the risk of severe hypoglycemic episodes. The use of beta blockers in diabetes is not without controversy, and a balance between the cardiovascular benefits, blood pressure reducing capabilities, or the other indications for use in the individual must be balanced against risks of hypoglycemic unawareness. In situations where severe neuropathy is interfering with sensation and hypoglycemic awareness, looser blood

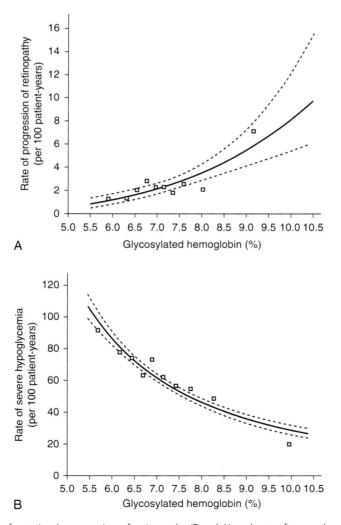

FIGURE 5.3 Risk of sustained progression of retinopathy (Panel A) and rate of severe hypoglycemia (Panel B) in patients receiving intensive therapy according to their mean glycosylated hemoglobin values during the DCCT trial. (Reproduced from The effect of intensive treatment of diabetes on the development and progression of long-term complications in insulin-dependent diabetes mellitus. *New Engl J Med.* 1993;329:977-986.)

glucose control may be necessary to balance risks and benefits considering both short- and long-term goals for diabetes management. In addition, pancreatic damage may also limit glucagon production, and this counter-regulatory hormone may not be produced normally to help reverse hypoglycemia.

Symptoms of hypoglycemia typically occur when plasma glucose levels fall below 55 mg/dL; however, there is variability in when an individual will experience symptoms. Patients with poor glucose control who usually run higher serum glucose levels may experience symptoms at a level above 55 mg/dL. On the other hand, the glucose level in patients with tight control may drop significantly lower before they become symptomatic. Other factors, including the rate of drop in glucose level, can influence the glucose reading at which patients become symptomatic.

Management of hypoglycemia is multifaceted and includes acute management of low glucose levels, management of symptoms when present, and longer term management of blood glucose and activities during recovery.

Based upon symptoms and glucose level, several approaches can be considered. A measured low glucose in the absence of symptoms should prompt defensive action, including carbohydrate consumption and adjustment of insulin dose in the short term, especially if by continuous infusion. Activities that require full concentration such as driving should be deferred until the glucose level is normal and stable.

When symptoms develop, a two-stage approach is needed for short- and long-term glucose management. A short-acting carbohydrate such as glucose tablets or fruit juice should be administered immediately to patients who are alert enough to swallow. Patients who are taking insulin will generally have glucose tablets on hand with their diabetes testing supplies. Because the insulin or oral diabetes drug causing hypoglycemia is likely longer acting than an oral glucose dose, a complex carbohydrate such as a slice of bread should be consumed as well for longer term control. Patients should not drive or engage in other activities that may involve risk to themselves or others until the glucose level is stable and their risk for hypoglycemia returns to baseline.

Hypoglycemia is considered severe when a patient requires assistance. For conscious patients, oral glucose remains an option as long as there is minimal risk for aspiration. Patients who are lethargic or unconscious should be treated with glucagon injection if available; many diabetic patients carry glucagon, and emergency kits in healthcare and other public facilities often include glucagon. Formal medical care is typically required, and an unconscious patient should trigger a call for an emergency medical response. In a community setting, after a 911 call, responding paramedics will initiate a continuous infusion of intravenous glucose to combat the ongoing risk for hypoglycemia.

Chronic complications of diabetes are often grouped into microvascular and macrovascular conditions. However, there are a number of other long-term risks, many of which are infectious.

MICROVASCULAR DISEASE

Diabetic microangiopathy refers to damage of small-caliber blood vessels in the setting of hyperglycemia, and includes diabetic retinopathy, nephropathy, and neuropathy. All forms may share a similar pathogenesis which is likely multifactorial, and may be the result of metabolic changes related to chronic hyperglycemia, although exact mechanisms are unknown. Protein glycation and the formation of advanced glycation end products (AGEs) as well as impaired autoregulation of blood flow are likely important contributing factors, and numerous studies have linked higher HbA_{1c} levels with development and progression of diabetic microvascular disease.[13-16] The end result of diabetic microvascular disease is tissue hypoxia and ischemia with potential loss of tissue and organ function, for example, the development of permanent retinal photoreceptor damage, renal failure, and sensory polyneuropathies or loss of digits or limbs.

Diabetic Retinopathy

Diabetic retinopathy is the most common microvascular complication in diabetes with a prevalence as high as 40% among insulin-dependent diabetics, although fortunately the prevalence of

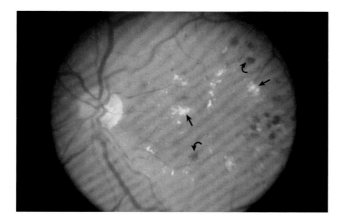

FIGURE 5.4 Diabetic retinopathy. Ocular fundus of a person with background diabetic retinopathy. Several yellowish "hard" exudates (straight arrows) and several retinal hemorrhages (curved arrows) are present. (Reprinted from Strayer DS, Saffitz JE, Rubin E. *Rubin's Pathology: Mechanisms of Human Disease.* 8th ed. Philadelphia, PA: Wolters Kluwer; 2019.)

sight-threatening disease is much less (10%).[17] Patients with type 1 diabetes are at a higher risk of developing diabetic retinopathy as compared to patients with type 2 diabetes, their eye disease may occur earlier in life, and they may develop more severe eye disease. Disease duration is the most important risk factor for diabetic retinopathy, as good metabolic control alone will not prevent retinopathy, but rather delays its onset. Retinopathy rarely develops within 5 years of diabetic onset but rises to 50% after 10 years and 90% after 30 years.[13] In addition to poor glycemic control and disease duration, risk factors for diabetic retinopathy include pregnancy, diabetic nephropathy, and the presence of comorbid cardiovascular disease risk factors such as hypertension, hyperlipidemia, smoking, and obesity.

Diabetic retinopathy is classified into nonproliferative and proliferative disease states, with or without macular edema. Nonproliferative diabetic eye disease is characterized by the formation of retinal microaneurysms, dot/blot hemorrhages, cotton wool spots (swollen retinal nerve fiber layer), "beading" of retinal venules, and the formation of intraretinal microvascular abnormalities (IRMAs; fine arteriolar-venous shunts) (**FIGURE 5.4**).

Proliferative disease carries a significant risk for vision loss and involves the ischemia-driven formation of new retinal blood vessels (neovascularization) which are prone to leakage and vitreous hemorrhage, and the formation of fibrovascular membranes which are prone to tractional retinal detachment (**FIGURE 5.5**). Iris and anterior segment angle neovascularization may also occur in proliferative diabetic retinopathy and impart risk for neovascular glaucoma. Macular edema occurs

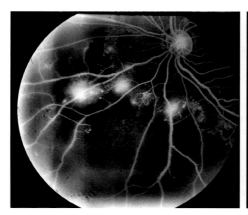
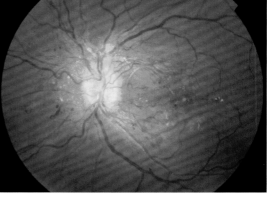

FIGURE 5.5 Left: Frame from a fluorescein angiogram in a case of proliferative diabetic retinopathy showing new vessels (areas of intense dye leakage) next to nonperfused area, which appears black at the lower right of the image. Right: Proliferative diabetic retinopathy with macular edema, hard exudate, and neovascularization of the disc (NVD). (Left, From Das A. *Therapy for Ocular Angiogenesis.* Philadelphia, PA: Wolters Kluwer; 2010. Right, From Fineman MS. *Color Atlas & Synopsis of Clinical Ophthalmology.* 3rd ed. Philadelphia, PA: Wolters Kluwer; 2018.)

in both nonproliferative and proliferative disease states and results from exudative leakage of fluid from retinal vessels; it is the most common cause for vision loss in diabetes and may be accompanied by retinal exudates (lipoprotein and lipids). Diabetic papillopathy/papillitis uncommonly occurs alongside diabetic retinopathy and typically presents as bilateral anterior optic disc edema; it may be a variant of anterior ischemic optic neuropathy, although visual prognosis is often better (acuity 6/12 or better in 80% of cases, also considering comorbid diabetic retinopathy).[13]

The widely accepted classification of diabetic retinopathy is based on the modified Airlie House description in the Early Treatment Diabetic Retinopathy Study (ETDRS)[18] (**TABLE 5.4**). Examiners grade retinopathy based on the presence of nonproliferative and proliferative diabetic signs in comparison with standard photo examples, as well as the presence or absence of clinically significant macular edema (CSDME). Management guidelines are determined by the level of retinopathy and whether or not CSDME is present. In recent years, the advent of optical coherence tomography (OCT) imaging has allowed for the visualization of macular edema even prior to stereoscopically evident thickening by clinical fundus exam, and new definitions of center-involved diabetic macular edema (CI-DME) and non–center-involved diabetic macular edema (non–CI-DME) are used in clinical trials studying modern treatments for macular edema.[19]

TABLE 5.4 Early Treatment Diabetic Retinopathy Study (ETDRS)[15] Classification of Diabetic Retinopathy

Classification	Definition	Management
Nonproliferative diabetic retinopathy (NPDR)		
None	No retinopathy	Observe in 12 mo
Mild NPDR	H/Ma < standard photo 2A	Observe in 12 mo
Moderate NPDR	H/Ma > standard photo 2A and/or mild CWS, VB, intraretinal microvascular abnormality (IRMA)	Observe in 6 mo
Severe NPDR	IRMA in 1+ quadrants > standard photo 8A or VB in 2+ quadrants > standard photo 6B or H/Ma in 4+ quadrants > standard photo 2A	Observe in 4 mo
Very severe NPDR	Two or more signs consistent with severe NPDR	Observe in 2 mo
Proliferative diabetic retinopathy (PDR)		
Early PDR	NVD or NVE not meeting high-risk characteristics	Retina specialty care within 1 mo—consideration of treatment vs close observation
High-risk PDR	NVD > standard photo 10A or mild NVD with fresh vitreous or preretinal heme or moderate NVE with fresh vitreous or preretinal heme	Retina specialty care within 24-48 h—prompt treatment
Clinically-significant macular edema (CSDME)		
CSDME	Retinal thickening at or within 500 μm of fovea or hard exudates at or within 500 μm of fovea with adjacent retinal thickening or retinal thickening 1 disc area in size at least partially within 1 disc diameter of fovea	Retina specialty care within 2-wk period—consideration of treatment vs close observation

CWS, cotton wool spots; H/Ma, hemes/microaneurysms; NVD, neovascularization of the disc; NVE, neovascularization elsewhere; VB, venous beading.

Patients with mild-to-moderate nonproliferative eye disease without macular edema may be regularly monitored without treatment intervention beyond systemic glucose control. It is important to recognize that a subset of patients (10%-15%) with diabetic retinopathy will show transient worsening of retinopathy in the early stage of intensive glycemic control, but this does not outweigh the long-term benefits of metabolic control and has no impact on visual outcomes.[8] Intravitreal drugs targeting vascular endothelial growth factor (anti-VEGF) alone or in combination with laser photocoagulation are well established for the treatment of diabetic macular edema, and have also found a role in the treatment of proliferative diabetic retinopathy, where they may have similar efficacy to traditional pan-retinal photocoagulation without the undesirable side effect of peripheral vision loss, although may require more frequent monitoring for recurrent disease.[19,20] Pan-retinal photocoagulation, focal and grid laser photocoagulation, intravitreal triamcinolone, and pars plana vitrectomy (PPV) remain beneficial treatment options for proliferative diabetic retinopathy and/or macular edema. For all diabetic patients, blood glucose control is imperative for minimizing the risk of retinopathy. The historic Diabetes Control and Complications Trial (DCCT) showed that, over a 6.5-year period, a median hemoglobin A_{1c} level of 7.2% reduced the incidence of diabetic retinopathy by 75% and reduced the progression of retinopathy by 54%.[13] Besides glucose control, control of comorbid disease states among diabetics is also very important. Multifactorial risk reduction with intensive treatment of hyperglycemia, hypertension, hyperlipidemia, and nephropathy (particularly at early stages of disease) has been shown to prevent both microvascular and macrovascular complications in type 2 diabetes. Hypertension control among diabetics has been especially emphasized since the United Kingdom Prospective Diabetes Study (UKPDS) showed that good blood pressure control decreases the incidence of retinopathy and slows the rate of retinopathy progression.[21] Interestingly, more recent studies involving more intensive blood pressure control (ie, <140/80) have actually failed to show an effect on retinopathy outcomes, possibly because both control and treatment groups demonstrated relatively good blood pressure control to begin with, or because longer term follow-up is required to demonstrate a protective effect of more aggressive hypertension control.[22] Nonetheless, the evidence is clear that all patients with diabetes should be counseled on control of their comorbid conditions to minimize the risk of microvascular diabetic disease.

Advanced imaging modalities such as spectral-domain OCT (SD-OCT), enhanced-depth imaging OCT (EDI-OCT), and OCT angiography (OCT-A) are emerging as useful tools for studying the pathogenesis of diabetic retinopathy and may also prove useful for clinical risk stratification and management decisions, especially because subclinical retinal changes and changes in choroidal thickness among diabetics are detectable by these modalities even prior to the development of funduscopic diabetic retinopathy.[23,24]

Diabetic Cataract

Clinical studies have shown that cataract development occurs more frequently and at an earlier age in patients with diabetes as compared to nondiabetic patients (**FIGURE 5.6**). Data from the Framingham Eye study[25] indicate a three- to fourfold increased prevalence of cataract in patients with diabetes younger than 65 years, and up to a twofold excess prevalence in patients older than 65 years. The risk is increased in patients with longer duration of diabetes and in those with poor metabolic control.

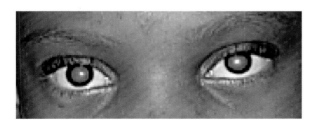

FIGURE 5.6 Bilateral total cataracts in a diabetic patient. (From Wilson ME. *Pediatric Cataract Surgery: Techniques, Complications and Management.* 2nd ed. Philadelphia, PA: Wolters Kluwer; 2014.)

Diabetic lens opacification occurs as a direct consequence of hyperglycemia. The aqueous humor glucose level is about half the serum level. Under normal conditions, when glucose enters a cell, hexokinase converts it into glucose-6-phosphate for use in metabolic processes. However, when large amounts of glucose are present in poorly controlled diabetes, hexokinase becomes saturated and the excess glucose is converted to sorbitol (via the polyol pathway). Sorbitol cannot cross cell membranes, and as a large molecule, its osmotic effect draws water into lens cells, opacifying and swelling the lens. In the short term, this effect is seen with poorly controlled serum glucose as changes in refractive error.

Nephropathy

Nephropathy is a leading cause of kidney failure in diabetes. There is an inverse relationship between glucose control and the development of nephropathy.[12] Renal disease typically begins with the onset of proteinuria and progresses. Between 20% and 40% of patients with diabetes will develop chronic kidney disease, with estimates varying between populations studied.[26] Despite increased use of medications for glucose control and renin system antagonists (such as ACE inhibitors) that can reduce the risk of progressive proteinuria, the incidence of diabetic kidney disease has, unfortunately, followed closely with the incidence of diabetes[27] without a proportional decline. When patients are first diagnosed with type 1 diabetes, since the onset of the insulin defect is recent, microvascular disease (including diabetic kidney disease) is not expected to be present. Typically, it is about 10 years after diagnosis that kidney disease develops. In type 2 diabetes, because there may be a long preclinical phase of prediabetes and sometimes undetected diabetes, diabetic kidney disease may be present at diagnosis and appropriate evaluation includes measuring renal function (with a serum creatinine) and assessment for urine protein (including microalbumin).

Diabetic nephropathy is responsible for a substantial number of cases of advanced renal failure in industrialized countries. Patients diagnosed with advanced kidney disease are at higher risk for cardiovascular disease, heart failure, and death. Healthcare costs also increase substantially for patients with end stage kidney disease. Considering the substantial impact on individuals, the public health, and healthcare costs, screening and prevention of chronic kidney disease is important. For patients with normal renal function, annual testing for urine microalbumin is recommended. Early detection of microalbumin should prompt initiation of preventive interventions including therapy with antagonists of the renin system (ACE inhibitors or angiotensin receptor blockers), a reassessment of blood glucose management with a goal to improve control if appropriate, and aggressive management of blood pressure, as hypertension is a significant risk factor for progression of diabetic kidney disease. Smoking is also a risk for many vascular conditions, and diabetic kidney disease is no exception. Counseling, medications, and referrals should be provided to smokers as appropriate. Administration of x-ray contrast material may also increase the risk of kidney injury, especially in patients with established kidney disease, and measures to limit exposure and mitigate the risk when contrast imaging is medically necessary are important considerations. While mild microalbuminuria may regress with ACE inhibitor or ARB treatment, over time it may reappear, with proteinuria often progressing. Thus, ongoing monitoring and continued assessment of treatment targets is appropriate.

More advanced stages of diabetic kidney disease can lead to end-stage renal disease which typically requires dialysis or renal transplantation for long-term management.

Neuropathy

Diabetes is the most common cause of peripheral neuropathy. It is estimated that about 50% of patients with diabetes will develop neuropathy.[28] Long-standing hyperglycemia results in damage to peripheral nerves through several postulated mechanisms. As noted above, the metabolic abnormalities that lead to hyperglycemia result in nonenzymatic glycosylation, and the end products of glycosylation are likely toxic to nerves. Small vessel vascular disease, as occurs in the eye and kidney, can also lead to nerve infarctions with loss of function. As with other microvascular manifestations of diabetes, neuropathy is not present at diagnosis with type 1; in contrast, a patient with years of prediabetes, and possibly some time with undiagnosed type 2 diabetes, can present with neuropathy at diagnosis. Less commonly, patients without known glucose impairment who present for evaluation of neuropathy may be found to have impaired glucose tolerance on evaluation. Although some patients may not notice symptoms, impaired nerve conduction is typically present on sensitive tests of neurological function, such as nerve conduction studies, in patients with longstanding diabetes. For patients who do experience symptoms, different syndromes of neuropathy can occur, with some manifestations resulting in permanent neurological impairment, while others may be transient. In addition to direct effects on neurological function, neuropathy can also cause secondary effects, such as increased infection risk from foot trauma when sensation is diminished and difficulty with glucose control when autonomic neuropathy impacts digestion and nutrient absorption.

A peripheral symmetrical polyneuropathy is most commonly seen clinically with sensory loss and at times, painful sensations in the distal extremities, so-called *stocking and glove* distribution, may be present. Longer axons are impacted initially, resulting in sensory impairment in the distal toes, progressing proximally over time. Less often, fingers can be affected as well as the neuropathy progresses proximally to also involve ankles and lower legs. Large peripheral nerve fibers are involved, resulting in sensory loss, manifest as tingling or numbness. More severe involvement can lead to asymptomatic trauma, with dislocations, fractures, and the development of the deformities of Charcot foot (**FIGURE 5.7**). Severe neuropathy can also result in motor dysfunction and permanent deformities from soft tissue involvement, leading to the claw foot. The consequences of sensory loss and deformity include pressure sores and trauma. Ulceration can develop (**FIGURE 5.8**) that in turn can lead to infection (including osteomyelitis, or bone infection), gangrene, and risk for amputation. Risk factors for these advanced complications include poor glucose control and longstanding diabetes with other disease complications. Hyperglycemia impairs leukocyte function for infection-fighting, and poor circulation from comorbid peripheral vascular disease impairs delivery of leukocytes to fight infection and erythrocytes to deliver oxygen for healing. Neuropathy can thus have serious health consequences.

When the small fibers that transmit pain are affected, a painful neuropathy develops, with symptoms often described as a sharp, lancinating pain, typically in the lower extremities. Painful neuropathy symptoms can impair sleep and function.

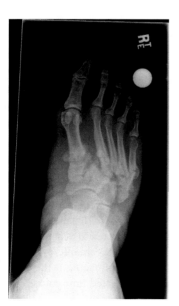

FIGURE 5.7 Imaging demonstration of neuropathic (Charcot) foot on radiograph. AP x-ray views of the right foot demonstrate extensive Charcot-type arthropathic changes at the tarsometatarsal joints with bone destruction, fractures, fragmentation, and dislocations. Owing to sensory deficiencies associated with the underlying diabetic neuropathy, pain is not always present, so the patient keeps ambulating. (From Positano RG. *Systemic Disease Manifestations in the Foot, Ankle, and Lower Extremity*. Philadelphia, PA: Wolters Kluwer; 2017.)

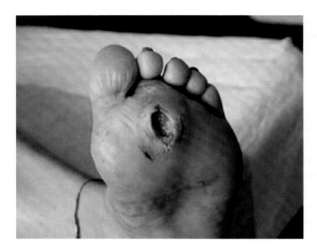

FIGURE 5.8 Left foot ulcer in a patient with diabetic peripheral neuropathy. (From Zgonis T. *Surgical Reconstruction of the Diabetic Foot and Ankle.* 2nd ed. Philadelphia, PA: Wolters Kluwer; 2017.)

While generally irreversible, evaluation for other causes of peripheral neuropathy (including nutritional deficiencies and infectious causes) should be undertaken to identify comorbid risk factors that are potentially treatable. In addition, measures to prevent progression should be reviewed; in patients with poor disease control, improved glucose control may slow progression. Smoking is an important risk factor as well, and counseling and referral for cessation is always appropriate for smokers.

Early detection and counseling are also important. A foot examination is recommended at every primary care and endocrinology encounter to assess for skin breakdown, impaired circulation, sensory loss, early infection, and any other abnormality for which treatment and counseling can be implemented. Patients with diabetes should be counseled never to walk barefoot, especially outside such as at the beach. Patients with neuropathy, poor foot grooming or established skin or toenail problems should be referred to podiatry for specialized care and management.

Autonomic neuropathy can involve several organ systems and may trigger other secondary clinical issues. Gastrointestinal manifestations can include gastroparesis or gastric atony with unpredictable responses to meals. Nausea, emesis, and delayed gastric emptying can be especially challenging for patients on insulin who can develop hypoglycemia when insulin is taken in preparation for calories to be consumed, but then the food is vomited or digested unpredictably slowly. Lower GI symptoms such as constipation or diarrhea can occur from colonic involvement. Cardiovascular neuropathy can result in silent ischemia (Chapter 3); thus, any adult patient with diabetes who presents for acute care with any possible ischemic cardiovascular symptom (eg, nausea, left arm pain) should have an electrocardiogram (ECG) at a minimum to rule out ischemia. Impairment in vascular tone inhibits reflex responses to change in posture (ie, distal vasoconstriction) resulting in postural hypotension with standing up. Genitourinary involvement can impair bladder emptying, resulting in an increased risk for urinary tract infections, which is further exacerbated when glycosuria is present. Male sexual dysfunction can also be a complication of both autonomic and sensory neuropathy.

Management requires awareness of the neuropathy, and measures to address the effects need to be individualized to the patient's specific symptoms, overall goals of therapy, and capabilities in diabetes management.

Mononeuropathy usually presents with acute functional loss of a single nerve and usually improves over time. Cranial or peripheral nerves can be involved. The cranial nerves of ocular motility are involved most often, specifically III, IV, and VI (**FIGURE 5.9**). Patients present with acute diplopia that may worsen over the first few weeks, although resolution is ultimately expected to occur, usually within 90 days. Although more than 40% of all cranial nerve III, IV, and VI palsies are microvascular in nature,[29] other causes of cranial neuropathy should be pursued with neuroimaging if there are multiple cranial nerves involved or if resolution does not occur within the expected time course.

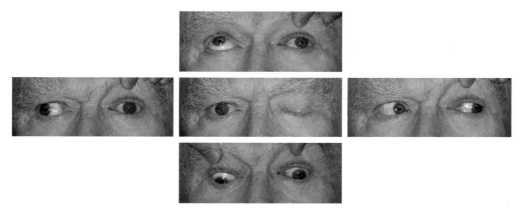

FIGURE 5.9 A 65-year-old man with a diabetic (vasculopathic) left third-nerve palsy. There is a pupil-sparing loss of all third-nerve function. (From Biller J. *Practical Neurology*. 5th ed. Philadelphia, PA: Wolters Kluwer; 2017.)

The median nerve (at the wrist) is the most frequent site of peripheral nerve involvement. Evaluation should rule out other causes of nerve dysfunction (eg, compression or a concurrent vasculitis). Treatment consists of supportive measures to compensate for motor dysfunction, such as prismatic glasses for diplopia or wrist support for median neuropathy.

Less frequently, diabetic amyotrophy can develop involving a lumbar spinal nerve root. Proximal weakness and pain occur in the region of the nerve distribution. Short-term management centers on supportive care and pain control when necessary. Diabetic amyotrophy is also typically self-limited and will improve over time.

MACROVASCULAR DISEASE

Macrovascular complications occur in large arteries where atherosclerosis leads to thrombosis and occlusion or embolization. As reviewed in the cardiovascular section (Chapter 3), there are three main domains for large vessel atherosclerotic disease: cardiovascular disease, cerebrovascular disease, and peripheral vascular disease. The incidence of these conditions is increased in patients with diabetes and further increases when comorbid risk factors are present, including smoking, hypertension, and dyslipidemia. Both coronary artery disease and cerebrovascular disease account for 65% of deaths in people with diabetes, and the rate of these conditions is between two and four times higher than the general population without diabetes. The incidence of comorbidities like hypertension and diabetes is also increased in people with diabetes.

While there are interventions and other treatments for many of these conditions, prevention remains critical. For patients with diabetes, the goal is to achieve a level of disease control that is appropriate for the individual, while also identifying and managing risk factors such as smoking, hypertension, and dyslipidemia. Pharmacologic management is important, but the critical role of lifestyle factors including healthy eating, exercise, and smoking cessation cannot be overemphasized.

DERMATOLOGICAL AND INFECTIOUS DISEASE

Dermatological conditions including infections and conditions caused by diabetes are estimated to occur in at least 30% of patient with diabetes during their lifetimes.[30]

The skin is a critical barrier that prevents infection, and many dermatological conditions in diabetes either reflect infection, or increase the risk for developing an infection if untreated.

Hyperglycemia and other metabolic changes in diabetes contribute to an increased risk for infections. Multiple factors often contribute to clinical presentations; for example, if a patient with neuropathy steps on a splinter but feels no pain, the splinter remains impacted which results in an infection. The higher risk for vascular disease impairs circulation, limiting the ability to fight this infection. A cycle like this can lead to severe local and systemic complications such as osteomyelitis, systemic infections, and, when severe, sepsis or amputation can result. For these reasons, the foot examination is an important component of medical care for any patient with diabetes. Patients should also be encouraged to examine their feet daily and care for any compromises in skin integrity as soon as possible. Early detection of neuropathy, poor grooming, skin breaks, and mild infections can direct interventions that prevent serious, if not devastating, and costly complications.[26]

One of the most common skin conditions is fungal or mycotic infection. When presenting on the feet and between the toes, it is called tinea pedis. Tinea pedis can present with skin breakdown, often with symptoms of pruritus. While tinea is a localized skin infection, the secondary skin breakdown allows for bacterial entry and increases the risk for a local and systemic bacterial infection. Treatment with topical antifungals is generally a simple, safe, and effective treatment. Genital mycotic infections can present as vaginitis in women or balanitis in men. The presence of glycosuria, seen with poor glucose control or with SGLT-2 inhibitors, increases the risk. Both can be treated with topical antifungal medications, although an oral dose of fluconazole is often preferred due to convenience. As with other conditions related to poor glucose control or drug-related effects, recurrent infections should prompt a review of treatments.

Cellulitis is a more serious infection of skin and subcutaneous soft tissue that results from an interruption in the integrity of the skin as a barrier to bacteria. The trigger for cellulitis can be common and minor skin problems including cuts, a splinter, a paronychia (ingrown nail), tinea, or even dried, cracked skin. Cellulitis requires systemic antibiotics for treatment, and a seemingly mild infection can rapidly progress if untreated or inadequately treated. As foot cellulitis can involve multiple bacteria, a broad-spectrum antibiotic or a combination of antibiotics may be required. Severe cellulitis can lead to serious local complications, systemic infection, and life-threatening sepsis (Chapter 9).

Insulin injections are generally given in regions of adequate subcutaneous fat, including the anterior abdomen, thighs, and upper arms. To avoid complications, insulin injection sites or the location of an insulin pump needle should be alternated. When the same location is used repeatedly, atrophy or hypertrophy of the subcutaneous fat can occur. Called lipoatrophy and lipohypertrophy,[31] respectively, these conditions can result in erratic and unpredictable insulin absorption leading to both hyperglycemia and more frequent hypoglycemic episodes (**FIGURE 5.10**).

Necrobiosis lipoidica is a rash that is associated with type 1 diabetes and occurs in females more often than males. While occurring in fewer than 1% of patients with diabetes, this rash can be difficult to manage and has important cosmetic implications for those patients in whom it develops. Typically occurring on the lower, anterior legs, or pretibial regions, areas of redness enlarge with central atrophy and telangiectasia (erratic, superficial blood vessels) developing. More severe involvement is marked by ulcer formation. While diabetes control is emphasized, good control will not always improve the rash. Often, patients are referred to a dermatologist for local treatments, which include topical and injected corticosteroids.

TREATMENT OF DIABETES

Several important medical studies have made critical contributions to our understanding of diabetes treatment. Two studies performed and published decades ago[12,32] informed medical science about the long-term management of diabetes. Both demonstrated that tighter blood glucose control improved outcomes for patients with diabetes, and at the same time, showed an inverse correlation between the risk for hypoglycemia with tight control. In contrast, a more recent study looking at older patients with type 2 diabetes and cardiovascular disease demonstrated that tight control was associated with

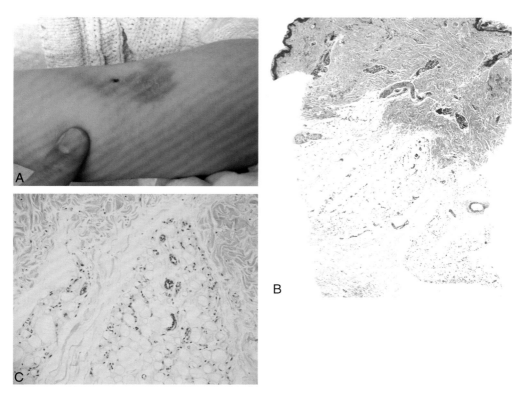

FIGURE 5.10 Localized lipoatrophy. A, Localized depression on the thigh. B, Shrunken, retracted fat lobules. C, Shrunken, retracted adipocytes with mucin and prominent capillaries. (From Elder DE. *Lever's Histopathology of the Skin.* 11th ed. Philadelphia, PA: Wolters Kluwer; 2014.)

more adverse health outcomes.[33] Thus, diabetes treatment goals need to consider a balance of risks and benefits for the individual patient such as age, medical literacy, patient preference, and other medical risks and comorbidities.

There are a growing number of options for managing diabetes including newer insulins, novel delivery systems for injected drugs, and multiple oral drugs for type 2 diabetes.

For type 1 diabetes, the requirement for insulin also requires tracking and adjusting for meals, snacks, exercise, alcohol, illness, and many other factors to which people without diabetes never give a second thought. Type 2 diabetes also requires a focus on factors such as diet, exercise, and weight control as well as adherence to any prescribed medications. In both types of diabetes, complications may require further treatment and can also impact patients' ability to adhere to their lifestyle and diabetes regimens.

Insulin is necessary in all patients with type 1 diabetes and may also be required to manage type 2 diabetes, either alone or with oral and injected medications.

Insulin has been available for the treatment of diabetes since 1922, revolutionizing the treatment of the previously fatal type 1 diabetes. Several formulations of insulin are now available, and as of publication, they are all delivered by injection. While much research has been invested to create other delivery methods, only a temporarily marketed inhaled formulation has been released. The older forms of insulin are regular and NPH (neutral protamine Hagedorn) which were available for decades as the short- and long-acting formulations, respectively. Newer insulins include very short-acting lispro and aspart as well as very long-acting glargine, detemir, and degludec. With currently available insulin formulations, better control and lower risks for hypoglycemia can often be achieved. Type 1 diabetes control requires either multiple daily insulin injections or the use of an insulin pump, which can improve glucose control and enable better short-term management of insulin delivery in

TABLE 5.5	Commonly Used Insulins			
Insulin	**Type**	**Onset**	**Peak**	**Duration**
Insulin glulisine	Rapid acting	15 min	1 h	2-4 h
Insulin lispro	Rapid acting	15 min	1 h	2-4 h
Insulin aspart	Rapid acting	15 min	1 h	2-4 h
Regular (human) insulin	Short acting	30 min	2-3 h	3-6 h
NPH insulin	Intermediate acting	2-4 h	4-12 h	12-18 h
Insulin detemir	Long acting	Several hours	No peak	24 h
Insulin glargine	Long acting	Several hours	No peak	24 h
Insulin glargine U-300	Ultra-long acting	6 h	No peak	Up to 36 h

response to activities and meals. Many patients with diabetes type 2 who require insulin can often achieve satisfactory control with a single daily injection of a long-acting insulin, with oral medications helping to meet short-term glucose management.

Insulin is injected subcutaneously and absorbed into the blood. It can also be administered intravenously by medical professionals such as paramedics responding to a hypoglycemic patient, or in a hospital setting. The various subcutaneous insulin preparations have different mechanisms to control absorption, including added proteins to slow absorption (eg, NPH) or modifications in the insulin molecule, so-called insulin analogues. Key factors in insulin selection and timing of injection include the onset, peak, and duration of action. As **TABLE 5.5** illustrates, a range of insulin types are available. The goal for insulin management in type 1 diabetes is to time the peak of short-acting insulin injections with calorie intake, while a long-acting insulin controls background or basal needs. Very quick absorption is ideal for premeal insulin, enabling the patient to prepare a meal, estimate the carbohydrates, check a blood glucose (which determines if a correction factor needs to be added for hyperglycemia) and administer the insulin dose just before eating. Slow, steady absorption is the goal for long-acting or basal insulin, which releases in the background to prevent an insulin-deficit state (which can trigger ketone release), while avoiding a spike in insulin absorption, which can trigger hypoglycemia if not occurring together with calorie intake. Intravenous insulin results in an immediate response, and regular insulin is used.

The major risk with insulin use is hypoglycemia. Patients who take insulin should monitor their blood glucose level regularly; in the case of type 1 diabetes, typically multiple times per day. Continuous glucose monitoring can be used to help predict patterns of blood glucose and can predict hypoglycemia risk. However, because it relies on passive diffusion of glucose from blood to subcutaneous tissue, there is a delay between continuous blood glucose monitor readings and the actual blood glucose level; thus, it is not a replacement for blood glucose checks.

Weight gain is typically seen when insulin is initiated. While some patients may cut back on insulin doses to avoid weight gain, the resulting hyperglycemia is not healthy. Referrals for diabetes education, nutritional guidance and often emotional support should be provided. Insulin injection sites must be alternated to avoid development of lipoatrophy or hypertrophy as noted above.

Type 2 diabetes can also be managed with oral and injected medications as well as with insulin. Oral medications are usually initiated after lifestyle approaches through diet and exercise do not get a patient to goal. When patients present with more advanced diabetes, oral medication, insulin, or an injected noninsulin drug may be initiated at diagnosis (**TABLE 5.6**).

Metformin is the only drug currently available in the biguanide drug class in the United States. It is generally considered the initial drug of choice when starting a patient on medication to treat

33. ACCORD Study Group. Long-term effects of intensive glucose lowering on cardiovascular outcomes. *N Engl J Med.* 2011;364:818-828.

34. Knowler WC, Barrett-Connor E, Fowler SE, et al. Reduction in the incidence of type 2 diabetes with lifestyle intervention or metformin. *N Engl J Med.* 2002;346(6):393-403.

35. Brett AS. Sulfonylureas for patients with type 2 diabetes: still an option. *NEJM J Watch.* 2020. https://www.jwatch.org/na50710/2020/01/16/sulfonylureas-patients-with-type-2-diabetes-still-option.

36. Vilsbøll T, Christensen M, Junker AE, Knop FK, Gluud LL. Effects of glucagon-like peptide-1 receptor agonists on weight loss: systematic review and meta-analyses of randomised controlled trials. *Brit Med J.* 2012;344:d7771. doi:10.1136/bmj.d7771.

37. Zheng SL, Roddick AJ, Aghar-Jaffar R, et al. Association between use of sodium-glucose cotransporter 2 inhibitors, glucagon-like peptide 1 agonists, and dipeptidyl peptidase 4 inhibitors with all-cause mortality in patients with type 2 diabetes: a systematic review and meta-analysis. *J Am Med Assoc.* 2018;319:1580. doi:10.1001/jama.2018.3024.

38. Lee M, Sun J, Han M, et al. Nationwide trends in pancreatitis and pancreatic cancer risk among patients with newly diagnosed type 2 diabetes receiving dipeptidyl peptidase 4 inhibitors. *Diabetes Care.* 2019;42:2057-2064. doi:10.2337/dc18-2195.

39. Pasternak B, Ueda P, Eliasson B, et al. Use of sodium glucose cotransporter 2 inhibitors and risk of major cardiovascular events and heart failure: Scandinavian register based cohort study. *Brit Med J.* 2019;366:l4772. doi:10.1136/bmj.l4772.

40. Zelniker TA, Wiviott SD, Raz I, et al. SGLT2 inhibitors for primary and secondary prevention of cardiovascular and renal outcomes in type 2 diabetes: a systematic review and meta-analysis of cardiovascular outcome trials. *Lancet.* 2018;393:P31-P39. doi:10.1016/S0140-6736(18)32590-X.

41. Neal B, Perkovic V, Mahaffey KW, et al. Canagliflozin and cardiovascular and renal events in type 2 diabetes. *N Engl J Med.* 2017;377(7):644-657. doi:10.1056/NEJMoa1611925.

42. Lago RM, Singh PP, Nesto RW. Congestive heart failure and cardiovascular death in patients with prediabetes and type 2 diabetes given thiazolidinediones: a meta-analysis of randomised clinical trials. *Lancet.* 2007;370:1129-1136.

43. Loke YK, Singh S, Furberg CD. Long-term use of thiazolidinediones and fractures in type 2 diabetes: a meta-analysis. *Can Med Assoc J.* 2009;180:32-39.

Endocrinology

David M. Shein and Rachel C. Druckenbrod

LEARNING OBJECTIVES

Normal homeostasis relies upon a complex interplay of the endocrine system with organs, physiologic systems, and the environment. In disease, a multitude of symptoms and clinical findings typically occur. A solid understanding of the endocrine system can turn seemingly disparate clinical findings and symptoms into a syndrome, the cause of which can be identified and treated. Many endocrine disorders involve the eyes directly and indirectly, including through neurological mechanisms that affect vision.

Sections 1-3 address function and diseases of the pituitary gland, adrenal glands, and thyroid gland, respectively, with thyroid eye disease (TED) included in Section 3. Section 4 covers calcium homeostasis, which involves the interplay between parathyroid hormone, vitamin D, serum calcium, and a range of other physiologic and environmental factors. The most common disease state affected by calcium is osteoporosis, though unlike the other hormone deficiencies reviewed above, osteoporosis is a complex disease, and not merely parathyroid hormone deficiency.

KEY CONCEPTS

Normal function and diseases of
   Pituitary gland
   Adrenal glands
   Thyroid gland

Parathyroid glands
   Calcium homeostasis
   Vitamin D
   Osteoporosis

SECTION 1: PITUITARY

The **pituitary gland** is a key component of the endocrine system. This section will cover growth hormone, prolactin (PRL), gonadotropins or sex hormones, and antidiuretic hormone (ADH). Normal states as well as hormone excess and deficiency will be reviewed.

The pituitary gland is suspended beneath the brain by the pituitary stalk or infundibulum, and rests on the sphenoid bone in a depression called the sella turcica (Turkish saddle) due to its appearance. The pituitary gland is divided into two sections, the anterior pituitary which comprises about two-thirds of the gland, and the posterior pituitary or neurohypophysis, comprising the other third. The stalk delivers dopamine to the pituitary and supports a rich venous supply that delivers trophic hormones (**FIGURE 6.1**). It also carries ADH or arginine vasopressin (AVP) to the neurohypophysis. Key neurologic and vascular structures are located in close proximity to the pituitary gland, and abnormalities in the pituitary that cause it to enlarge can cause physical symptoms before hormonal derangement is appreciated. The proximity of the pituitary to important vascular structures (the cavernous sinuses and the carotid arteries) is an important consideration for medical diseases and surgical procedures (Chapter 15).

Importantly for the optometrist, the optic chiasm sits above the pituitary gland, and cranial nerves III (oculomotor), IV (trochlear), and VI (abducens) are located on either side of the pituitary within the cavernous sinuses; thus visual impairment from chiasmal compression, and diplopia or Horner syndrome due to cavernous sinus invasion, can be initial manifestations of pituitary enlargement. Less-common neuro-ophthalmologic manifestations of pituitary adenoma include see-saw nystagmus, visual hallucinations (Charles Bonnet syndrome), and the "hemifield slide" phenomenon (diplopia due to breakdown of sensory fusion from absence of overlap of nasal-temporal fields in each eye, in the setting of dense bitemporal field loss).[1] Macroadenomas (the larger pituitary tumors) are much more likely to impact the cavernous sinuses and/or chiasm, since the chiasm sits about 10 mm above the pituitary gland and the cavernous sinuses sit just laterally on either side (**FIGURE 6.2**). Neuro-ophthalmological examination in the setting of known or suspected pituitary mass should include measurement of central visual acuity, color vision and/or contrast sensitivity, confrontation visual fields, pupillary examination, assessment of cranial nerves III, IV, and VI, dilated examination of the optic nerves, and automated or Goldmann visual field examination.

Retinal ganglion cell fibers travel to the optic chiasm via the optic nerves and maintain a predictable organization, with nasally derived retinal fibers decussating contralaterally at the chiasm and temporally derived retinal fibers traversing the ipsilateral aspect of the chiasm. Thus, chiasmal compression by a sellar mass classically results in bitemporal visual field loss from compression of the decussating nasal retinal fibers, though other patterns of visual field loss are also possible.[1] Depending on how the chiasm is fixed above the pituitary gland in the anteroposterior plane (for example, directly above the

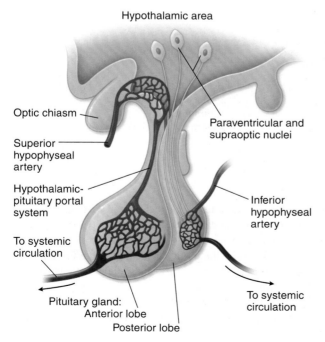

Hypothalamic area

Optic chiasm

Superior hypophyseal artery

Hypothalamic-pituitary portal system

To systemic circulation

Pituitary gland:
Anterior lobe
Posterior lobe

Paraventricular and supraoptic nuclei

Inferior hypophyseal artery

To systemic circulation

FIGURE 6.1 Anatomy of the pituitary gland and vasculature of the hypothalamic-pituitary axis. (Reprinted from Golan DE. *Principles of Pharmacology*. 4th ed. Philadelphia, PA: Wolters Kluwer; 2016.)

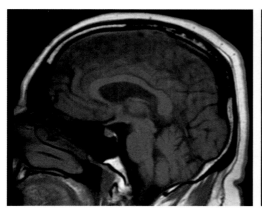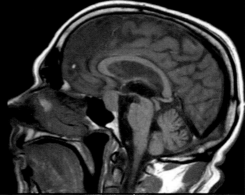

FIGURE 6.2 T1-weighted sagittal MRI scans showing normal pituitary gland (left) and pituitary macroadenoma with chiasmal compression (right). (Image credit: Rachel Druckenbrod, OD [VA Boston Healthcare System].)

gland, "prefixed" [in front of the gland], or "postfixed" [behind the gland]), there may be relatively denser inferior versus superior field loss within the temporal field. Occasionally only one quadrant (superior or inferior) of the temporal field is affected, resulting in bitemporal quadrantanopsia. A so-called junctional scotoma (central field loss in one eye and temporal field loss in the other) may result from compression of the prechiasmal optic nerve on only one side by an anteriorly positioned sellar mass. Uncommonly, a unilateral temporal field defect may result from a pituitary adenoma. Central vision is usually decreased in all cases of pituitary chiasmal compression due to the large proportion of foveomacular fibers within the chiasm. Prognosis for visual recovery after decompression of the chiasm depends on duration and severity of the compression and whether there is optic atrophy, though on average more than 75% of patients show improvement in central vision, visual fields, or both. Patients who undergo chiasmal decompression (eg, via transsphenoidal surgery) often experience a dramatic improvement in vision within 24 hours, and those treated medically (eg, with bromocriptine) notice improvement within 24 to 72 hours. A majority of improvement occurs within 4 months. Patients are less likely to show improvement beyond 6 to 12 months (**FIGURE 6.3**).

The nearby hypothalamus plays an important role in the regulation of pituitary function. Trophic hormones from the hypothalamus stimulate the release of stimulatory hormones from the anterior pituitary gland. To facilitate this close communication, the hypophyseal portal system, a network of veins, carries hormones from the hypothalamus directly to the pituitary gland (**FIGURE 6.1**).

Pituitary hormones are involved in a feedback loop that stimulates release when hormones are needed and provides negative feedback when physiologic needs are met (**FIGURE 6.4**). In the case of most pituitary hormones, that normal loop begins with hypothalamic hormones which are trophic (stimulatory) toward the pituitary gland. Thus, trophic hormones secreted by the hypothalamus stimulate the pituitary gland to produce a stimulatory hormone which acts on the target gland via hormone receptors. This may trigger release of another hormone (eg, thyroxine) or modulation of homeostatic functions (eg, salt and water balance). Once adequate hormone is available, the hypothalamus decreases trophic hormone release.

Multiple factors can disrupt this system, and pituitary dysfunction is named by convention to indicate the level or region of interruption. When a gland itself is either hyperactive or hypoactive, the disorder is primary. For example, hypothyroidism due to thyroid gland dysfunction is termed *primary hypothyroidism* (**FIGURE 6.5**). When defective signaling fails to stimulate an otherwise normal gland, the disorder is secondary. An example of *secondary hypothyroidism* is with deficiency of pituitary-derived thyroid-stimulating hormone (TSH). In the least common situation, impaired trophic hormone release by the hypothalamus results in a tertiary disorder. Deficient

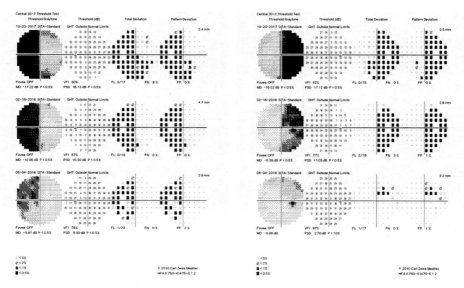

FIGURE 6.3 Improvement of visual field loss from pituitary macroadenoma causing chiasmal compression, status post endoscopic transsphenoidal resection. Top: Presurgical bitemporal visual field loss; middle: improvement in visual fields 2 months after surgery; bottom: further resolution of visual field loss 6 months after surgery. (Image credit: Rachel Druckenbrod, OD [VA Boston Healthcare System].)

thyrotropin-releasing hormone (TRH) from the hypothalamus failing to stimulate the pituitary and thyroid glands results in *tertiary hypothyroidism*. This terminology is important in the diagnosis and management of endocrine disorders.

Anterior pituitary hormones can be divided into two major types based upon structural characteristics. The polypeptide hormones are growth hormone, adrenocorticotropic hormone (ACTH), and PRL. The glycoprotein hormones are heterodimers, sharing a common alpha subunit, and each has a distinct beta subunit. These hormones are TSH, luteinizing hormone (LH), and follicle-stimulating

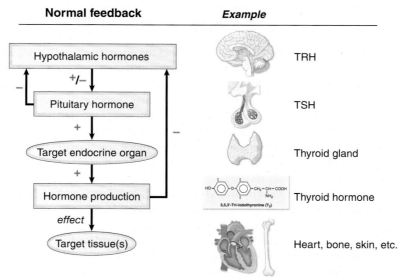

FIGURE 6.4 Pituitary-hypothalamic feedback loop. TRH, thyrotropin-releasing hormone; TSH, thyroid-stimulating hormone.

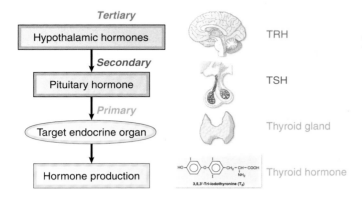

FIGURE 6.5 An example of primary versus secondary and tertiary endocrine disease. TRH, thyrotropin-releasing hormone; TSH, thyroid-stimulating hormone.

hormone (FSH). Other hormones, including human chorionic gonadotropin (HCG), also share a common alpha and distinct beta subunit.

Symptoms of pituitary abnormalities typically come to clinical attention with one (or more) of the three main modes of presentation:

- Local growth
- Excess hormone secretion
- Hormone deficiency

Local growth can result in compression of adjacent nervous structures, often impacting vision as noted above. Tumors often present with extrasellar extension (beyond the confines of the sella turcica), impairing vision and ocular motility, as well as causing headache, dizziness, and nausea (Chapter 15). Hormonal abnormalities present as hormone excess or deficiency (or both simultaneously). Pituitary microadenomas (measuring less than 10 mm) are more likely to present with symptoms of hormone excess, while macroadenomas (measuring 10 mm or greater) are more likely to cause symptoms of compression.[2] The differential diagnosis for pituitary insufficiency includes tumor invasion, local infection, infiltration, trauma, bleed, or iatrogenic (caused by medical treatments) including surgical or radiation injury.

Craniopharyngiomas, which arise from remnants of Rathke pouch, occur in the region of the sella turcica and typically present with symptoms of extrasellar extension. While representing a minority of brain tumors (about 5% of brain tumors in children and fewer in adults), these benign tumors are important to consider in the differential diagnosis of a sellar mass. On imaging, they may appear part solid and part cystic with calcifications within the tumor. Local excision is the treatment of choice.[3]

GROWTH HORMONE

Growth hormone is a polypeptide hormone secreted by the pituitary gland. Release is triggered by hypothalamic growth hormone–releasing hormone (GHRH) and by gut hormones responding to nutrient intake and fasting. Growth hormone secretion is inhibited by hypothalamic secretion of somatostatin. The key target tissue for growth hormone is the liver, which in turn produces insulin-like growth factor-1 (IGF-1). IGF-1 acts on target tissues including the bone, where it impacts growth. IGF-1 is also a counterregulatory hormone for insulin, stimulating glucose release; levels of IGF-1 increase in response to hypoglycemia. High levels of IGF-1 (such as in states of growth hormone excess) cause glucose intolerance and may result in type 2 diabetes mellitus (Chapter 5). IGF-1 feeds back to the hypothalamus to downregulate GHRH production and decrease growth hormone release. Growth hormone is secreted cyclically, and a random growth hormone level is typically of limited value for diagnosis.

States of growth hormone excess cause either gigantism or acromegaly (**FIGURES 6.6** and **6.7**). The former occurs if the growth hormone excess occurs during childhood before the epiphyses of the

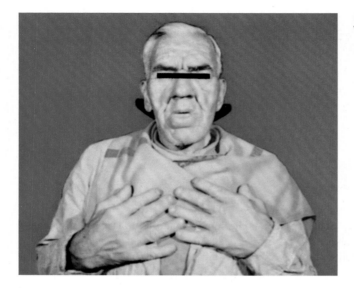

FIGURE   6.6 Acromegaly. (From Weber J, Kelley J. *Health Assessment in Nursing.* 2nd ed. Philadelphia, PA: Wolters Kluwer; 2003.)

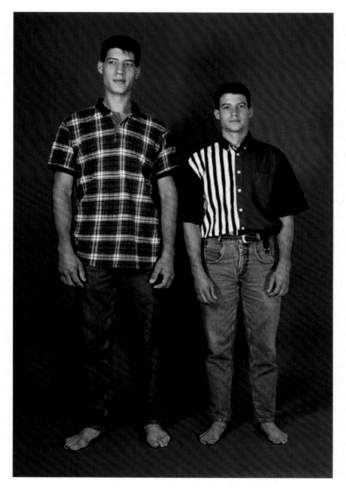

FIGURE 6.7 Gigantism. (From Porth C. *Essentials of Pathophysiology.* 4th ed. Philadelphia, PA: Wolters Kluwer; 2014.)

bones (the regions of growth) have closed; the result is excess linear growth. Later in life, acromegaly results with the overgrowth of bones and soft tissues in hands, face, and other areas. Due to the metabolic effects of growth hormone and IGF-1, hypertension and diabetes are often present with acromegaly and gigantism. In addition, myopathy with weakness and cardiomyopathy also occur.

The most common cause of growth hormone excess is oversecretion from a pituitary tumor. These tumors are often mixed, and other hormones such as PRL may also be secreted in excess. Options for evaluation include measuring IGF-1 after an oral glucose load to suppress growth hormone or sequential sampling of growth hormone levels over time. Since glucose will normally have a suppressive effect on growth hormone secretion (as IGF-1 is a counterregulatory hormone responding to low glucose), an inappropriately high growth hormone level after the glucose load suggests hormone excess. When pituitary overproduction of growth hormone is confirmed, brain imaging is necessary to assess the pituitary gland. When available, MRI is the preferred imaging modality (Chapter 15). Treatment options for tumors include surgery or radiation; medical therapy is used for suppression.

Growth hormone deficiency also manifests differently in children and adults. In childhood, short stature and fasting hypoglycemia are present. In adults, deficiency results in decreased fat metabolism with loss of lean body mass and increased fat deposition. There is also loss of bone mass and metabolic abnormalities in lipids and glucose. Growth hormone deficiency in children and adults is treated with hormone replacement therapy.

PROLACTIN

PRL is a polypeptide hormone secreted by the pituitary gland. PRL control differs from the other pituitary hormones. Instead of a stimulatory hormone, dopamine release by the hypothalamus inhibits PRL release. When dopamine levels drop, PRL secretion increases. This can occur not only with physiologic triggers but also with injury to the vascular structures in the pituitary stalk by preventing delivery of dopamine, therefore disabling its inhibitory effect. PRL acts on the breast, and suckling stimulates release. TRH also stimulates PRL release, and in some cases of hypothyroidism, when trophic hormone levels are elevated, PRL levels can increase as well.

Syndromes of PRL excess result in menstrual irregularity, galactorrhea (breast milk production), male impotence, and osteoporosis. Hyperprolactinemia can cause infertility. Physiologic PRL elevation occurs with pregnancy and delivery as well as nipple stimulation. A number of drugs, including those acting on the central nervous system, can trigger an increase in PRL. PRL-secreting pituitary tumors, and as noted above, injury or compression of the pituitary stalk, cause hyperprolactinemia. Suspicion for hyperprolactinemia based upon symptoms is evaluated with a serum PRL level. The initial evaluation of hyperprolactinemia should exclude medication-induced hormone excess and hypothyroidism. When there is suspicion for a pituitary lesion, brain imaging with CT or MRI is appropriate.

PRL-secreting pituitary tumors are the most common pituitary tumors. In premenopausal women, smaller microprolactinomas are more commonly diagnosed due to the impact on menstruation and fertility. In postmenopausal women and in men, larger tumors that cause compression of other structures present more commonly; thus tumors are typically larger at diagnosis. Treatment for pituitary prolactinomas may begin with dopamine agonists that lower the level and control tumor size. Larger tumors and those not responding to medical management can be treated surgically or with radiation therapy.

PRL deficiency is uncommonly diagnosed, and the only well-defined symptom is absent lactation.

GONADOTROPINS

LH and FSH are glycoprotein hormones. These gonadotropins act on the ovary and testes. Release is stimulated by gonadotropin-releasing hormone (GnRH), which is secreted in a pulsatile manner by the hypothalamus. The pulsatile secretion is necessary for normal function, and steady high levels of GnRH agonists will suppress pituitary gonadotropin release. Inhibin, secreted by the ovary and testes, also suppresses pituitary gonadotropins.

In women, the menstrual cycle is driven by changes in gonadotropin levels and is typically divided into three phases. During the follicular phase, FSH prompts maturation of an ovarian follicle containing an oocyte and the endometrium proliferates to support a pregnancy. During the ovulatory phase, a surge in LH prompts release of the oocyte and creation of the corpus luteum, which secretes progesterone. If fertilization does not occur, the luteal or secretory phase occurs as the corpus luteum involutes and progesterone secretion drops. During this phase, the endometrium is shed with bleeding lasting up to 7 days.

Amenorrhea refers to the absence of menstruation. Amenorrhea can be subdivided into primary, when no menstruation occurs by age 15, and secondary, when previous menstruation ceases for either a three-cycle interval or longer than 6 months. Amenorrhea is typically caused by failure of the ovaries to ovulate, which can be due to primary ovarian failure or secondary ovarian failure, in which case a normal ovary is not stimulated in a physiologic, cyclical manner. Secondary amenorrhea is seen more often in clinical practice, and there are a number of considerations in the differential diagnosis.

A patient history to elicit signs and symptoms of hormone excess or deficiency includes questions about galactorrhea, hirsutism (excess hair growth) and acne, weight change, excessive sweating, and palpitations. Examination should include height, weight and BMI determination, blood pressure, and a complete multisystem examination including a gynecological examination. The lab evaluation of amenorrhea includes ruling out pregnancy (by checking urine or serum for HCG). Gonadotropin levels assess for primary ovarian failure. Elevated levels point to primary ovarian failure as the cause of the amenorrhea. Causes of secondary amenorrhea include menopause, autoimmune disease, and iatrogenic causes such as ovarian surgery or cytotoxic cancer chemotherapy. Primary amenorrhea is most often associated with a genetic diagnosis, most commonly gonadal dysgenesis. Other causes of primary amenorrhea include endocrine conditions such as the polycystic ovarian syndrome or chronic anovulation, hypopituitarism, and congenital adrenal hyperplasia (see below). Anatomic considerations such as an imperforate hymen can be suggested by history and confirmed during examination. Some girls experience a constitutional delay in puberty, which is considered normal. Other secondary medical causes such as severe illness or very low body weight can also explain primary amenorrhea when present.[4]

Causes of secondary amenorrhea include hyperprolactinemia, for which a PRL level can be diagnostic; and thyroid dysfunction, with either hypo- or hyperthyroidism capable of disrupting normal menstruation. A TSH level is a good screening test and many labs will perform a reflex T4 level if the TSH is abnormal. Gonadotropin deficiency due to pituitary abnormalities (such as compression by a tumor) can be evaluated by checking FSH and LH levels. Androgen excess can occur from androgen-producing tumors, congenital adrenal hyperplasia, and polycystic ovarian syndrome. Each condition requires a detailed investigation.

Hypothalamic amenorrhea is seen in women with very low body weight and/or high levels of physical exertion. Starvation and eating disorders that result in very low body weight can be accompanied by amenorrhea. Very high levels of exercise, such as by competitive athletes, often trigger amenorrhea. Since these states are also accompanied by low levels of estrogen, there are additional risks such as development of osteoporosis[5] (see below). Geopolitical and societal causes of starvation, behavioral health needs of patients with eating disorders, and athletes' specific medical needs all require individualized attention. Medication use as a trigger should also be considered in the evaluation of amenorrhea and other menstrual irregularities.

In men, FSH stimulates spermatogenesis in the Sertoli cells while LH stimulates Leydig cells to produce testosterone. Abnormalities in patterns of gonadotropin secretion may manifest as erectile dysfunction (ED). This symptom is discussed more frequently in the clinical setting since the marketing of the phosphodiesterase-5 inhibitors such as sildenafil (sold under the brand Viagra). Public

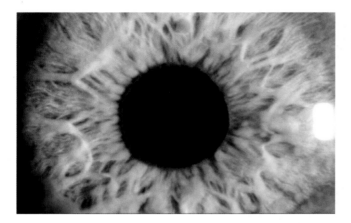

FIGURE 6.15 Lisch nodules of the iris in neurofibromatosis type 1. (Courtesy of R. Lewis, Baylor College of Medicine, Houston, Texas.)

Bilateral optic nerve gliomas are also pathognomonic when present, though unilateral optic nerve glioma may also occur in NF1. These usually present in childhood with slow-onset, painless proptosis, ophthalmoplegia, and vision loss with optic atrophy. Neuroimaging shows fusiform enlargement of the optic nerve(s) (**FIGURE 6.16**). Orbital lesions are possible (**FIGURE 6.17**), and larger gliomas in the region of the optic chiasm can also affect the pituitary gland leading to early or delayed puberty.

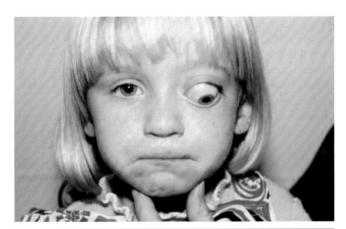

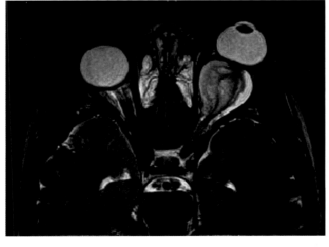

FIGURE 6.16 Unilateral left-sided optic nerve glioma in a 6-year-old girl with neurofibromatosis type 1, causing significant proptosis. Top: external appearance; bottom: T1-weighted axial MRI showing fusiform enlargement of the left optic nerve. (Top, From Penne RB. *Wills Eye Institute - Oculoplastics.* 2nd ed. Philadelphia, PA: Wolters Kluwer; 2011. Bottom, From Iyer RA, Chapman T. *Pediatric Imaging: The Essentials.* Philadelphia, PA: Wolters Kluwer; 2015.)

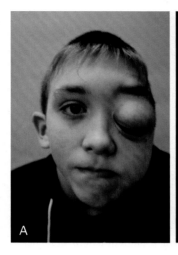
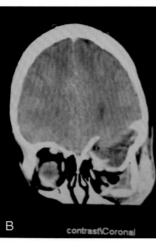

A

B contrast\Coronal

FIGURE 6.17 A, A 12-year-old boy with left orbital and mental nerve plexiform neurofibromatosis type 1, severe ptosis, and pulsatile exophthalmos. B, MRI demonstrated a plexiform tumor of the superior orbit and mental nerve, a large defect of the sphenoid greater wing, and prolapse of the temporal lobe into the orbit. (From Chung K, Gosain A. *Operative Techniques in Pediatric Plastic and Reconstructive Surgery.* Philadelphia, PA: Wolters Kluwer; 2019.)

Several other tumors occur with increased frequency in NF1, including pheochromocytoma as noted above, other central nervous system tumors, soft tissue sarcomas, and malignant peripheral nerve sheath tumors. A variety of abnormalities in bones can occur, including dysplasia, scoliosis, osteoporosis, and short stature. Learning disabilities, developmental delay, and seizures can also occur. Hypertension is also seen commonly, including at a younger age.

NF2 is also inherited in an autosomal dominant pattern, although a substantial number of cases occur from a de novo mutation in the individual without a family history. Nervous system abnormalities are common, including vestibular schwannomas and schwannomas of other cranial nerves, brain meningiomas, spinal tumors, and neuropathy.

Ocular findings are often the first manifestation of NF2 and commonly include juvenile cataracts in >50% of cases (posterior subcapsular, cortical, or mixed) (**FIGURE 6.18**) and epiretinal membrane. Optic nerve meningioma, optic nerve glioma, and Lisch nodules are less common, but do also occur in NF2.

Skin findings also occur in NF2, including pigmented plaque lesions, palpable subcutaneous nodules, and intracutaneous schwannomas.

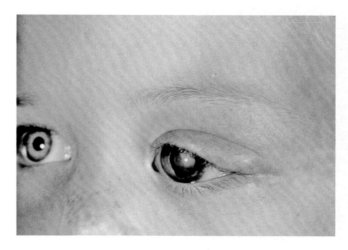

FIGURE 6.18 Plexiform neurofibroma of the left eyelid with characteristic S-shaped contour of left upper lid, cafe au lait spots in left temple, and buphthalmic left globe displaying an enlarged cornea, dilated pupil, ectropion iridis, and cataract. (From Gold DH, Weingeist TA. *Color Atlas of the Eye in Systemic Disease.* Baltimore, MD: Lippincott Williams & Wilkins; 2001.)

SECTION 3: THYROID

This section reviews normal thyroid physiology as well as the pathological states of goiter, hypo- and hyperthyroidism as well as Graves disease and ophthalmopathy, thyroiditis, and thyroid cancer.

The thyroid gland is located in the lower neck and is only visible when enlarged, such as a large goiter. The thyroid consists of two lobes (right and left) and a middle section, the isthmus. The thyroid gland has a rich blood supply to support its endocrine function. Nearby structures are important to consider with gland enlargement and by a surgeon performing thyroid surgery and include the recurrent laryngeal nerve (supplying the vocal cords), trachea, and esophagus. Dysphonia can occur with marked gland enlargement or as a surgical complication. Uncommonly, breathing or swallowing can be impacted as well, though this generally occurs only with marked thyroid enlargement in advanced thyroid cancer. The parathyroid glands (see next section) sit adjacent to the thyroid gland and can also be impacted by thyroid surgery (**FIGURE 6.19**).

The thyroid gland produces thyroid hormone, which requires iodine. Fish and seafood, dairy products, and some fruits, as well as iodized salt are typical dietary sources.[18] Iodine deficiency in developed countries is uncommon. The thyroid gland mostly produces thyroxine, T4. The other thyroid hormone, triiodothyronine, T3, is more biologically active and is generated by peripheral tissue conversion of T4. Preformed thyroid hormone is stored in the thyroid gland, and in the setting of acute thyroid gland injury such as infection or inflammation, the thyroid hormone stores can be released, causing acute hyperthyroidism.

Thyroid hormone is highly protein-bound, yet only free hormone (free T4, free T3) is active. Older lab assays could only measure total T4 and a process to estimate free T4 by measuring available thyroid binding sites was used to calculate a free thyroxine index. Most modern labs can measure free T4 directly and the total T4 measurement and free thyroxine index are rarely used today. T3 can also be measured; infrequently hyperthyroidism will occur due to excess T3, called T3 toxicosis. Most lab evaluations for thyroid function measure TSH and sometimes free T4. T3 tests are ordered less often, but may be assessed in the less common clinical situation of T3 toxicosis or for monitoring a T3 prescription.

The thyroid gland is under hypothalamic and pituitary control with TRH from the hypothalamus and TSH from the pituitary. Thyroid hormone provides negative feedback to the hypothalamus and pituitary to decrease stimulatory hormone release.

Thyroid disease can present at different levels of the hypothalamic-pituitary-thyroid axis. As with other hormonal conditions, both primary and secondary thyroid disease can be described. Thyroid gland disease, either hypofunction or hyperfunction, is considered primary. Pituitary hypo- or

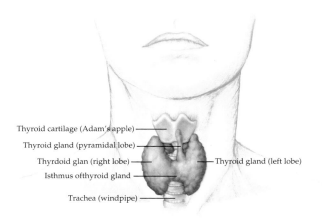

FIGURE 6.19 The thyroid gland is located in the anterior neck. Note the right and left lobes and the isthmus. (Asset provided by Anatomical Chart Co.)

Thyroid cartilage (Adam's apple)
Thyroid gland (pyramidal lobe)
Thyrdoid glan (right lobe)
Isthmus ofthyroid gland
Thyroid gland (left lobe)
Trachea (windpipe)

hyperfunction (a rare cause of thyroid dysfunction) would be considered secondary, and when hypothalamic dysfunction (also uncommon) affects the thyroid gland, it is termed tertiary.

Clinical examination for thyroid disease includes assessment of the thyroid gland by inspection of the anterior neck, then by palpation low down in the anterior neck, often done from behind the patient. A normal gland, or one with a relatively small nodule or asymmetry, can only be felt while the patient swallows, which elevates the thyroid gland above the upper sternum. Large nodules and significant thyroid enlargement can be palpated without swallowing and sometimes even seen with inspection of the neck. The ocular examination, as well as neurological, cardiac, and skin examinations are areas where the clinical effects of thyroid dysfunction can be detected. History is also important to elicit symptoms compatible with thyroid disease (FIGURE 6.20).

Goiter is defined as enlargement of the thyroid gland. It can be seen in all states of thyroid function including euthyroid, hyperthyroidism, and hypothyroidism. In regions of the world where iodine deficiency is more common, such as in mountainous regions of poor countries with limited seafood availability and few fortified foods, goiter due to iodine deficiency may be relatively common. Graves hyperthyroidism often causes thyroid enlargement as can other causes of thyroiditis. A multinodular gland may appear goitrous; however, on imaging, a nodular gland can be differentiated from a diffuse goiter. Thyroid cancer can also cause thyroid gland enlargement, but generally the enlargement is asymmetric and may be felt as a nodule; imaging and biopsy would differentiate a cancer from a benign nodule.

To assess for thyroid disease, measurement of serum TSH is a good screening test. When TSH is abnormal, adding a free T4 level is the next step in the evaluation. If pituitary function is normal, a low TSH level with a high free T4 indicates primary hyperthyroidism with TSH suppressed due to excess circulating thyroid hormone. A high TSH with a low thyroid hormone level indicates primary hypothyroidism. Both hypo- and hyperthyroidism can be subclinical, defined as an abnormal TSH with normal thyroid hormone levels. Subclinical disease is generally asymptomatic. In secondary and tertiary hypothyroidism, both TSH and measures of thyroid hormone are low. Normal thyroid function is referred to as euthyroid. The table lists several possible results from serum TSH and free T4 testing with the most commonly associated clinical diagnosis (TABLE 6.1).

All tissues in the body have thyroid hormone receptors. Thyroid function is a key regulatory factor, impacting functions as diverse as metabolism, cardiac rhythm, thermal regulation, and bone turnover. Normal thyroid hormone levels are critical for development, and hypothyroid infants that go untreated suffer impairment in brain development.

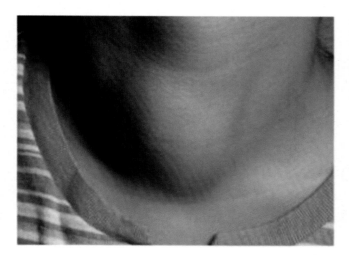

FIGURE 6.20 A large thyroid nodule involving most of the right thyroid lobe is clearly visible on physical examination. (From Pizzo PA, Poplack DG. *Principles and Practice of Pediatric Oncology.* 7th ed. Philadelphia, PA: Wolters Kluwer; 2015.)

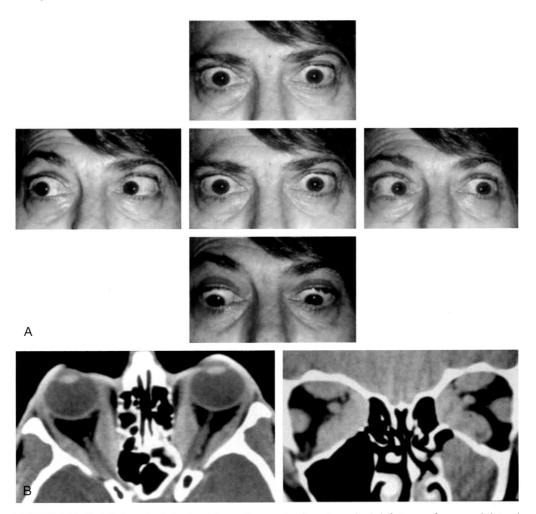

FIGURE 6.22 Ophthalmoplegia in thyroid eye disease. A, There is marked deficiency of upgaze, bilateral lid retraction, and bilateral proptosis. B, CT of the orbits shows enlargement of all extraocular muscles, with relative sparing of the lateral recti as is typical for thyroidopathy. (From Savino P, Danesh-Meyer H. *Neuro-Ophthalmology*. 3rd ed. Philadelphia, PA: Wolters Kluwer; 2018.)

(FIGURE 6.21 and 6.22). In the most severe cases, optic neuropathy with vision loss occurs due to optic nerve compression from swelling of the orbital contents. Fortunately, only about 5% of patients will experience optic neuropathy.

There can be dramatic and sometimes permanent alterations in the cosmetic appearance of patients which, along with the other chronic and debilitating symptoms of TED (discomfort and redness from dry eye, diplopia, blurry vision), may be truly life altering.

The natural history of TED involves an "active phase" where signs and symptoms may progress (typically lasts for 1 year for nonsmokers, 2-3 years for smokers), followed by a spontaneous "quiescent phase" of disease inactivity and stability. Disease activity level may be assessed at the time of diagnosis and thereafter using the Clinical Activity Score (CAS; TABLE 6.3), though there are other commonly used methods as well. Early intervention during the active phase is important to minimize the duration and severity of the disease. Management of TED involves systemic management of the thyroid dysfunction (as discussed later in this chapter), in addition to targeted ophthalmic treatments. Patients with moderate to severe TED should not be treated with radioiodine therapy

TABLE 6.3   Examination Elements of the Clinical Activity Score (CAS) for the Assessment of Thyroid Eye Disease[27,a]

Initial and subsequent assessments
Retrobulbar eye pain over the past 4 wk
Pain with eye movement over the past 4 wk
Redness of the eyelids
Redness of the conjunctiva
Swelling of the eyelids
Chemosis of the conjunctiva
Swollen caruncle
Subsequent assessments
Increase in proptosis ≥ 2 mm
Decreased eye movements $\geq 5°$
Decreased vision ≥ 1 Snellen line

[a]Each element is worth 1 point. A score of 3 or more suggests active thyroid eye disease.

as a means to achieve a euthyroid state, since this can worsen the eye disease.[28] Most patients with TED suffer mild to moderate disease, and ophthalmic treatment involves supportive care for dry eye disease (artificial tears and ointments, topical cyclosporine, moisture goggles) and lifestyle modifications such as smoking cessation, low-sodium diet, and stress reduction. Prism glasses may be prescribed for diplopia. Severe orbitopathy, especially with optic nerve involvement, requires more aggressive management with oral or intravenous corticosteroids, surgical orbital decompression, and/or orbital radiotherapy. Once patients reach the quiescent phase, surgical correction of residual eyelid misalignment or strabismus may be pursued. Except in cases where urgent orbital decompression is needed during the active phase, it is important to demonstrate at least 6 months of disease inactivity before pursuing surgical interventions.

In 2020, the FDA approved the first pharmacologic immunotherapy for adults with active TED, known as teprotumumab. The drug is a human monoclonal antibody targeting the insulin-like growth factor-1 receptor (IGF-1R) and acts to significantly reduce proptosis in moderate and severe TED, without the need for surgical orbital decompression. Furthermore, the drug can be used earlier in the disease process, while still active, such that patient symptoms may be addressed earlier with potentially less overall morbidity. A phase 3 multicenter randomized, double-masked, placebo-controlled trial demonstrated the drug reduced proptosis by ≥ 2 mm in 83% of treated patients versus 10% of control patients, with a mean reduction in proptosis of 2.8 mm in the treated patients. It also achieved a reduction in the CAS ≥ 2 points in 78% (vs 7% of controls), CAS of 0 or 1 in 59% (vs 21%), and a reduction in diplopia symptoms in 68% (vs 29%).[29]

Other causes of hyperthyroidism include toxic adenomas and toxic multinodular goiter. In these cases, one or more regions of thyroid tissue experience a genetic change resulting in an "escape" from control by TSH. These regions become autonomous and secrete thyroid hormone continuously, eventually causing thyrotoxicosis. The development of toxic multinodular goiter is associated with regions of low dietary iodine and increases in frequency with age (**FIGURE 6.23**).

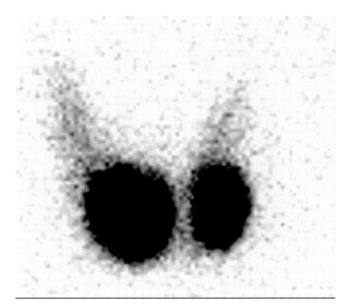

FIGURE 6.23 Hyperfunctioning nodules. I-123 scintigraphy of hyperfunctioning nodules. Two "hot" or autonomous nodules (right and left lower poles) that are producing supraphysiologic amounts of thyroid hormone appear as focal regions of increased I-123 activity in the lower pole of both the lobes. (From Werner SC, Ingbar SH, Braverman LE, Cooper DS. *Werner & Ingbar's The Thyroid*. 10th ed. Philadelphia, PA: Wolters Kluwer; 2012.)

Uncommon causes of hyperthyroidism include tumors, including cancers that secrete TSH. Secondary hyperthyroidism due to abnormal pituitary TSH production is also rare.

Hyperthyroidism increases the metabolic rate, resulting in weight loss, heat intolerance, and sweating. Menstrual abnormalities and impaired fertility are seen in women, and men have a higher risk for ED. Increased bone turnover is an important consequence of hyperthyroidism which increases the risk for osteoporosis and bone fractures (an important consideration to avoid treatment with excess levothyroxine). Tremor, insomnia, anxiety, and brisk reflexes are neuropsychiatric manifestations. Cardiovascular symptoms are common, including palpitations and increased heart rate. Risks for atrial fibrillation are increased with hyperthyroidism, especially in older adults.[30] More severe hyperthyroidism can cause fatigue and muscle weakness. Gastrointestinal symptoms of frequent bowel movements or diarrhea reflect quicker transit with less opportunity for water absorption. As noted above, TED is specific to Graves disease; similar dermatologic findings in the extremities of Graves dermopathy or pretibial myxedema are also antibody-mediated. Other dermatologic findings include thinning hair and hair loss.

Two important syndromes of hyperthyroidism are thyroid storm and apathetic hyperthyroidism. Thyroid storm is a thyrotoxic crisis, sometimes precipitated by infection, trauma, or surgery. Thyroid storm is life-threatening, requiring immediate recognition and prompt treatment. Fever is a hallmark of thyroid storm, and changes in mental status ranging from anxiety to delirium or psychosis occur. Cardiovascular manifestations are common, from tachycardia and other arrhythmias to heart failure, and when severe, vascular collapse. Apathetic hyperthyroidism is a syndrome occurring in older adults, for whom hyperthyroidism may only manifest as new onset of atrial fibrillation or heart failure. All patients with newly diagnosed atrial fibrillation and those with otherwise unexplained heart failure should have a TSH level checked to exclude thyroid disease as a trigger.

Subclinical hyperthyroidism is less common than subclinical hypothyroidism, but it is similarly identified by lab results and is typically asymptomatic. Low TSH with normal free T4 and T3 without symptoms or examination findings are consistent with hyperthyroidism. Subclinical hyperthyroidism can only be reliably diagnosed in patients without a concurrent serious illness which can affect thyroid function—termed nonthyroidal illness (which may occur in hospitalized patients). Subclinical hyperthyroidism can occur transiently in cases of thyroiditis and may also herald a future of overt hyperthyroidism in cases of hyperfunctioning nodules. A thyroid scan can help with the differential diagnosis and clinical approach to managing (see below).

Treatment for hyperthyroidism varies depending upon the cause. Antithyroid drugs (methimazole and propylthiouracil) can be used to quickly restore the euthyroid state. Longer term management can include radioactive iodine ablation or surgery to remove all or part of the gland, depending upon the clinical situation. Beta-blockers are often used for tachycardia and other tachyarrhythmias in hyperthyroid patients.

Imaging of the thyroid gland is often necessary as part of the evaluation of hyperthyroidism (overt and subclinical), thyroid nodules, and goiter. Ultrasound is used to evaluate the size of the thyroid gland and to assess for nodules and cysts. Assessment of hyperthyroidism as well as thyroid nodules can be done with a radioiodine uptake test. Radioactive iodine is used for imaging, and the pattern of uptake will help determine the nature of the condition. In the setting of Graves disease, the hyperthyroidism is characterized by diffuse thyroid gland uptake of radioactive iodine. A pattern of focal uptake in one or several localized areas of the gland suggests one or more autonomous thyroid nodules. Hyperthyroidism with no thyroid uptake suggests a thyroiditis with release of preformed thyroid hormone.

Nodules seen on an ultrasound that are "cold" on a scan (ie, no radioactive iodine uptake), especially those larger than 1 cm in size, are often referred for biopsy to exclude a thyroid cancer. Specialist referral is usually the next step for management of suspicious findings, and when needed, fine needle aspiration (FNA) with ultrasound guidance. FNA is done on an outpatient basis for lesions that are suspicious for thyroid cancer.

THYROID CANCER

There are four main types of thyroid cancer:

- Papillary carcinoma
- Follicular carcinoma
- Medullary carcinoma
- Anaplastic carcinoma

The prognosis for both papillary and follicular thyroid cancers is usually very good. Five-year survival rates for papillary cancer approach 100%, and for follicular cancer, 100% with localized disease and 97% overall.[31] Increasing rates of thyroid cancer diagnosis have been associated with thyroid screening programs, yet no improvement in long-term outcomes has been determined. As such, screening for thyroid cancer is discouraged.[32]

Medullary carcinoma is uncommon and results from malignant transformation of the parafollicular C cells that produce the hormone calcitonin. While most are sporadic (not genetic), a substantial minority of medullary carcinomas occurs in association with the inherited conditions that result in a predisposition to multiple endocrine neoplasia (specifically, the MEN2 syndrome). Five-year survival rates are 90% overall.

Anaplastic carcinoma occurs in older individuals and is often aggressive, carrying a very poor prognosis, with 5-year survival at 7% overall, but even for localized disease that number is 30%.[10]

Treatment for cancer is often surgical, though for some types of cancer adjunctive hormonal and radiation therapy may be given.

SECTION 4: CALCIUM AND OSTEOPOROSIS

This section will cover calcium homeostasis, including vitamin D, the parathyroid gland, and parathyroid hormone. It will also cover disorders of bone mineralization with a focus on osteoporosis.

hematologic malignancies such as multiple myeloma, lymphomas, and numerous solid tumors including lung, breast, and kidney cancers can trigger hypercalcemia as a paraneoplastic syndrome (Chapter 8).

Large amounts of vitamin D that may be produced through sun exposure or taking over-the-counter vitamins do not trigger hypercalcemia because activation to 1,25-dihydroxyvitamin D is controlled by the physiology of calcium homeostasis, including parathyroid hormone and the kidney. However, if the active 1,25-dihydroxyvitamin D is ingested (typically only available by prescription), then hypercalcemia can result.

Treatment of hypercalcemia depends upon both the degree of elevation and the cause. In the acute setting, when very high levels are causing significant symptoms, administering intravenous saline and loop diuretics will increase renal clearance of excess calcium acutely, and longer-term management can then be initiated. Long-term management focuses on treating the underlying condition causing hypercalcemia and monitoring. For cancer, therapy is directed as appropriate for the patient's clinical condition. Antiresorptive agents, such as the bisphosphonates used in osteoporosis (see below), can slow bone turnover and help lower calcium levels in malignancy. For abnormalities in the parathyroid glands, surgical intervention is curative. Ingestion of active vitamin D should be identified and stopped when present. Treatment of granulomatous disease, as well as restricting daily calcium intake may be needed for long-term management. Symptomatic band keratopathy may be treated with topical chelating agents, manual dissection, and/or excimer laser.

Hypocalcemia is seen infrequently, occurring most often with parathyroid gland injury in the setting of thyroid, parathyroid, and other head and neck surgery. Autoimmune parathyroid gland disease is a rare but potential cause of hypocalcemia. Vitamin D deficiency, while rare in developed countries, can cause the bone diseases of rickets in children and osteomalacia in adults. Symptoms of acute hypocalcemia differ from those of long-term hypocalcemia. Calcium plays a critical role in normal muscle function, and a rapid drop in the calcium level can cause muscular symptoms of tetany, repeated muscular contractions that can be felt as a cramp or spasm. On physical examination, the Chvostek sign can be seen by tapping the facial nerve anterior to the tragus of the ear to trigger facial spasm, seen as a twitch at the nose or lips. Abnormal cardiac function including serious arrhythmias can also result.

Though rare, hypocalcemia is an important cause of papilledema, particularly chronic cases in which no alternative cause has been identified or cases with atypical features (eg, acute vision loss).[42,43] Optic disc swelling from hypocalcemia is responsive to calcium supplementation, and visual parameters can return to normal (see Chapter 12 for discussion of papilledema). Other ophthalmic manifestations of hypocalcemia include cataract (most common; usually posterior subcapsular), corneal abnormalities (epitheliopathy and Salzmann-like peripheral nodules), extraocular motility abnormalities, photophobia, blepharoptosis, and alopecia of the eyebrows.[44]

Hypocalcemia after thyroidectomy is not uncommon, and levels usually return to normal over time. Surgeons and endocrinologists are aware of this risk, and postoperative monitoring for clinical signs of hypocalcemia and lab testing are routine. Oral calcium administration and assuring adequate vitamin D are usually adequate for managing. Vitamin D deficiency and hypoparathyroidism are both treated with calcium and vitamin D replacement. Acute hypocalcemia can be treated with intravenous calcium.

OSTEOPOROSIS

Bone consists of a three-dimensional matrix that is mineralized with calcium pyrophosphate to give the skeleton strength. Osteoporosis occurs when both the matrix and the bone mineral (chiefly calcium) are decreased (**FIGURE 6.26**). Measures of bone mineralization are used to assess bone strength and can be determined by bone density testing. A lower bone density reflects lower mineralization, and the resulting decrease in bone strength is strongly correlated with a higher fracture risk.

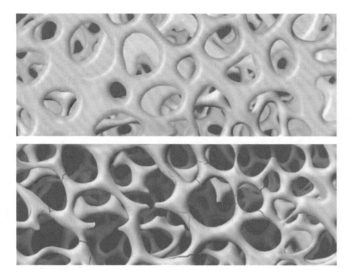

FIGURE 6.26 Normal bone mineralization (top) in contrast to poor bone mineralization in osteoporosis (bottom). (Asset provided by Anatomical Chart Co.)

Osteoporosis is defined at a point where the fracture risk is significantly elevated. It is seen more commonly in women as compared with men; however, men can develop osteoporosis. In the presence of risk factors, this condition should also be considered in men.

Bone density increases through early growth and puberty. Most adults reach their peak bone mass around the age of 30 years. Men tend to achieve a higher peak bone mass as compared with women, one factor that contributes to a lower frequency of osteoporosis in men. By the age of 40, most adults have begun a slow loss of bone mass, approximately 1% per year. However, withdrawal of sex steroid hormones will accelerate bone loss. Women experience this hormone level change at the time of menopause, and for about 5 years afterward, bone loss accelerates. Men do not normally experience abrupt sex hormone withdrawal with accelerated bone loss, another reason for the disparity in the incidence of osteoporosis between women and men. A noteworthy exception is an increased risk of men undergoing anti-androgen therapy for prostate cancer treatment. The longer average lifespan of women in the United States also increases their likelihood of osteoporosis. Since bone density continues to decline in older age, longevity is associated with progressively lower bone density and increasing fracture risk (**FIGURE 6.27**).

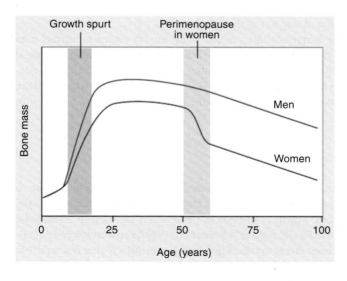

FIGURE 6.27 Typical pattern of bone strength through the lifespan. Peak bone mass is achieved in the third decade, followed by a slow decline; a period of accelerated loss is seen in women after menopause. (Reprinted with permission from Golan DE. *Principles of Pharmacology*. 3rd ed. Philadelphia, PA: Wolters Kluwer; 2011.)

Osteoporosis is seen frequently in older populations, and associated fractures can have serious impacts on health, longevity, and function. One in ten women carries this diagnosis at age 60, increasing to 2 of every 3 women at the age of 90. The lifetime risk for sustaining a fracture related to reduced bone strength caused by osteoporosis is about 50% for women and about 20% for men. Mortality rates for hip and spine fractures in older adults are alarming, with about 50% of women and 40% of men dying within 5 years of a hip fracture.[45] Many previously independent patients are unable to return to their prior degree of function, requiring an ambulatory aid, increased help at home, or a move to a different setting, such as long-term care.

Screening for osteoporosis is recommended for women 65 years and older at average risk. Earlier screening should be considered in people with an elevated risk due to significant risk factors like chronic glucocorticoid use and rheumatoid arthritis (see below). While routine screening of men is not recommended because of insufficient evidence that measurement translates into improved health outcomes, men can develop osteoporosis, particularly when risk factors are present. Accordingly, bone measurement should be considered in the appropriate clinical setting for men at risk.[46]

Bone density is most commonly measured with dual-energy x-ray absorptiometry or DEXA. Unlike a typical x-ray which produces a qualitative image, DEXA is a quantitative test. Transmission of radiation through the bone is measured and a determination of bone mineralization can be made. Results are reported with two number scores, based upon a comparison with adult peak bone mass (T-score) and age-matched cohort (Z-score). Based upon the T-score, the more useful measure clinically, a standard deviation from mean is calculated and osteoporosis is diagnosed when the T-score is 2.5 standard deviations or more below mean peak bone mass (written as T −2.5). Scores between T −1.0 and T −2.5 standard deviations (below peak bone mass) are referred to as osteopenia, and any score above −1.0 is considered normal. Other methods to determine bone density are used, most often ultrasound for a calcaneus bone density. The predictive value of the standard DEXA measurement, typically performed at both the spine and hip, is more robust.

Bone density results are predictive of fracture risk, with lower scores predicting higher risk.[47] However, many other factors also influence an individual patient's overall risk of sustaining a fracture. Gait impairment and dementia may increase the risk for a fall. Medications and lifestyle factors that impact bone strength, cause sedation, reduce muscle tone, and impair balance are also important considerations. Together with the medical management of osteoporosis and concurrent health risks, environmental measures to reduce the risk of falls are important. Grab bars in bathrooms, removing throw rugs and extension cords, balance training classes, and exercise or physical therapy can be implemented to lower fall risk and improve long-term health. Social supports from family, friends, and the community are also important factors for health, safety, and well-being.

Many diseases of the endocrine system can compromise bone density, including:

- Hypogonadism (including menopause and hormone-disrupting cancer therapies)
- Hyperthyroidism
- Hyperprolactinemia
- Hyperparathyroidism
- Vitamin D deficiency
- Glucocorticoid excess (iatrogenic or diseases)
- Growth hormone deficiency

Medications can impact bone density, most commonly the glucocorticoids which are used for a myriad of conditions and via a range of routes from oral and intravenous systemic therapy to inhaled, topical, and ocular. Long-term systemic use is clearly linked to a higher risk of fracture. Inhaled glucocorticoids are used for asthma and chronic obstructive pulmonary disease (Chapter 14), and bone impacts from inhaled use have been studied. Results demonstrate no documented impact on fracture risk at lower doses, though a small increase in the risk of bone density decline is seen from cumulative high-dose use.[48] Certain seizure medications and the injected blood thinner heparin are among the other medications where long-term use is linked to an increase in the risk for osteoporosis.

Other conditions, including eating disorders, low body mass index, tobacco use, and immobilization, are additional risk factors for osteoporosis. The corollaries, including higher body mass index and weight-bearing exercise, are protective. In addition, balance exercises such as tai chi improve balance and muscle tone, which can decrease the risk for falls[49] that often trigger bone fractures. A positive family history of osteoporosis or a spine or hip fracture in an older relative also increases an individual's risk. Men who experience withdrawal of sex hormones, as often occurs with anti-androgen therapy in prostate cancer treatment, can develop both acute symptoms of hormone withdrawal such as hot flushes and long-term risks to bone density, similar to the experience of women during menopause.

While bone density determinations correlate with fracture risk, it is possible to fine-tune the risk estimate with the use of a risk calculator that considers other factors. In clinical practice, the FRAX tool is often used. It considers bone mineral density, age, gender, family history, and medication use among the factors in its calculation. The aggregate risk assessment can be helpful in determining the approach to managing a low bone density, from lifestyle measures to medications. The FRAX tool is available online.[50]

Research and drug development are continuing to expand the range of options available to treat osteoporosis. Medical treatments generally fall into three main categories: estrogen replacement, bisphosphonates, and specific antiresorptive agents.

Since the loss of estrogen at the time of menopause corresponds to an acceleration of bone density loss, administering estrogens at the time of menopause can lower fracture risk. While postmenopausal estrogen has proven beneficial in decreasing fracture risk, it is also associated with specific harms including an increased risk of breast cancer, stroke, cardiac and vascular diseases and is not routinely used for this indication any longer (Chapter 1).[51] Selective estrogen receptor modulators (SERMs) were designed to maximize the benefit of estrogen on improving bone density, while lowering its other risks, for example, by inhibiting the carcinogenic effect of estrogen on breast tissue. SERMs can be used for osteoporosis prevention and treatment; however, other prevailing estrogenic effects may still pose a risk, including that of vascular thrombosis.

Bisphosphonates are considered first-line drugs for most patients with osteoporosis at high enough risk to warrant drug therapy. This drug class includes agents that can be administered orally or intravenously. The drug is incorporated into the bone and inhibits bone resorption. These drugs have been shown to improve bone density and decrease fracture risk. Oral absorption is poor and esophageal irritation is a significant risk; thus the drugs must be taken on an empty stomach with a full glass of water. Because of their long half-life, some can be taken as infrequently as once a month. Intravenous administration once yearly is also an option, especially with more severe osteoporosis. The bisphosphonates, especially at high doses used in cancer treatment for bone metastases, have been associated with bone complications including a rare form of hip fracture and necrosis of the jaw with dental work. Patients who take a bisphosphonate are thus typically treated for a limited time, such as 5 years, to preserve bone density without causing excess drug accumulation. The drug may be temporarily stopped in advance of invasive dental work.

For patients who cannot tolerate or have other contraindications to bisphosphonate use, several other options including salmon calcitonin, a parathyroid hormone analogue, and a bone resorption inhibitor are also available for osteoporosis treatment. Each choice has specific benefits and drawbacks, and treatment decisions should be individualized, often in consultation with a specialist.

REFERENCES

1. Gittinger JW Jr. *Tumors of the Pituitary Gland.* In: *Walsh & Hoyt's clinical neuroophthalmology.* Vol 2. Lippincott Williams & Wilkins; 2005:1532-1543.

2. Molitch ME. Diagnosis and treatment of pituitary adenomas: a review. *J Am Med Assoc.* 2017;317(5):516-524. doi:10.1001/jama.2016.19699.

Clinical Manifestations

While epigastric abdominal pain or dyspepsia is a typical symptom of these ulcers, many ulcers are asymptomatic and others present with bleeding as their initial clinical finding. Signs and symptoms of symptomatic peptic ulcers include epigastric pain that can be related to meals (either improved or worsened with eating) and typically improves with use of antacids and acid-suppressing drugs. Bleeding can present with a mild asymptomatic anemia if slow bleeding is detected early, with symptoms of anemia when significant blood loss has occurred, with melena (black-colored stool with a tarry consistency) due to digested blood, or acutely with emesis of blood, so-called coffee grounds emesis due to the appearance of the clotted blood. Symptoms of anemia (Chapter 8) include lightheadedness and fatigue with findings that include pallor of skin and mucous membranes. Perforated ulcers are a medical emergency and present with severe, acute abdominal pain resulting from perforation of the stomach or duodenum with gastric acid leakage into the peritoneal cavity. With current advanced understanding of peptic ulcers and the availability of potent drugs to prevent and treat, both the overall incidence of peptic ulcers and perforation are seen less frequently.[11]

Diagnosis

The goals for the clinical evaluation of suspected peptic ulcer disease include confirming a diagnosis, determining triggers, and initiating curative measures. Generally, either an upper GI x-ray study or upper endoscopy is required to confirm the presence and location of the ulcer or ulcers (as there may be multiple). Further diagnostic evaluation may include endoscopic biopsies to look for malignancy and infection; other tests can also be used to look for *H. pylori* infection. History can be useful to determine medications or other clinical factors that may be causative or contributory.

Prognosis and Treatment

The key to ulcer treatment is identifying the triggers and mitigating them. These include *H. pylori* treatment, measures to limit risk with NSAID use, and treating an associated malignancy. Treatment with acid-suppression therapies is often necessary, including long-term use to prevent recurrence.

INFLAMMATORY BOWEL DISEASE

This section will cover ulcerative colitis and Crohn disease, two similar disease entities with important differences. Whether these conditions represent a continuum of a single condition or separate diseases with overlapping manifestations is a matter of debate. There are many similarities, but also important differences in clinical and pathological findings.

Description and Pathogenesis

Ulcerative colitis (UC), by definition, is limited to the colon, and a colectomy is curative. Inflammation in UC is limited to the mucosa and submucosa and, unlike in Crohn disease, fistulas do not occur.

Crohn disease is marked by transmural inflammation, extending from the mucosa to the serosa. Serosal inflammation can impact adjacent structures, erode through other hollow organs, and cause abnormal connections, or fistulas. Crohn disease can also involve any portion of the GI tract, often with uninvolved mucosa, called skip lesions, between regions of inflammation. While small bowel and large bowel are involved most commonly, the upper GI tract can also be involved and anal fistulas may form. Inflammation can also recur in any region after surgical resection of inflamed bowel in Crohn disease.

The pathogenesis of these conditions is poorly understood; however, there is evidence of inappropriate activation of the mucosal immune system. Inflammatory cytokines including interleukins and tumor necrosis factor (TNF) are involved in active disease and are important targets for therapy. There is a component of genetic susceptibility with higher concordance between monozygotic twins versus dizygotic twins, as well as an association with a higher risk in first-degree relatives. Onset is typically between ages 15 and 30 years, although children may also be affected. Rates are highest in North America and Northern Europe.

Clinical Manifestations

Ulcerative colitis typically presents with diarrhea that may be bloody and accompanied by symptoms of fecal urgency and pain in the abdomen or rectum. Systemic symptoms can occur and include fever, malaise, and weight loss. Ulcerative colitis can vary in both its presentation and its manifestations over time. Some patients experience severe disease, while for others it is mild. Treatments are often successful at inducing remission, although there is always a risk for recurrence.

Because Crohn disease can involve any portion of the GI tract, presentations are more variable than with ulcerative colitis. The majority of symptoms are related to the bowel, either small bowel alone, colon alone, or a combination. Involvement of the upper GI tract is less common. In addition to symptoms of colonic inflammation as can be seen with ulcerative colitis, malabsorption due to small bowel involvement can be seen in Crohn disease (**FIGURE 7.6**). Malabsorption can result in weight loss, fatigue, and symptoms of nutrient deficiencies including iron, vitamin B12, and the key fat-soluble vitamins A, D, E, and K. Vitamin A deficiency causes night blindness and conjunctival drying (xerosis). Iron deficiency causes anemia and fatigue. Vitamin B12 deficiency results in pernicious anemia, along with white blood cell abnormalities and neurological symptoms (Chapter 8). Serosal involvement, as seen with transmural inflammation in Crohn disease, can cause fistulas between portions of the GI tract or other organs such as the bladder. Passing of air with urinating, pneumaturia, is never normal and could be an indication of a fistula between bowel and bladder (colovesical fistula). Fevers can also occur with inflammation.

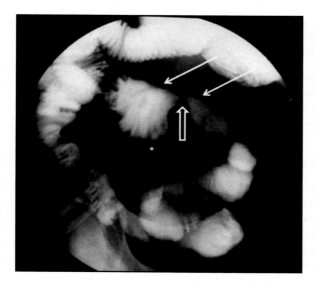

FIGURE 7.6 Small bowel inflammation in Crohn disease on fluoroscopy. Thin arrows highlight flattened bowel wall due to ulceration and chronic inflammation. Thick arrow identifies the presence of a stricture. (Photo credit: David Shein, MD.)

Extraintestinal Manifestations

GI disorders can be accompanied by extraintestinal manifestations, ie, inflammatory disorders that occur in other organs. The eyes, skin, and joints are the most common locations with inflammatory bowel disease and occur more commonly in Crohn disease, with more extensive ulcerative colitis involvement, in females, and in smokers.[12]

Ocular manifestations occur in about 10% to 20% of patients with inflammatory bowel syndrome.[13,14] Episcleritis is most common, followed by nongranulomatous anterior uveitis. Scleritis occurs less commonly but should be carefully distinguished from episcleritis given the risk for disease progression and vision loss if inadequately treated. Other serious inflammatory ocular disease states are rare but possible, including peripheral ulcerative keratitis; intermediate, posterior, or panuveitis; retinitis or choroiditis; retinal vasculitis; optic neuritis; and orbital inflammation. Clinical features of ocular inflammation in inflammatory bowel disease are generally nonspecific and indistinguishable from other causes of eye inflammation, though the (usually) bilateral presentation and chronic or recurrent nature are indicative of the underlying systemic disease process. Anterior uveitis in inflammatory bowel syndrome is typically bilateral and chronic, although may also present as an acute unilateral uveitis, particularly when patients are HLA-B27 positive.[14] Episcleritis also tends to present bilaterally, although unilateral cases are reported. While uveitis does not tend to mirror systemic disease activity, episcleritis and scleritis may flare along with intestinal or other extraintestinal symptoms.[15] *(Uveitis, episcleritis, and scleritis are also discussed in Chapter 11.)*

Secondary ocular complications may arise as a consequence of inflammatory bowel disease treatment or the chronicity of disease, for example, cataract (from topical steroid use) or neovascular glaucoma (from chronic uveitis). As mentioned previously, night blindness and xerophthalmia (**FIGURE 7.7**) may occur from vitamin A malabsorption due to bowel inflammation or status-post bowel resection.

Uncommon secondary complications like idiopathic intracranial hypertension and papilledema (from oral steroid taper or in association with other oral medications used in the treatment of GI inflammation, eg, sulfasalazine), and optic neuritis (associated with some anti-TNF-alpha biologic medications, eg, infliximab) have also been reported. All patients with chronic, recurrent, or bilateral uveitis or episcleritis, or any case of scleritis, should be asked about bowel symptoms which may suggest underlying systemic disease. Inflammatory eye disease related to active inflammatory bowel flare will resolve with resolution of the acute bowel inflammation. Eye disease that persists or arises independent of bowel inflammation is treated with topical corticosteroids, sub-Tenon corticosteroid injection, or oral corticosteroids (depending on severity). The use of oral NSAIDs may be beneficial for eye disease in some cases (eg, scleritis) but can also exacerbate GI symptoms, so a gastroenterologist should be consulted. Eye disease refractory to corticosteroids may require oral immunosuppressive agents, such as azathioprine, or biologic agents, such as infliximab and adalimumab.[16]

Several patterns of articular involvement, or arthritis, are described in association with inflammatory bowel disease including an axial pattern of involvement that includes spine and sacroiliac joints, as well as a pattern of peripheral joint involvement. While reports of incidence vary, about 10% of patients with inflammatory bowel disease have some degree of joint involvement.[17] The presence of ocular disease in the setting of inflammatory bowel disease increases the chances of articular involvement. The joint manifestations in patients with inflammatory bowel disease may precede a diagnosis of inflammatory bowel disease in as many as 2/3 of patients. Subclinical bowel disease has been found in a substantial number of patients who first present with spondyloarthritis (Chapter 11).

The two most frequent dermatological manifestations are erythema nodosum and pyoderma gangrenosum.

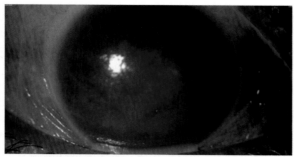

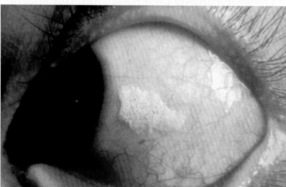

FIGURE 7.7 Extreme conjunctival drying (xerophthalmia) as can occur in vitamin A deficiency. Top: Extreme corneal dryness (xerophthalmia) can occur with vitamin A deficiency; bottom: Bitot spot of the temporal conjunctiva. (Top, Reprinted with permission from Nelson LB. *Harley's Pediatric Ophthalmology.* 6th ed. Philadelphia, PA: Wolters Kluwer; 2013. Bottom, Courtesy of Clare Gilbert.)

Erythema nodosum occurs in about 5% of patients with inflammatory bowel disease; however, there are other causes for erythema nodosum, and patients with bowel disease represent less than 5% of the overall population of patient with erythema nodosum.[18] The dermatological findings typically develop on the extremities, consisting of lesions that are tender, raised, and red to purple in color. The anterior legs are the most common location (**FIGURE 7.8**). Erythema nodosum typically flares when bowel symptoms are active, and treatments that treat the inflammatory bowel disease usually also improve the skin lesions.

Pyoderma gangrenosum is an uncommon extraintestinal manifestation, affecting fewer than 1% of patients with inflammatory bowel disease. However, up to 25% of patients with pyoderma gangrenosum have inflammatory bowel disease.[19] It is more common in women, seen more with Crohn disease versus ulcerative colitis, and occurs at younger ages when associated with inflammatory bowel disease. Lesions can be single or multiple and often occur on the legs, at sites of trauma or at sites of prior surgery, including around a stoma after bowel resection. Lesions often appear pustular; however, on culture, no pathogens grow (**FIGURE 7.9**). When seen in association with inflammatory bowel disease, the skin disease does not follow severity of the underlying bowel disease and is often treated separately, typically warranting a referral for specially consultation with a dermatologist.

Hepatic complications are uncommon but important due to their potential severity.

Primary sclerosing cholangitis (PSC) is an inflammatory disease affecting the bile ducts both within and outside of the liver. Pruritus or itching, along with fatigue, are common symptoms. Liver enlargement and jaundice may be noted on exam. Laboratory tests reveal an elevation in the alkaline phosphatase level. Over time, liver failure develops and patients often require liver transplantation.

Prognosis and Treatment

Adherence to a strictly gluten-free diet is necessary, and a referral for formal nutrition counseling can be helpful. Increasingly, prepared foods are marked with indicators of gluten content, and gluten-free foods are more frequently marketed. However, one study demonstrated that many gluten-free foods had a higher sugar content,[18] so attention to nutritional information and consumption of whole foods, such as fresh vegetables and fruits, is an important part of disease management. Progress is monitored both clinically and with antibody levels. Normalized IgA antibody levels confirms disease remission.

NONCELIAC GLUTEN SENSITIVITY

Many patients with GI symptoms, but without confirmed celiac disease, empirically limit gluten intake from their diet, and a substantial percentage notice an improvement in the underlying symptoms that prompted the dietary change. Research into this phenomenon has revealed several key findings. It is likely that there are people without celiac disease who cannot tolerate gluten in their diet[27] due to mechanisms that are not well understood. This condition is often called nonceliac gluten sensitivity. Other research focused on dietary elimination of a range of poorly absorbed sugars, so-called FODMAPs (Fermentable, Oligo-, Di-, Monosaccharides, And Polyols). The FODMAPs include fructans that are found (along with gluten) in wheat. Eliminating FODMAPs and not gluten correlated with symptom improvement,[28] leaving open the question of whether other components of common gluten-containing foods are responsible for the nonceliac gluten sensitivity symptoms in some people. Many patients with this condition are also diagnosed with functional disorders such as the irritable bowel syndrome (see below). Importantly, for celiac disease to be diagnosed, a proper medical evaluation should occur; thus, people with empiric symptom improvement on a gluten-free diet cannot formally be diagnosed with celiac disease.

In general, patients with nonceliac gluten sensitivity can be counseled to adhere to a diet that results in the fewest symptoms while also meeting their nutritional requirements. Referral to a nutritionist who specializes in this field can often be helpful to support patients and work with them to optimize their diet for symptom control and proper nutrition.

FUNCTIONAL BOWEL DISEASE

Description and Pathogenesis

The conditions covered in the prior sections of this chapter all include diagnostic indicators of disease, whether on physical examination, endoscopy, imaging, laboratory test, or pathological examination. In contrast, the defining feature of a functional disorder such as irritable bowel syndrome (IBS), the focus of this section, is that of a clinical diagnosis; no definitive features on testing, imaging, etc are present for diagnostic confirmation. To make the diagnosis, the clinician must consider the clinical criteria and employ a thoughtful approach to the diagnostic evaluation to balance the costs and inconvenience of testing with the importance of making the proper diagnosis.

Functional GI disorders including IBS represent the single largest cause for referrals to gastroenterologists in the United States.[29] IBS is estimated to occur in more than 10% of people worldwide, although only about 1/3 seek care for their symptoms.[30] IBS tends to be diagnosed at younger ages and is more commonly seen in women.

The pathogenesis of IBS is uncertain, and there may be a range of causes across a population with symptoms that can be diagnosed as IBS. While anxiety and depression occur more often in patients with IBS, for many patients the chronic bowel symptoms predate (and may thus contribute to) the development of the behavioral health comorbidities. Alterations in gut motility, gut sensory function, and the gut microbiome all have some supporting data, but the associations are not robust enough to definitively implicate any of these potential factors in the pathogenesis of the syndrome.[31]

Clinical Manifestations

The hallmark features of IBS include abdominal pain and abnormal stool patterns that predominantly consist of diarrhea, constipation, or alternating combinations of diarrhea, constipation, and normal stools. To establish a diagnosis of IBS, clinicians commonly employ the Rome criteria[32]:

1. Abdominal pain that occurs at least once weekly for at least 3 months
2. Pain occurs in relationship to one of the following:
   - Bowel movements
   - A change in stool frequency
   - A change in stool consistency

Diagnosis

In younger patients without significant comorbid medical conditions or significant risks for other conditions, a laboratory evaluation can be performed to exclude findings to suggest another condition that would require additional diagnostic evaluation. Findings that are inconsistent with IBS are those suggesting inflammation, bleeding, or malabsorption, including weight loss, anemia, vitamin deficiencies, rectal bleeding, or emesis. For patients at higher risk for other severe GI disorders such as inflammatory bowel disease or colon cancer (based upon age or family history), additional investigation is typically pursued before IBS can be diagnosed.

Prognosis and Treatment

While IBS has not been associated with a higher morbidity compared to unaffected control populations, it can cause substantial distress and a proper diagnosis for symptom management and reassurance is important. Symptoms of IBS may change over time, both with improvement or worsening, and often with a shift in the nature of the symptoms, for example, changing from diarrhea to constipation-predominant symptoms. Clinicians should remain aware that other conditions can also occur in patients with IBS, and with a change in symptoms that may indicate another GI condition (eg, new onset of rectal bleeding or unexplained weight loss) additional evaluation should be pursued.

The approach to managing milder symptoms begins with dietary guidance. While eliminating foods or food components that commonly trigger IBS symptoms (eg, dairy, gluten, or FODMAPs as noted above) may help, many patients need an individualized approach to find and eliminate specific triggering foods. A food diary and referral for nutrition counseling can be helpful. Other possible symptom triggers, including stress, should also be considered and addressed, including nonpharmacologic approaches such as stress management counseling or cognitive behavioral counseling. Mind-body approaches as well as reassurance have been found to offer more benefit versus placebo. A number of medications, including over-the-counter fiber additives and antidiarrheals when needed, can be helpful for symptom management. Peppermint oil has also been shown to offer benefit for some patients.[33] For patients with more severe or refractory symptoms, a number of prescription pharmacologic agents are available and can be helpful to reduce symptoms and improve quality of life.

A common feature for diagnosis and treatment of the above conditions is that of a partnership between patient and clinician. From the risk of recurrent peptic ulcer disease to exacerbation and remission in inflammatory bowel disease and IBS, or the long-term need for substantial dietary management in celiac disease, clinicians must partner with patients to treat, support, and understand patients' individual needs and preferences.

REFERENCES

1. Moayyedi P, Eikelboom JW, Bosch J, et al. Pantoprazole to prevent gastroduodenal events in patients receiving rivaroxaban and/or aspirin in a randomized, double-blind, placebo-controlled trial. *Gastroenterology*. 2019;157:403-412.

2. Saltzman R, Bjorkman D. Unraveling the safety profile of proton-pump inhibitors. *NEJM J Watch*. 2019.

3. Moayyedi P, Eikelboom JW, Bosch J, et al. Safety of proton pump inhibitors based on a large, multi-year, randomized trial of patients receiving rivaroxaban or aspirin. *Gastroenterology*. 2019;157(3):682.e2-691.e2. doi:10.1053/j.gastro.2019.05.056.

4. Graham DY, Malaty HM, Evans DG, Evans DJ Jr, Klein PD, Adam E. Epidemiology of *Helicobacter pylori* in an asymptomatic population in the United States. Effect of age, race, and socioeconomic status. *Gastroenterology*. 1991 100 1495-1501.

5. Eusebi LH, Zagari RM, Bazzoli F. Epidemiology of *Helicobacter pylori* infection. *Helicobacter*. 2014;19:1-5. doi:10.1111/hel.12165.

6. Graham DY, Agrawal NM, Campbell DR, et al; NSAID-Associated Gastric Ulcer Prevention Study Group. Ulcer prevention in long-term users of nonsteroidal anti-inflammatory drugs: results of a double-blind, randomized, multicenter, active- and placebo-controlled study of misoprostol vs lansoprazole. *Arch Intern Med*. 2002;162:169-175.

7. Hernández-Díaz S, Rodríguez LAG. Association between nonsteroidal anti-inflammatory drugs and upper gastrointestinal tract bleeding/perforation: an overview of epidemiologic studies published in the 1990s. *Arch Intern Med*. 2000;160(14):2093-2099. doi:10.1001/archinte.160.14.2093.

8. Griffin MR, Piper JM, Daugherty JR, Snowden M, Ray WA. Nonsteroidal anti-inflammatory drug use and increased risk for peptic ulcer disease in elderly persons. *Ann Intern Med*. 1991;114 257-263.

9. Sugano K, Kinoshita Y, Miwa H, Takeuchi T; Esomeprazole NSAID Preventive Study Group. Randomised clinical trial: esomeprazole for the prevention of nonsteroidal anti-inflammatory drug-related peptic ulcers in Japanese patients. *Aliment Pharmacol Ther*. 2012;36:115-125.

10. Rostom A, Dube C, Wells G, et al. Prevention of NSAID-induced gastroduodenal ulcers. *Cochrane Database Syst Rev*. 2002;(4):CD002296.

11. Lassen A, Hallas J, Schaffalitzky de Muckadell OB. Complicated and uncomplicated peptic ulcers in a Danish county 1993-2002: a population-based cohort study. *Am J Gastroenterol*. 2006;101:945-953.

12. Karmiris K, Avgerinos A, Tavernaraki A, et al. Prevalence and characteristics of extra-intestinal manifestations in a large cohort of Greek patients with inflammatory bowel disease. *J Crohns Colitis*. 2016;10(4):429-436.

13. Hopkins DJ, Horan E, Burton IL, Clamp SE, et al. Ocular disorders in a series of 323 patients with Crohn's disease. *Br J Ophthalmol*. 1974;58:732-737.

14. Thomas AS, Lin P. Ocular manifestations of inflammatory bowel disease. *Curr Opin Ophthalmol*. 2016;27:552-560.

15. Harbord M, Annese V, Vavicka SR, Allez M, et al. The first European evidence-based consensus on extra-intestinal manifestations in inflammatory bowel disease. *J Crohns Colitis*. 2016;10(3):239-254.

16. Mady R, Grover W, Butrus S. Ocular complications of inflammatory bowel disease. *Sci World J*. 2015;2015:438402.

17. Karreman MC, Luime JJ, Hazes JM, Weel AE. The prevalence and incidence of axial and peripheral spondyloarthritis in inflammatory bowel disease: a systematic review and meta-analysis. *J Crohns Colitis*. 2016;11(5):631-642.

18. Farhi D, Cosnes J, Zizi N, et al. Significance of erythema nodosum and pyoderma gangrenosum in inflammatory bowel diseases: a cohort study of 2402 patients. *Medicine (Baltimore)*. 2008;87:281-293.

19. Ashchyan HJ, Butler DC, Nelson CA, et al. The association of age with clinical presentation and comorbidities of pyoderma gangrenosum. *JAMA Dermatol*. 2018;154:409-413. doi:10.1001/jamadermatol.2017.5978.

20. Ekbom A, Helmick C, Zack M, Adami HO. Ulcerative colitis and colorectal cancer. A population-based study. *N Engl J Med*. 1990;323(18):1228-1233.

21. Hoffenberg EJ, MacKenzie T, Barriga KJ, et al. A prospective study of the incidence of childhood celiac disease. *J Pediatr*. 2003;143:308-314.

22. Aggarwal S, Lebwohl B, Green PHR. Screening for celiac disease in average-risk and high-risk populations. *Therap Adv Gastroenterol*. 2012;5(1):37-47.

23. Benjamin Lebwohl B, Cao Y, Zong G. Long term gluten consumption in adults without celiac disease and risk of coronary heart disease: prospective cohort study. *BMJ*. 2017;357:j1892.

24. Elliott C. The nutritional quality of gluten-free products for children. *Pediatrics* 2018;142(2):e20180525. doi:10.1542/peds.2018-0525.

25. Pizzimenti J, Pelino C. Hold the Gluten, Please. *Review of Optometry*. May 15, 2013. Accessed November 18, 2019. https://www.reviewofoptometry.com/article/hold-the-gluten-please.

26. West J, Logan RF, Smith CJ, Hubbard RB, Card TR. Malignancy and mortality in people with coeliac disease: population based cohort study. *BMJ*. 2004;329:716-718.

27. Biesiekierski JR, Newnham ED, Irving PM, et al. Gluten causes gastrointestinal symptoms in subjects without celiac disease: a double-blind randomized placebo-controlled trial. *Am J Gastroenterol*. 2011;106:508. doi:10.1038/ajg.2010.487.

28. Biesiekierski JR, Peters SL, Newnham ED, Rosella O, Muir JG, Gibson PR. No effects of gluten in patients with self-reported non-celiac gluten sensitivity after dietary reduction of fermentable, poorly absorbed, short-chain carbohydrates. *Gastroenterology*. 2013;145:320-328. doi:10.1053/j.gastro.2013.04.051.

29. Lacy BE, Patel NK. Rome criteria and a diagnostic approach to irritable bowel syndrome. *J Clin Med*. 2017;6(11):99. doi:10.3390/jcm6110099.

30. Canavan C, West J, Card T. The epidemiology of irritable bowel syndrome. *Clin Epidemiol*. 2014;6:71-80. doi:10.2147/CLEP.S40245.

31. Ford AC, Lacy BE, Talley NJ. Irritable bowel syndrome. *N Engl J Med*. 2017;376(26):2566-2578.

32. Lacy BE, Mearin F, Chang L, et al. Bowel disorders. *Gastroenterology*. 2016;150:1393-1407. doi:10.1053/j.gastro.2016.02.031.

33. Ford AC, Moayyedi P, Lacy BE, et al. American College of Gastroenterology monograph on the management of irritable bowel syndrome and chronic idiopathic constipation. *Am J Gastroenterol*. 2014;109(suppl 1):S2-S26.

8 Hematology and Oncology

Brianna Jones, Kenneth E. Rosenzweig, David M. Shein, and Rachel C. Druckenbrod

LEARNING OBJECTIVES

Hematology and oncology are often grouped together clinically, with many physicians specializing in both areas; this chapter adheres to that framework.

The hematologic system includes red blood cells, white blood cells, and platelets. In health, the hematologic system supports tissue oxygenation, infection fighting, and coagulation. In the setting of hematologic disease, the abnormalities can have far-reaching effects, including impacts on the ocular system. Hematologic disorders involve an excess, deficiency, or dysfunction in one or more cell types and may collectively be referred to as blood "dyscrasias," from the Greek, meaning "bad mixture." Related disorders of thrombophilia (increased clotting risk), bleeding disorders, and iron overload are included in this chapter.

Oncology is the study and treatment of cancer. The section will focus on the most common non-skin cancers, covering aspects of cancer including epidemiology, risk factors, prevention, screening, diagnosis and clinical findings, and treatment. This chapter highlights links to ocular manifestations of cancer. (Skin cancer is covered in Chapter 13; neurological manifestations of intracranial tumors are covered in Chapter 12.)

KEY CONCEPTS

Section 1: Hematology
Normal hematopoiesis and blood cell function
Lab testing in hematology
Abnormalities in blood cell counts
Bleeding and clotting disorders
Hemochromatosis
Section 2: Oncology
Epidemiology
    Etiology, diagnosis, treatment

Risk factors
Staging
Treatment
Overview of cancers
    Prostate
    Breast
    Colon and rectum
    Cervical
    Lung
    Wilms tumor

SECTION 1: HEMATOLOGY

Hematopoiesis, the formation of blood cells, begins with a **progenitor stem cell** in the bone marrow capable of differentiating into any of the key cell types—leukocytes, erythrocytes, or platelets (thrombocytes) (**FIGURE 8.1**). Under stimulation by factors that drive cell differentiation, the stem cells become increasingly differentiated and committed to a specific lineage as they mature. Both external factors and hematologic disease can increase or decrease one or more cell lines.

RED BLOOD CELLS

The key function of the **erythrocyte** is tissue oxygen delivery via **hemoglobin,** a metalloprotein with iron at its core. Each molecule of normal adult hemoglobin is a tetramer containing two alpha- and two beta-globin chains, each with an iron binding heme portion (**FIGURE 8.2**). Alpha-globin is normally coded by four genes, two inherited from each parent. Beta-globin is coded by two genes, one from each parent. Abnormalities in globin genes can be inherited as a single gene mutation or as multiple defects (in more than one globin gene). Hemoglobin gene mutations, when inherited in a heterozygous state, are believed to offer protection against malaria and carry very limited or no significant clinical disease. When homozygous, these mutations contribute to sickle cell anemia or thalassemias of varying severity.

When oxygenated, each molecule of hemoglobin carries four oxygen molecules as oxyhemoglobin. When the oxygen is released to tissues, deoxyhemoglobin results. Oxyhemoglobin and deoxyhemoglobin absorb different wavelengths of light, the concept behind the pulse oximeter's transcutaneous oxygen saturation measurement.

Normal erythropoiesis in the bone marrow is stimulated by the protein erythropoietin, produced by the kidney in the setting of a reduced red blood cell mass or hypoxemia (low tissue oxygen delivery). Erythropoiesis results in the formation of **reticulocytes,** which are early and immature red blood cells that complete maturation in the circulation. Normal mature erythrocytes survive for about 120 days in the circulation. Thus, ongoing replacement from the bone marrow is essential for maintaining a normal cell count.

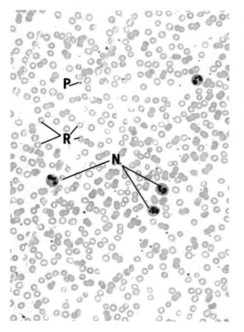

FIGURE 8.1 Blood smear. Human. Wright stain. ×270. This normal blood smear presents erythrocytes (R), neutrophils (N), and platelets (P). The apparent holes in the centers of the erythrocytes represent the thinnest areas of the biconcave discs. Note that the erythrocytes far outnumber the platelets, and they in turn are much more numerous than the white blood cells. Since neutrophils constitute the highest percentage of white blood cells, they are the ones most frequently encountered of the white blood cell population. (Reprinted from Gartner LP, Hiatt JL. *Color Atlas and Text of Histology.* 6th ed. Philadelphia, PA: Wolters Kluwer; 2013.)

Decreased iron absorption and/or increased iron losses are the mechanisms through which iron deficiency typically results. Dietary deficiency can occur in malnutrition; small bowel inflammation can trigger malabsorption such as with Crohn or celiac disease; intestinal parasites can cause malabsorption and iron loss. More often, iron loss is the result of bleeding. Heavy menstrual periods in younger women or increased bleeding around the time of menopause in middle age causes iron loss that may not be replaced in a typical diet. However, even moderate bleeding can result in iron deficiency when coupled with low dietary iron intake. Because gastrointestinal bleeding can be slow and asymptomatic, an appropriate evaluation to rule out a gastrointestinal cancer is an important part of the anemia workup in patients at risk due to age, family history, significant radiation exposure, or other risk factors. Simply replacing the lost iron with increased intake could mask the underlying abnormality and result in a missed chance to diagnose and treat a gastrointestinal malignancy at an earlier stage. Postpartum and after major surgical procedures, anemia may also be present due to blood loss, and temporary iron supplementation may be advised to avoid developing iron deficiency.[2]

In addition to anemia, iron deficiency can be accompanied by atrophic glossitis (tongue atrophy), stomatitis, esophageal disease with difficulty swallowing, and koilonychia (flattened, spoon-shaped nails). Pica, the eating of dirt and other nonfood items, is also associated with iron deficiency anemia for uncertain reasons.

Once a history and appropriate evaluation to exclude underlying treatable causes of anemia is completed, replacement with oral iron is typically initiated and follow-up blood counts and iron levels are obtained several weeks later to assure appropriate response to therapy (**FIGURE 8.5**).

Vitamin B12 deficiency results in a macrocytic anemia. Vitamin B12 and folic acid are cofactors in synthesis of DNA and myelin. Vitamin B12 is also essential to formation of the heme component of hemoglobin. Deficiency impacts erythrocyte and leukocyte maturation, as well as neurological function. Anemia, peripheral neuropathy, and memory loss are some of the symptoms that develop with vitamin B12 deficiency.

Vitamin B12 is water-soluble and is found in animal proteins including eggs, milk, and fish. Dietary deficiency is uncommon but can occur with vegan diets that are not properly balanced. Many cereals are also enriched with vitamin B12, which can be a good source for people who do not eat meat, fish, milk, or eggs. Vitamin B12 supplements are also available over the counter.[3] Folic acid is added to all grain products in the United States, making deficiency an uncommon clinical finding (**TABLE 8.1**).

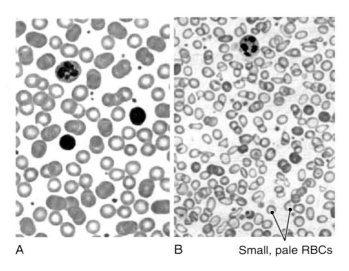

A   B   Small, pale RBCs

FIGURE 8.5 The blood in iron deficiency anemia. A, Normal blood smear. B, Blood smear in iron deficiency anemia. The red cells are small (microcytic) and pale (hypochromic). (From McConnell TH. *Nature of Disease*. 2nd ed. Philadelphia, PA: Wolters Kluwer; 2013.)

TABLE 8.1   Laboratory Abnormalities in B12 Deficiency

Macrocytic anemia

Normocytic anemia with increased red cell distribution width[a]

Low reticulocyte count

Leukopenia and/or thrombocytopenia (mild)

Hypersegmented neutrophils on blood smear

Low serum vitamin B12 level

Elevated serum homocysteine and methylmalonic acid

Presence of anti-intrinsic factor antibodies[b]

[a]If simultaneous iron deficiency is present.
[b]If autoimmune pernicious anemia is present.

Understanding the process of vitamin B12 absorption will elucidate the nature of clinical conditions that result in deficiency. Once ingested, vitamin B12 must be complexed to intrinsic factor (IF) for optimal absorption. In the stomach, ingested vitamin B12 binds to IF, which is secreted by the gastric parietal cells. In the distal ileum, the IF vitamin B12 is absorbed. Pernicious anemia is an autoimmune condition that results in parietal cell destruction. As a result, IF is not released and vitamin B12 absorption is impaired. Called pernicious, this condition can take years to come to medical attention due to the substantial stores of the vitamin in the liver. Lab testing will reveal antibodies to IF; however, the diagnosis can be made clinically and vitamin B12 replacement is convenient and inexpensive; thus, lab confirmation with antibody testing is often unnecessary. Inflammatory conditions of the small bowel such as Crohn or celiac diseases can also impair vitamin B12 absorption and cause deficiency. Weight loss surgeries that involve small intestinal bypass intentionally trigger malabsorption, impacting not only total calorie absorption but also many vitamins. Patients who have had stomach or small bowel resections (for example, due to cancer surgery or Crohn disease) are also at risk for vitamin B12 malabsorption. Postsurgical patients who have had these procedures are prescribed a daily multivitamin, and key vitamin levels, including B12, should be monitored periodically.

When vitamin B12 deficiency is initially diagnosed, parenteral replacement with subcutaneously injected vitamin B12 should be initiated to immediately provide this necessary cofactor for the hematologic and neurological systems. Autoimmune pernicious anemia is typically treated with parenteral replacement long term, either via nasal spray or monthly subcutaneous injection. Underlying conditions causing malabsorption due to small bowel inflammation should be treated as necessary to assure normal absorption of all nutrients; often, oral multivitamin supplements are added to the treatment regimen long term.

Clinical features of vitamin B12 deficiency may include typical symptoms of anemia. The anemia is macrocytic (increased MCV). Abnormalities in white blood cells characterized by hypersegmented neutrophils are visible on a blood smear. With progressive disease, pancytopenia, or reduced levels of all cell lines (red cells, white cells, and platelets), can occur.[4] Glossitis or tongue inflammation can also occur, marked by pain, atrophy, or both. The neurological symptoms of B12 deficiency often manifest as a symmetric peripheral neuropathy in the feet. Testing the vitamin B12 level is thus a standard part of the evaluation for a new onset of neuropathy. Gait disorders with ataxia can also develop due to degeneration of the dorsal columns in the spinal cord with more advanced deficiency.[5] Impaired cognition including impaired memory is also reported with longer term B12 deficiency.

When nutritional deficiencies or malabsorption results in deficiencies of both iron and vitamin B12 (microcytic and macrocytic, respectively), the result of an automated blood evaluation may suggest a normocytic picture. However, as noted previously, results of the RDW will be increased, suggesting a mixed picture. When vitamin B12 deficiency is clinically suspected but serum levels return borderline normal, elevation of the B12 metabolites homocysteine and methylmalonic acid (MMA) is diagnostic. Deficiency in levels of folate (vitamin B6) may occur alongside vitamin B12 deficiency, though folate deficiency is less common among individuals living in developed countries (**FIGURE 8.6**).

Rarely, ocular manifestations of B12 deficiency occur. Retinal hemorrhages have been reported with severe anemia due to vitamin B12 deficiency.[6] Bilateral optic neuropathy is the most common manifestation, and simultaneous tobacco and/or alcohol abuse may increase the risk for B12-associated optic neuropathy.[7,8] Patients present with painless, slowly progressive, bilateral central vision loss over a period of months, dyschromatopsia, and centrocecal visual field defects. The optic nerves may appear normal or demonstrate bitemporal pallor with thinning of the temporal retinal nerve fiber layer on optical coherence tomography, the severity of which is directly correlated with serum B12 levels.[9,10] Since vision loss may precede other symptoms in B12 deficiency, this clinical presentation should prompt serum B12 testing in all patients. Significant improvement in vision (and sometimes full recovery) can occur with appropriate and timely oral or parenteral B12 supplementation. Vitamin B12 acts as a cofactor in formation of succinyl CoA, an integral part of Krebs cycle. B12 deficiency decreases succinyl CoA levels, impairing oxidative metabolism and leading to depletion of ATP. Because of the unusually high metabolic demand of neurons in the papillomacular bundle, bitemporal optic nerve atrophy occurs, resulting in cecocentral and/or central scotoma (**FIGURE 8.7**).[10,11]

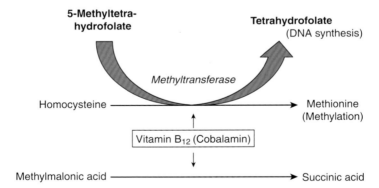

FIGURE 8.6 The methyltetrahydrofolate trap hypothesis: the relationship between folate and vitamin B12 in the pathogenesis of the megaloblastic anemias. Tetrahydrofolate is required for DNA synthesis. In bone marrow rapid cell turnover requires adequate supplies of tetrahydrofolate for normal cell maturation. Methyltetrahydrofolate is a metabolite involved in methyl group transfers including the synthesis of methionine from homocysteine, but is not functional in DNA synthesis. Cyanocobalamin (vitamin B12) is required to regenerate the tetrahydrofolate form, which is necessary for normal DNA synthesis and normal red cell maturation. In pernicious anemia (PA), the absence of B12 causes a deficiency of useable folate at the cellular level resulting in megaloblastic differentiation. B12 is also required for myelin synthesis and the conversion of methylmalonic acid (MMA) to succinate; buildup of MMA in the blood is now the preferred test for the diagnosis of PA. (From Landsberg L. *On Rounds: 1000 Internal Medicine Pearls*. Philadelphia, PA: Wolters Kluwer; 2015.)

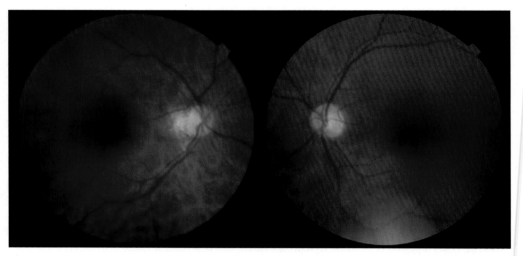

FIGURE 8.7 A 59-year-old Caucasian male with bilateral temporal optic nerve head pallor was found to have significant B12 deficiency from dietary insufficiency (B12 level <146 pg/mL). Folate was normal and intrinsic factor antibody was negative. (Photo credit Dr Druckenbrod.)

Sickle cell disease is characterized by a normocytic anemia caused by premature destruction of abnormally shaped circulating red blood cells. An inherited single gene mutation results in a defective beta-globin protein within the hemoglobin molecule, which leads to sickle-shaped cells that suffer physical cell damage as they circulate through the bloodstream and are targeted premature destruction by the body (FIGURE 8.8).

Sickle cell disease is the most common single gene disorder in the world. Substitution of glutamic acid for valine (Glu6Val) in the hemoglobin beta molecule results in hemoglobin S (HbS).[12] Homozygous disease, with HbS inherited from both parents, is marked by the formation of an abnormal hemoglobin which polymerizes in a low oxygen environment. The polymerized hemoglobin forms linear structures that deform the cell membrane, resulting in sickle-shaped cells, which are destroyed in the reticuloendothelial system, resulting in higher rates of hemolysis. These abnormally shaped, inelastic sickle cells also occlude capillaries and cause the range of symptoms and complications seen in sickle cell disease (FIGURE 8.9).

Sickle cell trait is the heterozygous state characterized by the inheritance of one HbS and one normal beta-globin gene for adult hemoglobin A (HbA) and does not typically result in clinical symptoms. However, certain situations can trigger symptoms in patients with sickle trait. A study of military recruits found a higher rate of rhabdomyolysis (muscle damage) with sickle cell trait but no increase in death.[13] A population study evaluating kidney function in sickle cell trait showed an association with declines in kidney function and chronic kidney disease, but no increase in end stage renal disease.[14]

Hemoglobin C (HbC) is an abnormal hemoglobin that results from a point mutation much like HbS, with a lysine substitution for the glutamic acid on the beta-globin chain. A single HbC mutation is typically asymptomatic, but inheritance of one HbC gene and one HbS gene (HbSC) results in a less severe form of anemia with a higher hemoglobin concentration. However, almost paradoxically, HbSC disease can result in more significant ocular symptoms, likely due to the higher hematocrit that increases the risk of impaired vascular perfusion in the small retinal arterioles.

Sickle cell disease occurs in several subpopulations, including African, Indian, and Middle Eastern groups. The severity varies due to a range of factors, including the ability to make fetal hemoglobin (HbF), which can lessen the severity of the sickle cell disease when present. Sickle cell disease can also occur with other beta-globin defects (thalassemia, see below), which will impact the clinical manifestations of each of these combined disorders.

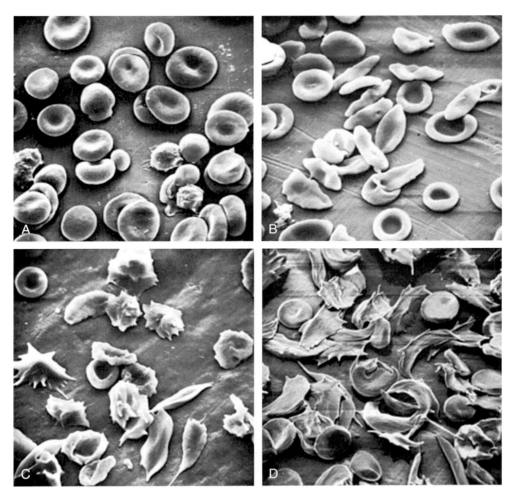

FIGURE 8.8 Erythrocytes from a patient with sickle cell anemia examined with scanning electron micros-copy. A, Oxygenated blood. Red cells appear normal except for one microspherocyte. Three leukocytes are evident in the field. B, Oxygenated irreversibly sickled cells are smooth in texture and outline but are ovoid or boatlike in shape. C, Partial deoxygenation causes the cells to assume bizarre shapes with spikes, spic-ules, and filaments that protrude from the cells. D, More complete deoxygenation causes the cells to assume sickled shapes with longitudinal surface striations. (From Greer JP, Arber DA, Glader BE, List AF, Means RT Jr, Rodgers GM. *Wintrobe's Clinical Hematology.* 14th ed. Philadelphia, PA: Wolters Kluwer; 2018.)

In addition to the hemolytic anemia, patients develop symptoms related to capillary occlusion including recurrent vaso-occlusive crises and suffer an increased risk for infections, ocular disease, and stroke. Episodes of acute pain from vaso-occlusive disease may involve the chest, back, extrem-ities, and/or abdomen. Pain severity ranges from mild to severe and patients may require opioid medications for adequate relief. Triggers can include cold, dehydration, stress, and menstruation. Since acute pain may accompany other serious complications (such as the acute chest syndrome or organ infarction), a thorough clinical evaluation is appropriate. Comprehensive care of patients may require behavioral health referrals, as frequent vaso-occlusive pain interferes with quality of life, activities of daily living, and may lead to symptoms of depression.[15]

Organ infarction due to capillary occlusion with sickled, inelastic erythrocytes impairs function across multiple organs. The spleen typically suffers multiple infarcts, and by adulthood, most patients with sickle cell disease have substantial loss of splenic function with the attendant increased risk

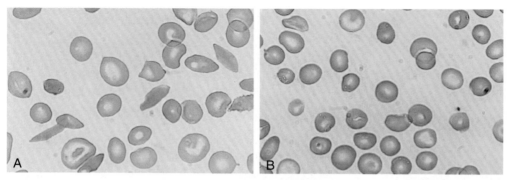

FIGURE 8.9 Blood smears of patients with hemoglobin (Hb) SS and Hb SC disease. A, Red blood cell morphology in sickle cell anemia (SCA) is characterized by sickled forms (dense elongated cells with pointed ends), target cells, ovalocytes, and polychromatophilia. B, Hb SC disease is characterized by target cells, relatively few sickled forms, and a small proportion of cells that contain dark blunt protuberances (hemoglobin "crystals"). (From Greer JP, Wintrobe MM. *Wintrobe's Clinical Hematology*. 13th ed. Philadelphia, PA: Wolters Kluwer; 2013.)

for infections, encapsulated bacteria such as pneumococcus in particular. Occlusion of pulmonary vasculature and bone marrow have serious repercussions including triggering the acute chest syndrome as noted below. Multiorgan failure is life-threatening and requires prompt exchange transfusion therapy.

Infection risk is increased in sickle cell disease due to complications such as hyposplenism, reduced tissue perfusion, and hypoventilation. Bacteremia, meningitis, and pulmonary infections are more common, and organisms include *Streptococcus pneumoniae*, *Haemophilus influenzae*, *Escherichia coli*, *Staphylococcus aureus*, *Mycoplasma pneumoniae*, and *Chlamydia pneumoniae*. Preventative measures such as pneumococcal vaccination, prophylactic penicillin in childhood, and education to seek prompt care when symptomatic are important in sickle cell disease.[16]

The acute chest syndrome is characterized by chest pain, cough, fever, and pulmonary infiltrate on chest x-ray. Dyspnea and hypoxia can also be present. In both children and adults, the acute chest syndrome can be life-threatening; thus proper management is critical. Triggers can include pulmonary conditions that impair oxygenation and trigger vascular occlusion, such as infection, asthma, and vascular occlusion due to other causes. Fat embolization from bone marrow infarcts can also trigger the acute chest syndrome, a clinical situation seen more commonly in adults.

Patients with sickle cell disease are at higher risk of stroke, which can occur at a young age. As many as 25% of patients will suffer stroke by the age of 45. Asymptomatic strokes may contribute to neurocognitive and behavioral deficits.[16] Both cerebrovascular occlusions and hemorrhagic stokes occur in patients with sickle cell disease. Management includes prompt diagnosis, determination of the stoke type, and hospital treatment.

There are numerous other systemic complications in sickle cell disease including renal, skeletal, cardiac, and hepatobiliary complications as well as skin ulceration, complications in pregnancy, impaired growth, and delayed puberty.

Sickle cell retinopathy occurs in 5% to 40% of patients and as noted it is more common with heterozygous (HbSC) disease.[17] It is an important recall that the internal diameter of most retinal capillaries is only around 6 μm. Hence, even a normal RBC, 7 μm in diameter, must be very flexible to navigate this vascular bed. Sickling results in stiff, inelastic red cells, making it difficult for them to pass through these capillaries. This leads to retinal ischemia and a subsequent neovascular response. Risk for retinopathy increases with age and may be asymptomatic. Regular screening with dilated retinal examinations should begin at age 10.[18] Retinal arteriolar occlusion creates dark red "sunburst" hemorrhages in the deep retinal layers, superficial pink-orange

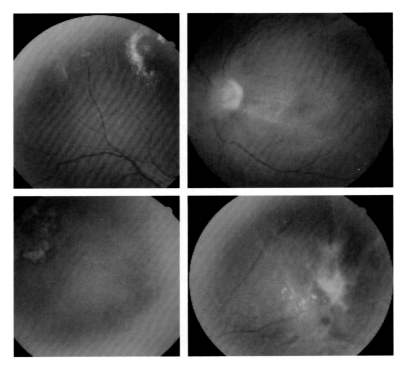

FIGURE 8.10 A 51-year-old African American male with peripheral retinal exudation (top-right), fibrotic retinal traction over the optic nerve (top-left), "salmon patch" peripheral retinal hemorrhage (bottom-left), and peripheral retinal traction causing retinal detachment (bottom-right) due to sickle cell (hemoglobin SC) disease. (Photo credit Dr Druckenbrod.)

"salmon patch" retinal hemorrhages, and proliferative retinopathy with characteristic "sea fan" neovascular structures in the mid-periphery of the retina.[19] Retinopathy is more prevalent in the mid-peripheral retina, though macular ischemia may importantly contribute to vision loss. Other mechanisms of vision loss include vitreous hemorrhage, retinal detachment and retinoschisis, and macular pucker and macular hole. Laser photocoagulation with or without adjunctive anti–vascular endothelial growth factor (VEGF) treatments is commonly used in treating proliferative vitreoretinal lesions. Vitrectomy and retinal detachment surgeries are necessary for advanced disease states (**FIGURE 8.10**).

Thalassemia occurs due to one or more genetic defects in the hemoglobin alpha and/or beta-globin genes. Normally, there is matched alpha- and beta-globin production for hemoglobin tetramer production. The defect(s) in thalassemia cause an imbalance in the relative amounts of the globin proteins, with excess globin proteins forming abnormal precipitates in the red cells and accelerating red blood cell destruction. Like sickle cell disease and G6PD (see below), patients with thalassemia minor (heterozygous disease) benefit from a lower risk of malaria, and populations with higher penetrance of thalassemia mutations are seen in regions of endemic malaria risk.

Beta-thalassemia occurs with an inherited defect in one or both of the beta-globin genes. The defect can be an absence mutation or one of decreased production. One or both copies of the beta-globin gene can be impacted. Presentations thus vary. Thalassemia minor results from reduced globin synthesis in only one of the genes and is typically identified in an asymptomatic patient with a chronic normochromic, microcytic anemia due to increased red blood cell destruction.

Alpha-thalassemias are diverse, as with four copies of the alpha-globin gene a large range of possible inheritance patterns are possible. When a single copy of a defective alpha-globin gene is defective, no symptoms result. More extensive genetic involvement can result in severe anemia requiring transfusions. When defects occur in all four genes, fetal death often results. Clinical findings can be aided by genetics to diagnose and determine the best approach to management.

Ocular complications in thalassemias (most commonly reported in beta-thalassemia) are distinct from, and less severe than, sickle cell disease. These include pseudoxanthoma elasticum-like angioid streaks, optic nerve drusen, and "peau d'orange" pattern dystrophy-like retinal pigment epithelium (RPE) changes. Vision is only affected if the macula is involved. Complications may be related to the hemoglobinopathy itself or to iron overload related to repeated blood transfusions. Desferrioxamine mesylate, a chelating medication used to treat iron overload in beta-thalassemia, may also cause ocular toxicity in the form of RPE damage (creating reduced visual acuity, visual field defects, or night blindness) as well as optic disc edema.[20]

G6PD deficiency is the result of an X-linked inherited disorder leading to a reduction in the enzyme glucose-6-phosphate dehydrogenase (G6PD) in erythrocytes. G6PD protects the cells from oxidative damage. Several populations from African, Asian, and Mediterranean countries are identified with a higher incidence of G6PD deficiency. It is likely that this geographic distribution which overlaps with regions of endemic malaria reflects a lower risk of malaria infection in individuals with lower G6PD levels.

The degree to which the G6PD enzyme production is diminished determines the clinical severity in any individual patient. As expected for an X-linked disorder, males are affected more commonly. Most affected individuals have mild forms of the disease without signs or symptoms until oxidative stress triggers hemolysis. The triggers include some foods (eg, fava beans), medications (including the antimalarial primaquine), and some infections.

Hemolysis can be mild in some patients who have a full recovery without medical intervention, and in others severe hemolysis occurs with an acute, severe reduction in the red cell count and complications such as kidney failure. Avoidance of triggering foods and medications is important. Individuals who are at high risk may be tested for the disorder in advance of treatment with potential drug triggers.

Autoimmune hemolytic anemias are caused by a diverse range of conditions including autoimmune diseases (such as lupus—Chapter 11), hematologic malignancies, infections (such as hepatitis C—Chapter 9), and as a reaction to some drugs. Depending upon the trigger, there are different mechanisms of action that cause the red cell destruction. Severity and approaches to treatment vary and the approach in any given patient depends upon the underlying cause.

ERYTHROID APLASIA

Normal red blood cell production can cease due to a range of causes. When the disruption is temporary in a patient with an otherwise normal hematologic system, recovery typically occurs with resolution of the trigger. In patients with underlying disorders of hemoglobin production, such as sickle cell disease, however, the transient aplasia can cause an aplastic crisis with severe anemia requiring transfusions until the bone marrow recovers.

In the setting of an anemia evaluation, a finding of decreased reticulocytosis indicates deficient bone marrow output of red blood cells. Causes to consider include[21]

- Infectious
- Autoimmune
- Malignant
- Iatrogenic
- Idiopathic

Significant infectious considerations include parvovirus B19, hepatitis viruses, and HIV infection.

Parvovirus B19 is also known as fifth disease or erythema infectiosum. It is a common viral illness of childhood and typically causes a rash on the torso and cheeks, the latter of which may appear as though the child has slapped cheeks. In children, the disease is typically self-limited and resolves without serious complications. When transmitted to an adult, arthralgias without joint inflammation and a transient aplastic anemia can occur. Parvovirus B19 infection during pregnancy increases the risk of adverse fetal outcomes (FIGURE 8.11).

While uncommon, autoimmune red cell aplasia with antibodies against erythrocyte precursors can develop. This type of red cell aplasia can be seen in the setting of other autoimmune conditions including systemic lupus, rheumatoid arthritis (Chapter 11), and inflammatory bowel disease (Chapter 7).

Red cell aplasia can also occur with malignancy, including solid tumors, leukemias, and lymphomas. The strongest association with red cell aplasia is for thymic tumors.

A variety of drugs can cause an aplasia, which typically recovers upon withdrawal of the offending agent. For many of these drugs it is a rare adverse event. This list includes immunosuppressants, some antibiotics (including ampicillin, sulfamethoxazole/trimethoprim, rifampin), the NSAID sulindac, and several anticonvulsants. Cancer chemotherapeutic drugs often suppress the bone marrow, and aplasia is a common adverse effect.

Systemic use of the antibiotic chloramphenicol is associated with a risk of aplastic anemia; since many antibiotics are currently available, with the exceptions of rare situations in which an alternative cannot be used, it has largely been eliminated from the arsenal of systemic antibacterial treatments. Ocular administration has also been traditionally avoided due to notoriety in leading to aplastic anemia.[22] However, large multinational controlled clinical trials have provided a basis to question this old adage.[23] While unable to completely exclude an association, at worst it is an exceedingly rare complication.

Polycythemia is marked by an increased circulating red blood cell mass. This can be a physiologic response or a marker of an underlying disease.

Chronic hypoxia triggers a physiologic increase in the red cell mass. This occurs in inhabitants at high altitude under normal circumstances or in response to underlying lung diseases with chronic hypoxia.

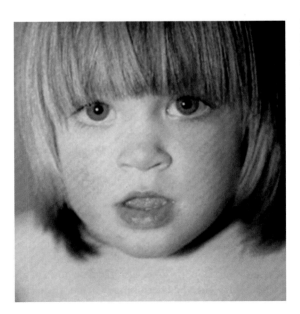

FIGURE 8.11 Parvovirus B19 slap cheek rash. Typical "slapped cheek" appearance of a child infected with parvovirus B19 ("fifth disease"). (From Kline-Tilford AM, Haut C. *Lippincott Certification Review: Pediatric Acute Care Nurse Practitioner.* Philadelphia, PA: Wolters Kluwer; 2015.)

Polycythemia vera is a myeloproliferative disorder, often related to the JAK2 mutation that results in clonal expansion of red blood cells. A defect in an early erythrocyte precursor results in uncontrolled proliferation and an increase in the red blood cell mass. It is often accompanied by lesser increases in platelets and white blood cells. The increased red blood cell mass results in increased blood viscosity, with slow flow in capillaries causing complications such as thrombosis and infarction. Although the platelet count may be increased, the platelets are abnormal and bruising and bleeding may also occur.

Early symptoms of polycythemia vera can include pruritus, headache, epistaxis, and easy bruising. More severe complications related to hyperviscosity include ophthalmic vascular occlusions (involving the ophthalmic, central retinal, or branch retinal arteries), which may be recurrent, cardiovascular events, and cerebral infarcts. Palpable splenic enlargement is often found on examination.

Treatment for polycythemia vera begins with phlebotomy and is monitored by periodic measurement of hemoglobin and hematocrit. Aspirin is given as well to decrease the risk of thrombotic vascular events. If the disease progresses, cytotoxic chemotherapy may be needed to suppress the abnormal cell proliferation. Polycythemia vera also poses a risk of transition to acute leukemia or myelofibrosis over time.

WHITE BLOOD CELLS

Leukocytosis and leukopenia may be physiologic or pathologic. Physiologic causes reflect responses to triggers such as some medications or infections; pathologic causes include leukemias. Leukopenia can be the result of bone marrow failure or rare autoimmune white blood cell destruction. The former is often caused by bone marrow infiltration such as by a tumor, and the latter can be caused by drugs or associated with other autoimmune conditions. Immunoglobulin production is also a key component of immune function, and disorders of immunoglobulin production can cause ocular disease.

Leukopenia may result from various causes. Drug-induced leukopenia is often seen with cytotoxic chemotherapy for cancer treatment and is generally accompanied by reductions in all cellular elements in blood, resulting in pancytopenia. Isolated leukopenia can be triggered by immunosuppressive drugs with treatment for autoimmune diseases and after organ transplants. Infrequently, other medications may trigger an immunologic response that results in leukopenia, including medications for epilepsy, hyperthyroidism, depression, and some antibiotics. Discontinuation of the offending agent typically results in resolution of the condition; although rare, fatal reactions can occur[24] (**TABLE 8.2**).

Bone marrow involvement in malignancy such as myelofibrosis, as well as metastatic disease to the marrow, can impair bone marrow cellular output. As with other processes that affect the bone marrow, a pancytopenia generally results with reductions in all three cell lines (white cells, red cells, and platelets).

Many viral infections are accompanied by leukopenia, including acute Epstein-Barr virus mononucleosis, often seen in teens and young adults; other viral triggers include HIV (Chapter 10) and viral hepatitis (Chapter 9). Overwhelming systemic bacterial infections, often with sepsis (Chapter 9), can also present with a low white blood cell count. Autoimmune disorders including systemic lupus erythematosus[25] and rheumatoid arthritis[26] can also be marked by low white blood cell counts, both due to the illness and treatment-related (Chapter 11).

Leukocytosis is commonly associated with acute infections, and fever may also be present. With acute bacterial infections, the increased white blood cell count is frequently accompanied by an increase in band neutrophils. Other conditions such as stress, major surgery, and chronic inflammation can cause leukocytosis.

Medications are another potential cause of leukocytosis, with glucocorticoids in particular causing a mild or moderate increase in the total white blood cell count. Since glucocorticoids are immunosuppressive agents and their use increases the risk of infection, the findings of leukocytosis in an ill patient taking a glucocorticoid can present a clinical challenge in determining whether the cause of the leukocytosis is due to glucocorticoid use, infection, or both.

TABLE 8.2   **Drugs Associated With Neutropenia (Excluding Chemotherapeutic Agents)[24]**
Antipsychotics
Clozapine
Anti-infectives
Dapsone, hydroxychloroquine, oxacillin, penicillin G, quinine, trimethoprim-sulfamethoxazole, vancomycin
Biological therapies
Infliximab, rituximab
Neurological agents
Lamotrigine
Antithyroid agents
Methimazole, propylthiouracil
Cardiovascular agents
Procainamide, Quinidine
Misc anti-inflammatories
Sulfasalazine

One of the most concerning causes of substantial leukocytosis is the presence of a hematologic malignancy.

Leukemias are malignant disorders characterized by uncontrolled proliferation of a leukocyte precursor in the bone marrow. The precursor may involve the myeloid lineage ("myelogenous leukemia," affecting monocytes or granulocytes) or the lymphoid lineage ("lymphocytic leukemia," affecting lymphocytes). Metastatic lesions can also develop. The white blood cell count is often markedly elevated and immature forms are typically seen on the white blood cell differential. In addition, as malignant leukocyte production takes over the marrow, red blood cell and platelet production is often compromised with anemia and thrombocytopenia accompanying the leukocytosis.

Broadly, leukemias can be characterized as acute or chronic. Early, undifferentiated precursors divide rapidly and cause acute leukemias that require prompt treatment for survival. Chronic leukemias are caused by slower proliferation of more differentiated cells and progress much more slowly. Because chronic leukemias can transform into acute leukemias, monitoring is an important part of their care. In general, children are diagnosed more commonly with acute leukemias and adults with chronic leukemias. There are a number of underlying conditions that predispose to the development of leukemia, including Down syndrome (trisomy 21). Presenting signs and symptoms of leukemia depend on the particular subtype, but generally patients with leukemia suffer constitutional symptoms such as fever, fatigue, malaise and night sweats, shortness of breath, easy bruising and bleeding, cutaneous pallor, lymphadenopathy, infections, and neurological symptoms if the central nervous system (CNS) is involved. Visual symptoms may accompany eye disease.

Ophthalmic complications in leukemia are common in acute more often than chronic leukemia and manifest as

- Primary infiltration of the retina/choroid/vitreous, anterior segment, or orbit by leukemic cells
- *Leukemic retinopathy* secondary to anemia, thrombocytopenia, and hyperviscosity (**FIGURE 8.12**)
- Opportunistic ocular infections
- Adverse effects from chemotherapy[27,28]

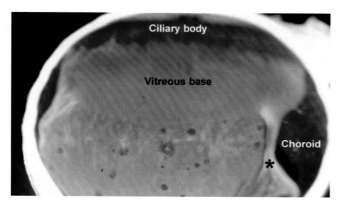

FIGURE 8.12 Lateral view of interior of postmortem eye from patient with leukemia (anterior segment at top). Numerous white-centered hemorrhages are evident. The patient had undergone vitrectomy for extensive vitreous hemorrhage. Residual heme is present in the remaining vitreous base. (With permission from Freddo T, Chaum E. Anatomy of the Eye and Orbit, Cptr 3, Wolters-Kluwer, 2018.)

Eye disease should respond to appropriate systemic therapy. Retinal complications are most common with reported prevalence of around 30% to 50%, though autopsy studies have found retinopathy at higher rates (80%-90%) in patients with severe disease. Leukemic retinopathy involves bilateral hemorrhaging at all retinal levels (usually in the posterior pole), cotton wool spots, Roth spots (white-centered hemorrhages), vitreous hemorrhage, venous dilation/tortuosity, retinal venous occlusion, and/or peripheral retinal ischemia with microaneurysms and neovascularization (more common in chronic than acute leukemia). Retinal infiltrates appear as gray/white or pink multi- or unifocal masses in the superficial retina (though any layer can be involved) and/or along the retinal vasculature. Choroidal infiltration is actually more common than retinal infiltration on histopathologic studies but is often less obvious to the clinical examination, unless accompanied by serous retinal detachment. Macular edema is uncommon, as is optic nerve infiltration with vitreous spillover (leukemic vitritis). CNS leukemia may result in papilledema or cranial nerve palsy causing diplopia. Anterior segment infiltration involving the iris, conjunctiva, or anterior chamber (which can mimic a uveitis) is also uncommon. Orbital leukemia presents with proptosis, eyelid edema, and chemosis and usually involves a mild diffuse infiltrate rather than a large mass, less commonly involving the lacrimal gland or extraocular muscles. Opportunistic globe infections resulting from immunosuppression include viral (CMV, VZV, HSV, measles, mumps), fungal (*Candida*, *Aspergillus*), bacterial, and protozoal sources. Various ocular side effects from chemotherapy have been reported, including corneal toxicity (eg, cytarabine), cataract (eg, dexamethasone, busulfan), and neuro-ophthalmic complications such as nystagmus and optic neuropathy (eg, vincristine). Retinopathy with decreased vision may be a presenting sign of leukemia (**FIGURE 8.13**) and isolated eye disease may uncommonly herald relapse in some patients with leukemia.

Lymphomas often present with lymph node enlargement or systemic symptoms such as night sweats, weight loss, and anemia. Lymphomas represent a clonal proliferation of lymphoid cells within the lymphatic system. As opposed to leukemias (which largely involved circulating populations of white cells), patients with leukemia develop palpable masses of malignant cells within one or more lymph nodes. There are two major categories for lymphomas: Hodgkin lymphoma and non-Hodgkin lymphoma, of which numerous subtypes exist. The key finding on pathologic examination of affected tissues in Hodgkin lymphoma is the Reed Sternberg cell. Non-Hodgkin lymphoma is more common, affects older patients on average, is often diagnosed at later stages, and generally carries a worse prognosis than Hodgkin lymphoma.

Almost all structures of the orbit, ocular adnexa, and globe may be involved in lymphoma, and disease may be primary or secondary. Though orbital/adnexal lymphoma comprises only 5% to 10% of all extranodal lymphomas, it is the most common orbital/adnexal malignancy.[29] In general, elderly patients are affected more often than the young. Both Hodgkin and non-Hodgkin subtypes exist, though B-cell non-Hodgkin tumors are by far the most common.[30] Orbital tumors are most

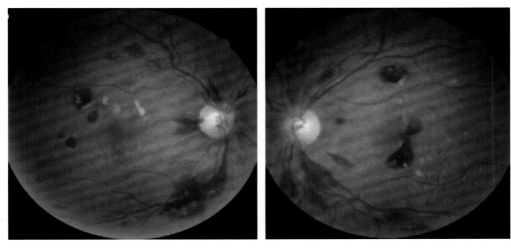

FIGURE 8.13 Leukemic retinopathy as the presenting sign of acute lymphocytic leukemia in a 26-year-old white male (WBC = 77.8 K/mm³, HCT = 22.7%, Plt = 57 K/mm³). (Photo credit Dr Druckenbrod.)

common, followed by conjunctival and eyelid tumors. Orbital tumors usually localize to the extraconal space (72%) and/or the lacrimal gland (51%) and a majority arise as primary disease without systemic involvement, generally with a good prognosis. Patients can present with unilateral proptosis, ophthalmoplegia and diplopia, eyelid swelling, periorbital pain, "salmon patch" pink conjunctival or eyelid masses, eyelid ptosis, and changes in visual acuity, typically over a period of months. All patients with orbital/adnexal lymphoma should have a full evaluation with a hematologist/oncologist for disease staging and to evaluate for the presence of simultaneous systemic disease. Local radiotherapy may be sufficient to treat isolated eye disease with an excellent prognosis, though chemotherapy and surgical excision may also be useful. Serial monitoring for development of systemic lymphoma is indicated for several years after a diagnosis of isolated ocular/adnexal lymphoma.

Primary intraocular lymphoma (PIOL) occurs as a subtype of primary CNS lymphoma, which is an uncommon subtype of B-cell non-Hodgkin lymphoma and is seen in immunocompromised patients, including advanced HIV. About 15% to 25% of primary CNS lymphoma involves the eye and up to 80% of isolated PIOL will go on to develop systemic CNS disease.[31] Full neurological assessment with cerebrospinal fluid analysis is indicated in all cases of isolated PIOL to assess for systemic CNS disease. PIOL presents as a bilateral intraocular inflammation primarily with vitritis, with or without anterior segment inflammation. Yellow, multifocal retinal infiltration may occur with lymphocytic cells accumulating between Bruch membrane and the RPE. A characteristic "leopard spot" pattern of fluorescence occurs on fluorescein angiography. PIOL may be initially mischaracterized as a chronic uveitis (eg, from sarcoidosis or viral etiologies) or other inflammatory chorioretinal disease and thus a high degree of suspicion is usually required for timely diagnosis. Lymphomatous ophthalmic disease is treated with systemic chemotherapy and/or ocular/orbital radiation.

Plasma cell disorders result from clonal proliferation of these immunoglobulin-secreting B cells. Immunoglobulin (IG) subtypes are IgA, IgG, IgD, IgE, and IgM. Under normal conditions, the range of IG subtypes is present with an expected ratio of each. Immunoglobulins are normally produced in a polyclonal fashion as they are generated independently by B cells in response to immunogenic exposures. In the setting of plasma cell disorders, excessive levels of one immunoglobulin type or the individual immunoglobulin heavy or light chains are secreted from a population of abnormally proliferating B cells, resulting in a monoclonal pattern. The overproduction of immunoglobulin is more striking than the number of proliferating B cells, and in fact many plasma cell disorders show leukopenia. When an evaluation reveals an excess of monoclonal immunoglobulins, it reflects an abnormal population of plasma cells. Monoclonal gammopathy of unknown significance (MGUS), which itself is not malignant, is considered a precursor to myeloma. However, not all patients with MGUS will progress to myeloma. There are factors that increase the risk of progression, including excess IgA or IgM secretion (as opposed to IgG), the latter of which carries a lower risk or progressing to myeloma. Higher levels of monoclonal protein as well as an increased immunoglobulin light chain level are adverse prognostic prognostic factors for progression to myeloma over time. On average, the 20-year risk of an individual with MGUS progressing to myeloma is about 20%. However, this can be stratified by risk: in a low-risk individual, that number is about 5%, whereas a high-risk individual carries a risk over 50%.[32]

Multiple myeloma is characterized by the progression of the monoclonal gammopathy to a malignancy, with an abnormal plasma cell population and the secretion of excess monoclonal IG or a portion of the IG molecule, most often light chains. Along with excess monoclonal IG proteins, interleukins and other hormones are elaborated to excess. It is typically seen in older adults, with a mean age at diagnosis of 66.[33]

Common findings in multiple myeloma include hypercalcemia from bone lesions or abnormal protein secretion that causes bone resorption; bone invasion from malignant plasma cell proliferation including plasmacytomas; anemia from bone marrow involvement or renal disease (usually normocytic anemia); and renal failure from deposition of the abnormal immunoglobulin. Systemic symptoms such as fatigue and weight loss frequently occur as well. The above symptoms are often the initial findings that lead to the diagnosis. In addition to bone, plasmacytomas can develop in areas such as the CNS. Bone pain, pathological fracture, or neurological findings due to nerve compression may also be a presenting symptom of multiple myeloma (**FIGURES 8.14** and **8.15**).

Waldenstron macroglobulinemia is a specific plasma cell disorder resulting in excess secretion of IgM. IgG and IgA, the most commonly secreted immunoglobulins in myeloma (in that order), are dimers, with two protein chains. IgM is a pentamer with five chains, making it a much larger molecule. In excess, it increases blood viscosity with slow flow resulting in poor perfusion and an increased risk of clots and ischemic events. Patients may present with epistaxis, easy bruising or symptoms related to anemia, lymphadenopathy, constitutional symptoms, as well as neurologic symptoms related to hyperviscosity including peripheral neuropathy, headache, dizziness, ataxia, tinnitus, vision changes, and mental status changes or alterations in consciousness in severe cases.

Plasma cell disorders may result in retinopathy due to hyperviscosity, anemia, and thrombocytopenia. The fundus examination may demonstrate bilateral dilated and tortuous retinal venules, retinal

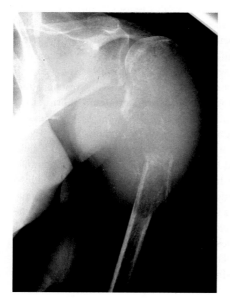

FIGURE 8.14 Anteroposterior radiograph of the proximal humerus in a patient with a plasmacytoma of the proximal humerus. Local treatment with irradiation was administered. (From Bucholz RW, Heckman JD, Rockwood CA Jr, Green DP. *Rockwood and Green's Fractures in Adults.* 5th ed. Philadelphia, PA: Lippincott, Williams & Wilkins; 2001.)

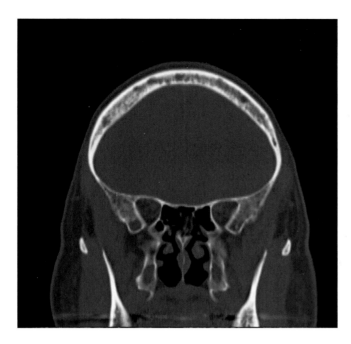

FIGURE 8.15 Coronal CT scan of the skull near the orbital apex demonstrating multiple lytic lesions in multiple myeloma. Lesions appear as "punched out" sections in the bone. (Image credit: D. Ginat, MD.)

venous occlusions, retinal hemorrhages, and exudation with or without macular edema. All patients with bilateral or sequential central retinal vein occlusion, especially younger patients, should undergo a workup that includes investigations for hyperviscosity syndromes such as plasma cell disorders. Retinopathy is present in 30% or more patients with Waldenstrom at the time of diagnosis and in 3% to 4% of patients with multiple myeloma, but since multiple myeloma is much more prevalent than Waldenstrom, it is a more frequent overall cause of hyperviscosity retinopathy[34] (**FIGURE 8.16**). Multiple myeloma may also lead to plasmacytoma deposition in and around the eye resulting in ciliary body or other uveal cysts, choroidal effusions, conjunctival and corneal deposits, orbital mass, or chorioretinal or optic nerve infiltration. Advanced multiple myeloma may rarely involve the CNS with

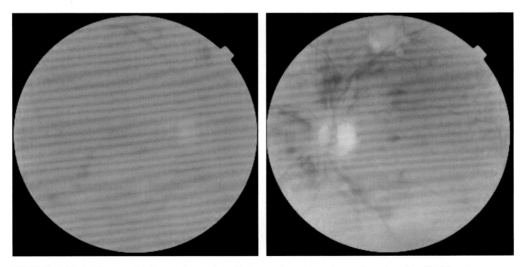

FIGURE 8.16 A 78-year-old Caucasian male with hyperviscosity retinopathy related to Waldenstrom macroglobulinemia. The right eye image is obscured by cataract. (Photo credit Dr Druckenbrod.)

diplopia from intracranial plasmacytoma causing one or multiple cranial neuropathies.[35] Ophthalmic disease in plasma cell disorders responds to systemic treatment of the hyperviscosity, which often involves RBC transfusion and several rounds of plasmapheresis, followed by disease-specific chemotherapy to target the underlying plasma cell proliferation.

The course of multiple myeloma is variable, as some patients progress rapidly and others have a course of disease with slower progression. The initial workup typically includes a comprehensive lab evaluation (including serum levels of calcium, creatinine, proteins; urine collection for protein evaluation; and a CBC), a bone marrow biopsy, and imaging studies including a skeletal survey to look for lytic lesions. Systemic chemotherapy is the most common treatment, with a range of regimens that can be selected based upon individual patient factors.

PLATELETS

Platelet disorders can be grouped into conditions of thrombocytopenia or thrombocytosis. Some platelet disorders demonstrate a normal platelet count, but dysfunctional cells lead to excessive bleeding.

Causes of thrombocytopenia include bone marrow failure and accelerated platelet destruction, typically antibody-mediated. Idiopathic thrombocytopenic purpura is an idiopathic, immune-mediated condition resulting in platelet destruction and an increased bleeding risk. It is typically treated with a course of immunosuppression and may resolve in its own.

Physiologic causes of thrombocytosis include inflammation, such as acute infection; reactive, such as during recovery from blood loss (surgery, trauma) and postsplenectomy. The spleen normally stores many platelets for rapid release in the event of bleeding, and patients who undergo splenectomy (often after trauma with splenic injury) lose this platelet store. More platelets remain in the circulation resulting in a high platelet count, typically without any symptoms.

Essential thrombocytosis (ET) results in an abnormal clonal proliferation of megakaryocytes. Patients with ET may experience both higher rates of thrombosis and hemorrhage. The malignant origins of the platelets make them ineffective; thus despite a high platelet count—sometimes as high as 1 million, about triple the normal upper limit—bleeding and bruising may paradoxically occur. Splenomegaly and erythromelalgia may also occur. Erythromelalgia is a syndrome of erythema, pain, and swelling that typically occurs in the hands and feet. Episodic vascular occlusion is the likely cause in ET; erythromelalgia can also occur in polycythemia vera. Similar to polycythemia vera, the JAK2 mutation is often responsible for the proliferation of the bone marrow precursor (**FIGURE 8.17**).[36]

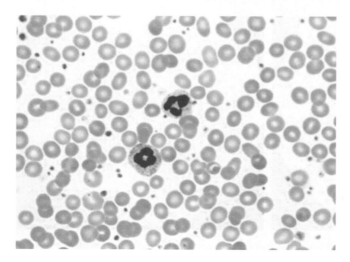

FIGURE 8.17 Essential thrombocythemia. Peripheral blood smear from a 50-year-old woman showing thrombocytosis. The platelets are fairly normal morphologically and no other significant abnormalities are noted on the smear. (From Orazi A, Foucar K, Knowles DM, Weiss LM. *Knowles Neoplastic Hematopathology.* 3rd ed. Philadelphia, PA: Wolters Kluwer; 2013.)

When there is an effective treatment for a disease, the prevalence increases if the incidence remains the same. Incidence and mortality rates are similar for an aggressive disease with limited treatment. In contrast, incidence exceeds mortality if there is early detection with effective treatment or with a less aggressive disease.

Cancer is defined as a disease caused by uncontrolled cell division with proliferation of abnormal cells. Cells are able to divide rapidly and evade both cell cycle control signals and programmed cell death. There are numerous environmental factors that contribute to the development of cancer beyond inherited genetic mutations. Many are well known, including tobacco smoking, sun exposure, and chemical carcinogens.

The most common cancers are skin, breast, lung, prostate, and colorectal. Lung cancer has the highest rate of mortality. Prostate cancer is the most common cancer among males, and breast cancer is most common in females. Skin cancer is the most commonly diagnosed cancer in the United States, but cases are not required to be reported in cancer registries (Chapter 13).

CANCER SCREENING

Cancer screening aims to detect premalignant or asymptomatic pre-invasive disease to initiate effective early treatment and reduce morbidity and mortality. Important factors to consider when recommending screening for a given cancer include

- Scope of the disease burden in the population
- Availability of effective screening to detect preclinical disease
- The availability of effective treatment
- Evidence of benefit for screening

In general, screening is recommended for prevalent cancers with high mortality that have an effective screening test and acceptable early therapy that has been shown to extend life. Ideally, both the duration and quality of life should be considered.

There are two major biases that impact the data used to determine the effectiveness of cancer screening tests: lead time bias and length time bias.

Lead time bias occurs when there is an earlier diagnosis of a cancer, but no effective treatment. This artificially appears to prolong survival without actually affecting cancer-related mortality. Only the time of diagnosis is advanced by screening; the time of death is not changed. Because people appear to live longer once diagnosed with disease, screening may appear to be effective. Lead time bias is generally associated with aggressive cancers.

Length time bias occurs in diseases that are by nature slow-growing and result in less mortality. The detection of this disease leads to more invasive diagnostic and therapeutic interventions, without a benefit in mortality. Screening can also lead to overdiagnosis, with detection of disease that is not progressive or lethal. It is also susceptible to selection bias as health-conscious patients may be more likely to participate in routine screening.[50]

CANCER RISK FACTORS

The etiology of cancer is multifactorial, with contributions from nonmodifiable factors (such as age, race/ethnicity, family history, and genetics) as well as a myriad of modifiable risk factors. Nonmodifiable risk factors, by definition, are not targets for cancer prevention or management. However, it is widely recognized that a large proportion of cancer is known to be preventable through modifiable risk reduction; in fact, the World Health Organization (WHO) has estimated between 30% and 50% of all cancer causes are preventable.[51]

Environmental exposures that damage DNA and increase risk for cancer development are known as carcinogens. These include chemicals, microbes, and radiation. The International Agency for Research on Cancer (IARC) has established a classification system for carcinogenic agents, and as of 2019, there are 120 agents designated as definitively carcinogenic to humans.[4] Carcinogenic microbes include viruses, bacteria, and parasites. Microbial carcinogenesis occurs through expression of proteins that affect cell cycle control regulators, tumor suppressor and proto-oncogenes, or as the result of a chronic inflammatory process. Notable microbes include *Helicobacter pylori* (gastric cancer), *Schistosoma haematobium* (bladder cancer), human papillomavirus (HPV) (cervical cancer), hepatitis B and C viruses (liver cancer), Epstein-Barr virus (lymphoma), and human T-cell lymphotropic virus type-1 (leukemia). An example of microbial-induced carcinogenesis is cervical cancer, which is most often caused by sexual transmission of HPV, a DNA virus. While over 150 subtypes of HPV exist, only a subset are known to have oncogenic capacity; subtypes 6, 11, 16, and 18 are most highly associated with cervical cancer.[2,3] High-risk HPV produces E6 and E7 proteins that cause destruction of p53 and Rb proteins. The loss of these tumor suppressor proteins leads to neoplastic transformation.

Chemical exposures are also well known to increase cancer risk. Exposure to asbestos, a widely used chemical in insulation in the United States before the 1980s, has been implicated in lung carcinoma and mesothelioma. Radon and radon decay products found in most soils and rocks have also been established as environmental carcinogens that cause lung cancer. Nonionizing ultraviolet B radiation from sunlight resulting in DNA damage has been associated with skin cancers, including basal cell carcinoma, squamous cell carcinoma, and melanoma. Ionizing radiation (radon, x-rays, gamma rays, and other high-energy radiation such as from nuclear reactor accidents) produces hydroxyl free radicals that increase risks of DNA damage and is associated with acute or chronic myeloid leukemia (CML) and thyroid carcinoma.

There are definitive links between increased cancer risk and certain lifestyle and dietary choices. Tobacco use is the most significant lifestyle risk factor linked to numerous cancers, including lung, esophagus, larynx, mouth, kidney, bladder, stomach, and cervix. It has been estimated that 20% of worldwide cancer death is associated with tobacco use.[52] Alcohol use is associated with head and neck squamous cell, esophageal, pancreatic, and hepatocellular carcinomas.[2] Obesity is associated with increased risk of developing colorectal, breast, endometrial, pancreatic, liver, and esophageal cancer, as well as others, likely mediated through metabolic and inflammatory mechanisms.[3] Sedentary lifestyle is also a risk factor and may contribute to an estimated 5% of cancer deaths.[53] While studies analyzing individual dietary components are less definitive, certain dietary patterns are associated with increased cancer risk, for example, those high in processed foods and red meat and low in fruits and vegetables.[54] Thus, cancer risk can be reduced with healthy lifestyle and dietary choices.[55]

CANCER STAGING

The **Tumor, Node, and Metastasis (TNM)** classification system is a standardized approach to staging cancer. This system was developed and is periodically updated by the American Joint Committee on Cancer (AJCC), a multidisciplinary organization formed in 1959 whose mission is to provide evidence-based guidance on cancer classification.[56] Using TNM classification, an overall cancer stage of 0 (in situ disease), I, II, III, or IV is then designated. There are also other staging systems specific to cancer type (eg, Gleason score for prostate cancer, FIGO for cervical cancer, BCLC for liver cancer, and the Ann Arbor staging system for lymphoma). Staging is important in predicting prognosis and determining appropriate treatments (**TABLE 8.3**).

Cancer is staged with information from clinical examination, radiographic studies, and surgery. Modern staging systems integrate molecular and biologic characteristics of tumors as well.

TABLE 8.3   Tumor, Node, and Metastasis Staging

T is the size and/or extent of the tumor
   T0 = no primary tumor, Tis = carcinoma in situ, T1-4 = increasing tumor size

N describes nodal involvement
   N0 = no regional node involvement, N1-3 = increasing number and/or extent of nodal
      involvement

M describes whether there are any distant metastases
   M0 = no metastasis, M1 = distant metastasis

CANCER TREATMENT

Major modalities to treat cancer include chemotherapy, surgery, radiation, and hormonal therapy. Generally, surgery and radiation are local therapies, while chemotherapy and hormonal treatments are systemic therapy. Recently advances have expanded available options to include targeted oncologic therapies and immunotherapy, which are profoundly altering the management of cancer.

Surgery

Surgery has been a cornerstone for the treatment of cancer since its inception. Surgery is central to the diagnosis and management of cancer and is often used in conjunction with other treatment modalities.[2] It has been used to diagnose, stage, cure, and debulk (reduce the tumor burden) solid tumors. Biopsy allows for tissue diagnosis, which is required for disease confirmation and treatment planning.

Radical oncologic surgeries are used with the intention of completely removing the tumor, adjacent involved structures, and lymph nodes. Local control is often improved with the procedure, but cure is not typically expected, especially with aggressive disease. For this reason, surgery is often combined with systemic therapies or radiation to allow for organ preservation, enhance complete surgical resection, and improve survival. Neoadjuvant therapies, such as chemotherapy or radiation treatment before surgery, aim to shrink very large tumors, rendering them operable.

Techniques for biopsy include punch, fine needle aspiration (FNA), core needle biopsy (CNB), incisional or excisional. Punch biopsy is reserved for superficial cutaneous or mucosal lesions. CNB has the advantage of maintaining the structural integrity of the tumor; but both FNA and CNB are predisposed to sampling error if the region of cancer is not properly sampled. Staging laparoscopy/laparotomy is less often used given advancements in imaging techniques, but it is still utilized in sites that are incompletely visualized with modern radiographic images (eg, peritoneal or omental disease in ovarian and gastric cancers). Nodal staging for solid tumors has also evolved to be less invasive and morbid (eg, sentinel node biopsy).

Radiation

Radiation oncology uses ionizing radiation to kill cancer cells and has been a mainstay of cancer treatment for over a century. Ionization is the process by which an atom loses a particle and becomes electrically charged. This ionization process causes indirect or direct cellular DNA damage, resulting in cell death. Cells that are rapidly dividing (in M phase) are particularly sensitive to DNA damage and thus cancer cells are more vulnerable to radiation damage as compared with normal cells. Additionally, cancer cells may have deficient DNA repair mechanisms, increasing their susceptibility to radiation damage. Because normal cells are also exposed to radiation with risk for damage, a therapeutic risk-benefit analysis is an important part of radiation therapy planning. Lowest possible doses and smallest exposure areas are indicated, and full radiation treatment doses may be divided (or "fractioned") out over a period of time to allow normal cells to heal.

Common forms of radiation used in cancer treatment include x-rays (most commonly), electrons, protons, gamma rays, and radioactive sources. External beam radiation therapy (EBRT) involves a linear particle accelerator to create a focused beam of radiation, commonly an electron beam or a photon (x-ray) beam, which is directed at the malignant tissue. Electron beam radiation is used to treat superficial tumors (eg, cutaneous lymphomas, skin cancers, breast cancer), while x-ray beams are used for deeper tissue penetration. Protons are an alternative form of radiation that allows for dose deposition at a very specific tissue depth, allowing for highly localized treatment. Proton therapy is thus an option for pediatric populations or retreatment of prior irradiated tissue as it minimizes dose outside of the targeted area. Gamma rays are produced by radioactive decay and are mostly utilized for CNS tumors, delivered in single-dose (or limited-dose) stereotactic radiation therapy protocols (eg, radioisotope Cobalt 60 used in the Gamma Knife system).

As opposed to EBRT, brachytherapy involves direct insertion of a radioactive treatment source into target tissue which delivers energy via radioactive decay. The advantage is high-dose radiation delivery to a target tissue with relative sparing of surrounding tissue, compared with EBRT. An example is prostate seed implantation directly into the gland. The Collaborative Ocular Melanoma Study (COMS) demonstrated the benefit of iodine-125 brachytherapy as an alternative to enucleation for uveal melanoma, establishing brachytherapy as a standard of care for these patients.[57] Systemic targeted radionucleotide therapy involves the use of radio-labeled molecules delivered intravenously to target specific tissues; an example is radiolabeled iodine-131 to target the thyroid gland.

Radiation Toxicity

The most common side effects of radiation include fatigue, skin effects, and myelosuppression. Toxic effects of radiation vary depending on targeted structures and surrounding organs at risk. Chest irradiation may result in inflammation of lung, premature coronary artery disease, or pericarditis. Abdominal radiation may lead to nausea, vomiting, esophagitis, dysphagia, or bowel changes. Pelvic irradiation leads to urinary or bowel irritative symptoms and sexual side effects. Due to the mechanism of action (ie, DNA damage), there is a slightly increased risk of secondary malignancy with radiation. While normal cells generally have better DNA repair mechanisms and different fractionation schemes allow normal cells to recover, there is still a risk of potential for carcinogenesis.[9]

Ophthalmic tissues are at risk for radiation damage with orbital, intraocular, paranasal sinus, and some CNS radiation treatments.[15,58] Damage may be expected in some cases (eg, retinal side effects after brachytherapy of a choroidal melanoma) and is directly dose-dependent. Minor tissue damage of both the anterior and posterior segment tissues generally begins to occur at doses around 25 to 30 Gy, with more severe and sometimes permanent effects after 50 to 60 Gy. Younger age, medical comorbidities such as diabetes and hypertension, and coadministration of chemotherapy increase risk for ocular damage. Eyelid side effects include lash loss, telangiectasia, hyperpigmentation, entropion/ectropion, trichiasis, and punctal stenosis. Conjunctival chemosis and edema may occur at lower doses, while contracture and symblepharon are possible at higher doses. Corneal insult ranges from superficial keratitis to edema, neovascularization, keratinization, and ulceration. Acute iritis may occur, and transient myopia is a less common but possible lenticular side effect. Cataract formation is a more common later-stage lens complication occurring on average 2 to 3 years after ocular and periocular radiation. The lens is especially radio-sensitive compared to other tissues, and changes always occur beyond radiation dose of 10 Gy.

Radiation retinopathy can be a vision-threatening complication with long-term consequences. With doses of 60 Gy, 50% of patients develop retinopathy, and up to 95% develop retinopathy after 70 to 80 Gy.[59] The COMS predicted with life table estimates that 43% of patients with uveal melanoma treated with brachytherapy have visual acuity of 20/200 or less 3 years later, due to chronic radiation–induced damage.[14] Transient retinal edema may develop in the acute phase (2-3 months) and usually resolves after several weeks. The most common form of radiation retinopathy is a more latent-onset disease (6 months-3 years or more) which is similar in appearance to diabetic microangiopathy. Vessel leakage with exudation, intraretinal hemorrhages, microaneurysms, macular edema, and retinal nerve fiber layer ischemia (cotton wool spots) are observed on fundus examination, and areas of retinal nonperfusion are seen on fluorescein angiography. In severe cases, perivasculitis, optic nerve edema, or retinal or optic nerve neovascularization with risk for tractional retinal detachment may occur. Treatment for proliferative radiation retinopathy is similar to proliferative diabetic retinopathy and may involve intravitreal injections of anti-VEGF and/or panretinal photocoagulation. Uncommonly, radiation-induced optic neuropathy results in permanent vision loss from optic atrophy. Hyperfractionation of radiation dose and proper shielding of the eyes minimize the risks of ophthalmic tissue toxicity (**FIGURE 8.20**).

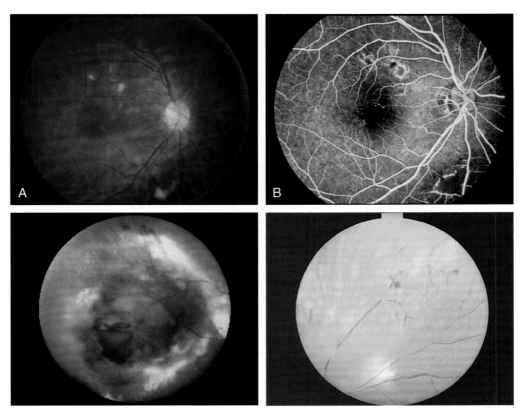

FIGURE 8.20 Radiation retinopathy examples. Top images: Radiation retinopathy after teletherapy. A, Cotton wool spots and small retinal hemorrhage are present in the posterior pole. B, Fluorescein angiogram corresponding to (A) at 25 seconds after injection. The cotton wool spots are hypofluorescent. Note the radiation-induced capillary telangiectasia at the fovea and below the inferior retinal vascular arcade where capillary nonperfusion is noted. Bottom-left: Radiation retinopathy surrounding a choroidal melanoma treated with brachytherapy. Marked lipid exudation is present at the necrotic tumor base. Bottom-right: Hard exudation, retinal sheathing, retinal hemorrhages, and telangiectases occurred in an eye with radiation retinopathy, neovascularization, and neovascular glaucoma. (Bottom-right, From Tasman W, Jaeger E. *The Wills Eye Hospital Atlas of Clinical Ophthalmology.* 2nd ed. Lippincott Williams & Wilkins; 2001. Top-left, Top-right and Bottom-left, From Fineman M. Retina. 3rd ed. Philadelphia, PA: Wolters Kluwer; 2018.)

Chemotherapy

Due to alterations in cell cycle signaling and division, cancer cells are susceptible to DNA damaging agents and are less able to repair this damage. Chemotherapy may be used alone or in combination with radiation or surgery depending on the type and stage of cancer. Chemotherapy can also be administered before surgery to shrink tumor size and improve surgical outcomes; this treatment is called neoadjuvant treatment.

The major classes of chemotherapy include alkylating agents, antimetabolites, microtubule targeting agents, topoisomerase inhibitors, and antitumor antibiotics, each with differential effects on the cell cycle. Cancer regimens often combine different classes to potentiate efficacy and minimize resistance and toxicity. Different routes of administration include intravenous (most common), oral, intraperitoneal, intrathecal, and intra-arterial and are employed based on specific characteristics of the cancer. Chemotherapy can also be used as a radiosensitizer to synergistically kill cells.

Chemotherapy Toxicity

As noted above, chemotherapy works on rapidly dividing cells such as mucosa, hair cells, and bone marrow. Common adverse effects include nausea, vomiting, diarrhea, alopecia, mucositis, and myelosuppression. Alkylating agents have dose-limiting bone marrow toxicity. Microtubule targeting agents have neurotoxicity. Cardiotoxicity is seen with anthracyclines, while pulmonary toxicity is seen with antitumor antibiotics like bleomycin.[58] **TABLE 8.4** provides examples of chemotherapy agents by class and outlines mechanisms action and common toxicities.

A variety of ocular toxicities have been described in association with many different systemic chemotherapies, most of which are mild in nature and reversible once chemotherapy is discontinued.[60,61] Often, ocular adverse effects are not sufficiently severe to warrant discontinuation of chemotherapy. While there are a few specified prescribing recommendations in the United States for ophthalmic evaluation and management surrounding some systemic chemotherapies (eg, BRAF inhibitors and

TABLE 8.4   Common Toxicities of Selected Chemotherapy Agents[8]

Class of Chemotherapy	Examples	Mechanism of Action	Common Toxicity
Antimetabolites	5-Fluorouracil, methotrexate, cytarabine, cladribine, aza-thioprine, 6-mercaptopurine	Purine/pyrimi-dine or folic acid analogs	Myelosuppression
Antitumor antibiotics	Bleomycin, dactinomycin, doxorubicin, daunorubicin	Intercalate DNA	Myelosuppression Bleomycin—pulmonary fibrosis Doxo/daunorubicin—cardiotoxicity
Alkylating	Busulfan, cyclophosphamide, nitrosourea, cisplatin	Cross-link DNA	Myelosuppression Cyclophosphamide—hemorrhagic cystitis Cisplatin—nephrotoxicity
Microtubule inhibitors	Paclitaxel, vincristine, vinblastine	Alter polym-erization of microtubules	Neurotoxicity
Topoisomerase inhibitors	Etoposide, irinotecan	Inhibit topoisomerase	Myelosuppression

THERAPY

The approaches to manage localized prostate cancer includes active surveillance, radical prostatectomy, or radiation. Advanced or higher risk patients often receive androgen deprivation therapy (ADT) and/or chemotherapy.

Active surveillance is often recommended for locally confined low-grade disease and patients with limited life expectancy. It consists of DRE and PSA every 3 to 6 months with routine biopsy in 1 to 2 years with treatment only if disease progresses. The goal is to avoid therapy when it will not improve life expectancy or quality of life. In contrast, watchful waiting forgoes curative treatment and is focused on symptom management. Watchful waiting is often reserved for elderly patients or patients with severe comorbidities.

Radical prostatectomy is generally performed in patients with locally confined disease without adverse features. Some centers use robot-assisted technology for prostatectomy, which can shorten the recovery and may decrease some surgical risks.[73] While appropriately selected patients generally tolerate surgery, there are higher rates of incontinence and erectile dysfunction compared with noninvasive approaches.

Radiation therapy can be delivered using external beam radiation or brachytherapy as noted above. These modalities are indicated for both locally confined and advanced disease or adjuvant/salvage treatment after prostatectomy. Brachytherapy carries a higher risk of urinary obstruction especially for larger prostates, but both techniques have less risk of impotence and incontinence versus prostatectomy. Prostate cancer often metastasizes to the bone, and external beam radiation may be used to alleviate painful bone metastases. A systemic calcium mimetic radioisotope (radium-223) with selective uptake in bone may be used for individuals with diffuse osseous metastatic disease.

Prostate cancer growth can be testosterone-driven, thus eliminating circulating testosterone with ADT used to treat high-risk, advanced, or recurrent disease. Common forms of ADT include luteinizing hormone-releasing hormone (LHRH) agonists or antagonists, androgen receptor antagonists, or surgical castration with orchiectomy. In advanced or metastatic prostate cancer that is not responsive to hormone therapy, chemotherapy (typically docetaxel) is used.[74]

BREAST CANCER

Breast cancer is the most frequently diagnosed cancer in women and second leading cause of cancer death in women. There were an estimated >200,000 new cases of invasive breast cancer in the United States with >40,000 cancer-related deaths in 2019.[2] Globally, there were more than 2 million new cases worldwide in 2018.[3] The strongest risk factor for breast cancer is age. Other risk factors include obesity, physical inactivity, alcohol consumption, estrogen exposure (early menarche, late menopause, nulliparity, postmenopausal hormone supplementation), personal or family history of breast or ovarian cancer, prior biopsy revealing atypical hyperplasia, and inherited genetic mutations (BRCA1/2, Li-Fraumeni, Cowden syndrome). BRCA mutation carries 40% to 85% lifetime risk of breast cancer and 25% to 65% lifetime risk of ovarian cancer. These genetic mutations are more commonly seen in women of Ashkenazi Jewish descent.[75]

SCREENING

There are several options for breast cancer screening. For average risk women, mammography (**FIGURE 8.22**), breast self-examination (BSE), and clinical breast examination are all options. MRI is sometimes recommended for women at higher risk. Differences across the medical literature, lay literature, and in guidelines reflect the presence of controversy regarding breast cancer screening modalities.

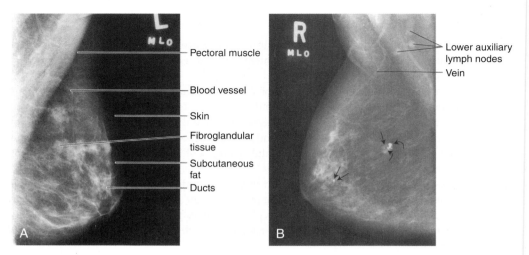

FIGURE 8.22 Mammograms. A, Normal mammogram, left breast. B, Mammogram of right breast showing lesions (arrows). In mammograms, fat tissue appears gray; breast tissue, calcium deposits, and benign or cancerous tumors appear white. (From Cohen BJ. *Medical Terminology*. 7th ed. Philadelphia, PA: Wolters Kluwer; 2013.)

According to USPSTF, for the average risk women, biennial mammogram is recommended between the ages of 50 and 74 and is optional between the ages of 40 and 49.[76] The ACS recommendations are substantially more complex, with routine mammography recommended starting at age 45.[77] The option of mammography for ages 40 to 45 should be offered and individualized. Screening should continue as long as the women is in good health with a 10-year life expectancy. Annual mammography is recommended until age 55, and biennial from then on, although women have the option to select annual mammography after the age of 55.

The value of screening in women who are between the ages of 40 and 49 is controversial and there are conflicting recommendations from different organizations. For example, the National Comprehensive Cancer Network and American College of Radiology recommend annual screening starting at age 40. In contrast, the USPSTF recommends informed decision-making with a health care provider from ages 40 to 49. The ACS recommends the option of screening for ages 40 to 45 and routine mammography starting at age 45. Studies examining the role of screening mammography in women aged 40 to 49 have had various flaws that make interpretation difficult. Other complicating factors include the fact that younger women have dense breast tissue, which can make abnormalities difficult to see on a mammogram. In any population, a lower risk of disease correlates with a higher risk of false positives on screening. Because women aged 40 to 49 have a lower risk of breast cancer, there are fewer cancers to detect and a corresponding higher rate of false-positive mammograms requiring repeat imaging, and often biopsy.[78] Additionally, breast cancer in younger women may grow faster, so it is possible that a new tumor can become clinically apparent during the interval between screening mammograms.[76,79] At the same time, a lethal cancer in a younger woman has a more significant impact on longevity. Thus, many guidelines recommend that decisions should be individualized.

According to USPSTF and ACS guidelines, the clinical breast examination and BSE are no longer recommended. The effectiveness of BSE was called into question with publication of results from a large study conducted in China, where an intervention group of working women were taught BSE technique and encouraged to perform self-examination regularly. The control group received no intervention. While there was no difference in breast cancer mortality, the intervention group experienced an increased rate of breast biopsies (about 50% more), leading experts to conclude that the benefit of BSE does not outweigh the risk of false-positive results.[80,81]

Screening recommendations change for women with genetic, familial, or exposure-related risk factors. For women with high lifetime risk (>20%-25%) (including those with known BRCA 1/2 mutations or a first degree relative with BRCA 1/2 but who have not had personal genetic testing, Li-Fraumeni or Cowden syndrome, or a history of chest radiation between ages 10 and 30), ACS guidelines[20] and ACOG guidelines[82] recommend annual screening MRI and mammogram as well as twice yearly clinical breast examinations, beginning around age 25. Several models are available for risk assessment calculation and are used to guide decisions such as more intense screening and preventive medications and surgery. Commonly used models include Gail, BOADICEA, and IBIS.[83]

DIAGNOSIS

The earliest stage breast cancer is asymptomatic and is diagnosed with screening mammography. Larger tumors can present with a lump or mass in the breast. Breast changes including nipple discharge, thickening, swelling, skin abnormalities, and rarely pain can occur. A classic sign of inflammatory breast cancer is peau d'orange, which is characterized by an inflamed, swollen breast with enlargement of pores and change in color. It is often confused with acute infectious mastitis, but inflammatory breast cancer does not improve with antibiotics.

Full workup includes a thorough history with a review of risk factors, specifically the gynecologic history (early menarche and late menopause are both risk factors), menopausal status, family history of breast or ovarian cancer, and use of hormone replacement. Physical examination should include evaluation of breast and lymph nodes. Imaging studies including mammography or ultrasonography should be acquired for patients with breast symptoms or an abnormal clinical breast examination. Bone scan and CT scan should be considered for large tumors, node positive, or symptomatic patients. Clinical staging using the TNM system is based on history, physical examination, and imaging studies.

A tissue diagnosis along with testing for estrogen receptor (ER), progesterone receptor (PR), and HER-2-neu status is required. Core biopsy of breast tissue or clinically enlarged nodes is an essential part of breast cancer workup. Sentinel lymph node biopsy is part of staging and involves injecting dye or tracer into the tumor. The first draining lymph nodes are biopsied and examined for tumor cells. If nodes are negative, it is generally assumed that the other levels of lymph nodes are negative. If tumor is present, further lymph node dissection is performed.[84]

TREATMENT

For locally confined disease, options include modified radical mastectomy versus breast conservation therapy with lumpectomy plus radiation, as established by a landmark clinical trial.[85] Modified radical mastectomy includes complete removal of breast tissue, pectoralis fascia, and levels I and II lymph nodes. Alternatively, lumpectomy or partial mastectomy is removal of only cancer-containing breast tissue. The decision to perform an axillary lymph node dissection is based on the results of sentinel lymph node biopsy.

Radiation is indicated after breast-conserving surgery and is generally delivered to the whole breast within 4-6 weeks of surgery or neoadjuvant chemotherapy. Partial breast irradiation is also offered for certain favorable subgroups of breast cancer. External beam radiation is also indicated for locally advanced disease after mastectomy if there are adverse features such as large primary tumors, positive lymph nodes, or close/positive tumor margins in resected tissue.

The decision to use chemotherapy is based on several adverse features including patients with tumor in lymph nodes, tumor markers including ER negative and HER2+, young age, or high oncotype DX genetic risk score (generated from a genomic test which analyzes activity of 21 genes which influence cancer activity and response to treatment). Chemotherapy is typically given prior to surgery or radiation (neoadjuvant) or after surgery or radiation (adjuvant).

Hormone therapy is another important aspect of breast cancer management and is beneficial for hormone receptor positive tumors. A 5-year course of adjuvant tamoxifen or raloxifene is generally indicated for ER/PR-positive tumors. However, 10 years of therapy has recently been shown to further reduce recurrence and mortality. Aromatase inhibitors (anastrozole, letrozole, exemestane) are used for postmenopausal women.[24]

COLORECTAL CANCER

Colorectal cancer is the third leading cause of cancer and cancer mortality in both males and females. In the United States, in 2019, there will be an estimated >140,000 new cases and >50,000 deaths related to colon and rectum cancer. The overall death rate and incidence of colorectal cancer is declining, which has been attributed to improved screening and treatments. There has been an emerging trend with an increase in incidence among individuals younger than age 55. Risk factors include obesity, physical inactivity, smoking, high fat and low fat diet, consumption of red or processed meat, alcohol, personal or family history of cancer, inflammatory bowel disease (with ulcerative colitis higher risk than Crohn disease), inherited genetic conditions (Lynch syndrome, familial adenomatous polyposis [FAP]), and type 2 diabetes.

FAP deserves special mention due to an increased colorectal cancer risk in association with hypertrophy of the RPE. An inherited genetic defect in the APC gene results in development of multiple polyps, resulting in a near-100% lifetime risk of developing colon cancer in affected patients, on average by age 40. Gastric and small intestine polyps can also be seen as part of the syndrome. Early and frequent surveillance for cancer is necessary, and colectomy may ultimately be performed as a preventive measure.

Extracolonic manifestations of FAP occur in 30% to 100% of patients and include stomach polyps, duodenal tumors, desmoid tumors (usually in the abdomen), nodular thyroid, and (uncommonly) hepatoblastomas and brain tumors.[86] There is a well-recognized association with congenital hypertrophy of the retinal pigment epithelium (CHRPE) on eye examination. While many patients without FAP have CHRPE, CHRPE associated with FAP is typically bilateral with multiple lesions in each eye (often described as "bear tracking") (**FIGURE 8.23**). The presence of four or more CHRPE lesions, or the presence of at least two lesions, one of which is large, has a sensitivity of 68% and a specificity of 100% for FAP.[87] The presence of multiple and/or bilateral CHRPE on eye examination should prompt

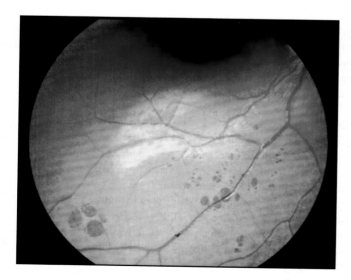

FIGURE 8.23 Multiple congenital hypertrophy of the retinal pigment epithelium ("bear tracking") on eye examination should prompt an assessment for colorectal cancer risk, due to its association with familial adenomatous polyposis. (From Fineman M. *Retina*. 3rd ed. Philadelphia, PA: Wolters Kluwer; 2018.)

a conversation to assess risk and make an appropriate referral (typically to a primary care physician). Questioning the patient about a family history of gastrointestinal cancers and any symptoms such as rectal bleeding can help assess the time frame for the referral; when there is a family history of gastrointestinal cancer, or in the presence of gastrointestinal symptoms, the referral should occur promptly together with communication to the provider.

Anatomic considerations are important in colorectal cancer. Layers of the colorectal tissue include (from inside to outside) mucosa, muscularis mucosa, submucosa, muscularis propria, serosa, and fat. Invasion of a tumor into the deeper layers will impact risk and affect treatment recommendations. The colon is divided into four parts: ascending (right), transverse, descending (left), and sigmoid colon. A lesion within 16 cm of the anal verge is considered rectal cancer. The rectum begins at the dentate line and extends to rectosigmoid junction. Encircling the lower third of the rectum is the mesorectum, which contains perirectal lymph nodes. The distinction between colon and rectal cancer is important due to differing treatment approaches.

SCREENING

For average risk patients (asymptomatic, no significant cancer family history, no personal risk factors such as prior polyps or IBD), USPSTF recommends screening beginning at age 50 and every 10 years if negative to the age of 75.[88] Both endoscopic and stool-based tests are commonly used in practice.[89] Colonoscopy is often recommended as the most robust screening test. The day before the procedure, a liquid diet and colon clean-out with a cathartic drug (laxative) is necessary.

The colonoscopy is usually performed under conscious sedation; a fiberoptic scope is advanced into the rectum and the entire colon is examined (**FIGURE 8.24**). Most polyps can be removed at that time and suspicious areas can be examined and biopsied. Sigmoidoscopy is a similar test, but only the rectum, sigmoid, and descending colon are examined. The benefit is that it is a simpler test and sedation is not required. The drawback is that the transverse and ascending colon are not examined, with potential for missed disease. A normal colonoscopy in an average risk patient does not require additional screening for another 10 years; a normal sigmoidoscopy should be repeated in 5 years. When adenomatous polyps are found on sigmoidoscopy, a full colonoscopy should be performed to follow-up and identify metachronous (occurring at the same time) polyps in the right colon. More frequent surveillance is also recommended (often at 5-year intervals) after removal of premalignant lesions.

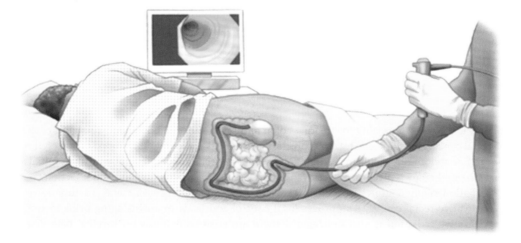

FIGURE 8.24 Colonoscopy. Patient is sedated, and a fiberoptic scope with a camera is advanced to the cecum. A thorough examination of the colonic mucosa occurs during withdrawal of the scope. Biopsies can be obtained for lesions and mucosal abnormalities. (From Lippincott Advisor [February 2016 release]. Philadelphia, PA: Wolters Kluwer; 2016.)

Some patients prefer simpler options for screening. Stool-based screening for blood includes the fecal occult blood test (FOBT) or fecal immunohistochemical test (FIT). Both evaluate a stool sample for small amounts of blood that are not visible. Stool DNA testing for mutations that are associated with colorectal cancer is also available, but as a newer test, long-term outcomes are unknown and its place in screening has not yet been firmly established. These tests all require a home stool collection that is sent to a lab, but differ in collection methods and lab processing. Abnormal results indicate either the presence of blood in the stool that may be from a bleeding cancer or DNA from mutations associated with colon cancer. In either situation, further evaluation with colonoscopy is necessary. Both false-positive and false-negative results are possible. Stool testing should be repeated annually and DNA tests at 3-year intervals.

CT scanning for colon cancer has been evaluated, yet is not widely accepted in practice at this time. In addition to usually requiring a colon clean-out, there is the drawback of radiation exposure. False-negative results occur, especially with smaller polyps that may not be seen, and false positives can also occur. Long-term outcomes are unknown, and as a newer test, the currently recommended screening interval is typically more frequent as compared with colonoscopy. Abnormal findings on imaging require a colonoscopy for follow-up, and thus another colon clean-out is necessary.

For high-risk conditions, colonoscopy is always the preferred method for screening and surveillance. While many organizations recommend that routine screening can cease at the age of 75, surveillance and follow-up of higher risk patients often continues when they are in good enough health condition to undergo the test and benefit from an intervention.

DIAGNOSIS

Most early stage colorectal cancer does not present with any symptoms and is discovered on routine screening. In the absence of screening, more advanced tumors present with symptoms such as rectal bleeding, new onset of constipation or diarrhea, stool caliber changes, abdominal pain, poor appetite, and weight loss. Colorectal cancer can also present with iron deficiency anemia (see above). If a patient's symptoms are suspicious for colorectal cancer, a colonoscopy with biopsy is performed (sensitivity and specificity of 95%). Workup should include a DRE, and blood tests including CBC, liver function testing (LFT), and the tumor marker carcinoembryonic antigen (CEA). The CEA level may be elevated in colorectal cancer; when high, it can be monitored during treatment to assess response, and post-treatment to assess for recurrence. An endoscopic ultrasound may be done to assess tumor extension and nodal involvement (for rectal cancer), and imaging typically includes CT scan of chest, abdomen, and pelvis to look for metastatic disease. Pelvic MRI may also be performed in certain situations to assess for the extent of involvement.[90]

TREATMENT

Surgery is the major modality for treating colon and rectal cancers. Importantly, surgical resection for rectal cancers must include total mesorectal excision with either low anterior resection (sphincter sparing) or abdominoperineal resection. Early stage colorectal cancer generally involves initial surgery. Chemotherapy is given in more advanced disease before and/or after surgical resection.

Radiation is often utilized preoperatively for the more advanced T3 and T4 tumors or for node-positive rectal cancer. It improves local control and leads to downstaging prior to surgery. Postoperative radiation is also indicated if there are positive margins on surgical pathology or other adverse features, but preoperative radiation is generally preferred. The role of radiation in colon cancer is controversial but has been used neoadjuvantly for locally advanced disease to allow resection.[91]

Paraneoplastic conditions result from immune and other chemical alterations induced by the cancer, affecting sites distant to the actual tumor. Those associated with lung cancer include the Lambert-Eaton myasthenic syndrome, demyelinating syndromes that can present as cancer-associated retinopathy (CAR) or encephalitis, as well as a hypercoagulable state (see above), often presenting with DVT or PE.

Neurological syndromes are uncommon, but when a patient at risk for lung cancer (usually a current or former smoker) presents with an otherwise unexplained retinopathy, neuromuscular or demyelinating condition, an evaluation for an underlying malignancy is a component of the evaluation (CAR is discussed later in the chapter). The Lambert-Eaton syndrome presents with muscle weakness, often seen in the proximal muscles of the extremities and manifesting as weakness climbing stairs or arising from a chair.

The diagnosis of lung cancer generally begins with an initial imaging study, often a chest x-ray or CT scan. Cross-sectional lung imaging, typically CT scan with or without PET scan, is employed to gauge the lesion and assess for metastatic disease. The brain is best assessed by cranial MRI when metastatic disease is a concern. Sequential lung CT scan imaging at 3- or 6-month intervals is employed in asymptomatic patients with screening-detected or an incidental finding of a very small lung lesion. Sequential scans assess for growth before an invasive procedure is done to obtain a tissue diagnosis. The use of PET scanning can add additional sensitivity to assessment of both primary cancers and metastatic disease. Tissue confirmation for suspicious lesions can be done via needle biopsy for peripheral lesions, endobronchial biopsy for airway lesions, or surgery with excisional biopsy or lobectomy for lesions that are not otherwise amenable to biopsy, often due to their location. For small malignant lesions without findings of lymphadenopathy or metastasis, excision may offer a reasonable chance of cure.

TREATMENT

Treatment of lung cancer depends upon the stage at diagnosis and the histology. When non–small cell cancer is localized in a patient able to proceed to surgery with low enough operative risk, then this is usually the best treatment option for long-term survival. Advances in understanding and treatment of cancer have enabled the molecular evaluation of tumor specimens. When so-called driver mutations are identified such as epidermal growth factor receptor (EGFR) or the anaplastic lymphoma kinase receptor (ALK), targeted therapies can be offered to these selected patients. In contrast, small cell lung cancer is most often advanced at diagnosis and it is uncommon that surgery is an option for treatment. Chemotherapy is used initially, with radiation added for local disease or for brain prophylaxis when chances of local treatment success are good. Immunotherapy, which simulates the body's immune system to attack cancer cells, has been found to be beneficial in lung cancer in patients with curable and metastatic disease.[99]

WILMS TUMOR

Wilms tumor (WT) is a malignant neoplasm of the kidney and there are approximately 500 new cases a year in the United States. The mean age at presentation is 2 to 3 years old. The most common presentation is an asymptomatic abdominal mass, but occasionally patients can have abdominal pain, hypertension, fever, or hematuria. The most common sites of spread are abdominal lymph nodes, lung, and liver.[100]

Most cases of Wilms tumor are sporadic, but approximately 15% of affected patients have a hereditary basis. *WT1* and *WT2* are two genes that are located on the short arm of chromosome 11. Mutations in these genes are associated with the development of several genetic syndromes. Given the rarity of this cancer, population-wide screening is not performed.

DIAGNOSIS

Wilms tumor most often presents with a renal mass; hematuria and secondary hypertension are less common modes of presentation.[101] It may also be diagnosed as part of the WAGR syndrome, consisting of Wilms tumor susceptibility, aniridia, genitourinary abnormalities, and developmental retardation. It is associated with a deletion in the *WT1* gene. Denys-Drash syndrome is linked to a point mutation on the *WT1* gene and can affect the development of the kidneys and genitalia. Beckwith-Wiedermann syndrome is linked to *WT2* and is associated with hypertrophy of isolated organs.[102]

The vast majority of Wilms tumors are considered to have favorable histology. Approximately 5% of Wilms tumor has anaplasia (either focal or diffuse), which confers a much worse prognosis. Additionally, clear cell and rhabdoid are variants with a poor prognosis.[103]

The evolution in the treatment of Wilms tumor represents the cooperation of many different oncologic specialties including pediatric oncologists, radiation oncologists, surgeons, and pathologists. In the United States, the National Wilms Tumor Study group and the Children's Oncology Group have conducted multiple landmark trials that have dramatically improved the survival in patients with this disease.

The staging system of WT is complex, but essentially, Stage I tumors are limited to the kidney and excised completely. Stage II tumors extend beyond the kidney and are also excised completely. In Stage III cases, there is residual disease after surgery due to either tumor that was unresectable or lymph node involvement. In Stage IV disease, there is distant spread to the liver or lung. Wilms tumor also has Stage V presentation, which is rare in the staging of cancers, which indicates bilateral renal involvement.

TREATMENT

Surgery and chemotherapy is a hallmark of treatment for all stages and histologies of Wilms tumor, except for low volume Stage I tumors which can be treated with surgery alone. In patients with favorable histology, radiation therapy to the tumor bed and abdomen is added for Stage III and IV patients and for Stage II patients with anaplastic, clear cell, and rhabdoid histologies. Although almost all patients receive chemotherapy, the regimens used become more aggressive (and therefore more toxic) as the stage and histology worsens. Vincristine and actinomycin-D are standard chemotherapies used.[104]

Stage I-III tumors with a favorable histology have a 4-year survival rate that ranges from 95% to 100%. Stage IV and V tumors with a favorable histology have a 4-year survival rate that ranges from 85% to 100%. Survival rates for tumors with focal anaplasia are lower and range from 70% to 95%. For tumors with a diffuse anaplastic histology, the survival rates range from 30% to 85% in different stage categories.[105]

OCULAR MANIFESTATIONS IN SYSTEMIC CANCER

Systemic cancer may affect the eye and visual system in several ways:

- Metastatic disease involving the globe, orbit, or efferent visual pathway
- Paraneoplastic disease involving the globe or efferent visual pathway
- Ophthalmologic side effects from systemic cancer treatment (discussed above)

Cancer Metastasis to the Globe, Orbit, and Efferent Visual Pathway

Cancer metastasis to the globe and orbit are uncommon, though important to recognize as they herald mortality. Uveal metastasis is more common than orbital metastasis and involves the choroid in a vast majority of cases (90%) and the iris (8%) and ciliary body (2%) in a minority. Choroidal, perimacular localization occurs most commonly because metastasis results from hematogenous spread, and the choroid (especially the foveal area) receives a majority of the overall blood flow to the globe.[106] A primary cancer diagnosis is usually already present or is quickly discovered with systemic workup; only 10% of cases do not reveal a primary tumor, and in these cases choroidal biopsy is an option. Breast cancer is the most common uveal metastasis (37%) followed by lung cancer (27%). Other cancers including renal, gastrointestinal, prostate, melanoma, and pancreatic are less common (<5% each). Uveal metastases are usually unilateral (80%) and lesions tend to be multiple in number (mean 1.7, range 1-29).[107] In the choroid, metastatic tumors of various primary type usually appear as deep foci of creamy, yellow infiltration, though orange and brown pigmentation is possible (the latter in cases of metastatic melanoma). It can be difficult to differentiate between primary and secondary choroidal melanoma; like all metastatic choroidal lesions, secondary melanoma often demonstrates a significant amount of subretinal fluid exudation in excess of lesion size, growth tends to be rapid (over weeks), and there may also be vitreous or multifocal retinal seeding, which are not typical features of primary melanoma (**FIGURE 8.26**). Fluorescein angiography shows late hyperfluorescence and ultrasonography shows echodensity (**FIGURE 8.27**). Subretinal fluid associated with metastatic choroidal lesions can lead to exudative retinal detachment (**FIGURE 8.28**), which creates a symptomatic decrease in visual acuity and/or positive visual phenomena, though many cases of choroidal metastasis are asymptomatic. Unfortunately, mean survival after diagnosis of uveal metastases is often less than 2 years. Treatment goals include improving visual acuity for best quality of life. Treatment options include observation, external beam radiation or brachytherapy, photodynamic therapy, intravitreal anti-VEGF, enucleation, and systemic chemotherapy.[67,68,106,107]

Metastatic tumors to the orbit constitute 1% to 13% of all orbital masses, and an estimated 2% to 3% of primary systemic cancer metastasizes to the orbit (**FIGURE 8.29**). More than 90% of cases occur unilaterally. Breast carcinoma (20%) is the most common to involve the orbit, followed by prostate (9%) and lung carcinoma (9%). Other cancer types such as gastrointestinal cancer, renal cancer, and melanoma are less common. Like uveal metastases, orbital metastases herald a poor prognosis and mean survival time after diagnosis of orbital metastasis is less than 2 years.[108] Symptoms most commonly include diplopia, palpable mass, pain, and proptosis or globe displacement. Enophthalmos is an unexpected sign which is characteristic for scirrhous breast cancer, a fibrotic tumor which causes contraction of orbital contents. Vision loss from optic nerve compression and gaze-evoked amaurosis are other possible symptoms with orbital metastases. In comparison with benign orbital tumors, symptom onset is abrupt. Signs may include ophthalmoplegia, ptosis, eyelid and/or conjunctival edema or congestion, resistance to retropulsion and/or a palpable mass, and relative afferent pupillary defect and optic nerve edema in cases of optic nerve compression. Contrast MRI of the orbit is the preferred imaging modality for most tumors though orbital CT can be helpful to demonstrate bone involvement in prostate cancer. Biopsy is indicated for tumor typing. Well-circumscribed orbital tumors may be amenable to complete excisional biopsy, while FNA is preferred for deeper or more infiltrative lesions. Tumors not amenable to surgical resection may respond to systemic chemotherapy and/or orbital radiation therapy.[69,108]

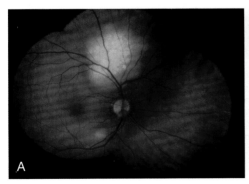 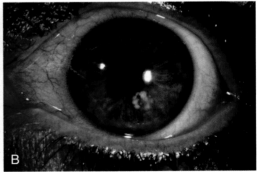

FIGURE 8.26 Choroidal (A) and iris (B) metastasis. A, Metastatic lung adenocarcinoma presenting as multifocal amelanotic choroidal lesions superior to the optic disc and in the inferonasal macula. Most choroidal metastases are amelanotic and occur posterior to the equator. They may be unifocal or multifocal. B, Small irregular iris metastasis from breast carcinoma. (A, From Fineman M. *Retina*. 3rd ed. Philadelphia, PA: Wolters Kluwer; 2018. B, From Shields JA, Shields CL. *Intraocular Tumors: An Atlas and Textbook*. 3rd ed. Philadelphia, PA: Wolters Kluwer; 2015.)

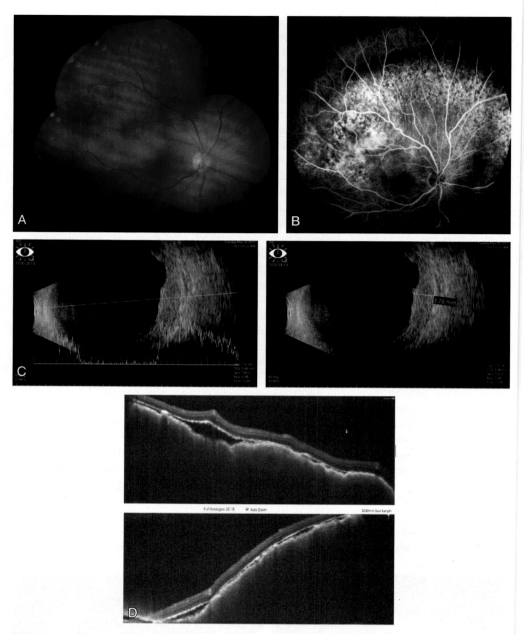

FIGURE 8.27 Choroidal metastasis. A 90-year-old woman developed (A) choroidal metastasis temporal to the macula. B, The fluorescein angiogram reveals diffuse retinal pigment epithelium (RPE) mottling without intrinsic vascularity to the tumor. C, Ultrasonography reveals a markedly thickened choroid on B-scan ultrasonography (left) and medium to high internal reflectivity on A-scan ultrasonography (right). D, Enhanced depth imaging optical coherence tomography shows a "lumpy bumpy" anterior tumor surface with overlying RPE atrophy. There is disruption of the ellipsoid zone. (Courtesy of Carol Shields, MD, Philadelphia PA USA.)

Since nearly every part of the brain is involved in vision in some way, metastatic cancer to the brain may impact the efferent visual pathway and create symptoms that present initially to an eye care specialist (**FIGURE 8.30**). Brain metastasis is usually diagnosed in the setting of a known cancer diagnosis, occurs in (overall) 20% to 30% of primary cancers, and heralds an unfavorable prognosis. Primary lung cancer is the most common tumor to metastasize to the brain, with lower incidences

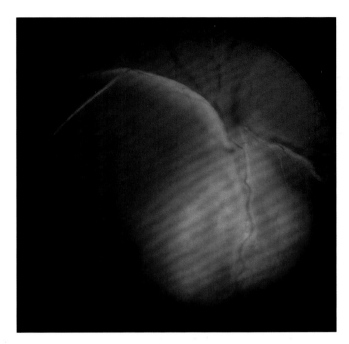

FIGURE 8.28 Choroidal metastasis from esophageal carcinoma. Note the extensive secondary retinal detachment that overlies the yellow tumor. (From Shields JA, Shields CL. *Intraocular Tumors: An Atlas and Textbook.* 3rd ed. Philadelphia, PA: Wolters Kluwer; 2015.)

reported for melanoma, breast, colorectal, and renal cancers, and even lower incidences for prostate cancer.[109] A majority of tumors (80%) develop in the cerebral hemispheres as opposed to the cerebellum (15%) and brainstem (5%); frontal and parietal lobe tumors are more common than temporal and occipital lobe tumors.[110] Large cell lung carcinoma may involve the occipital lobe more often than other cancer types.[111] Visual field loss (most commonly), diplopia, visual hallucinations, and visual perceptual disorders may all result and prompt patients to seek eye care. Eye examination may show signs of raised intracranial pressure, eye movement abnormalities, or nystagmus. Neuro-ophthalmological signs and symptoms in a patient with a history of cancer should raise strong suspicion for metastatic disease and prompt timely referral for neuroimaging (usually MRI with and without contrast) and systemic evaluation (Chapter 15).

Paraneoplastic Disease of the Globe and Efferent Visual Pathway

As mentioned previously, paraneoplastic syndromes result when a malignant neoplasm triggers an altered immune response and creates nonmetastatic disease effects elsewhere in the body. Patients may or may not carry an existing cancer diagnosis; in either scenario, the diagnosis of paraneoplasia is often challenging. Diagnosis may be aided in some cases by the presence of one or more paraneoplastic autoantibodies detectable in serum or CSF, though these are not always detected. Paraneoplastic disease of ocular tissues occurs in the form of CAR, melanoma-associated retinopathy (MAR), bilateral diffuse uveal melanocytic proliferation (BDUMP), and paraneoplastic optic neuropathy (PON).[112] CAR is the most common type and is discussed below. All of these conditions are rare. Other neurological paraneoplastic syndromes may involve the efferent visual pathways to create neuro-ophthalmological symptoms and signs including diplopia, ptosis, nystagmus, cranial nerve palsy, and deficits in pursuit and saccadic eye movements; examples include Eaton-Lambert myasthenic syndrome (mentioned previously), paraneoplastic opsoclonus-myoclonus syndrome, and paraneoplastic cerebellar degeneration.[113]

CAR is most often associated with small cell lung, breast, ovarian, endometrial, and cervical cancers, though many other cancer types have also been implicated. Paraneoplastic alterations in the immune system trigger autoantibodies which cross-react with retinal photoreceptors and result in outer retinal

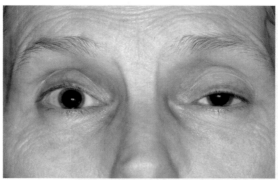

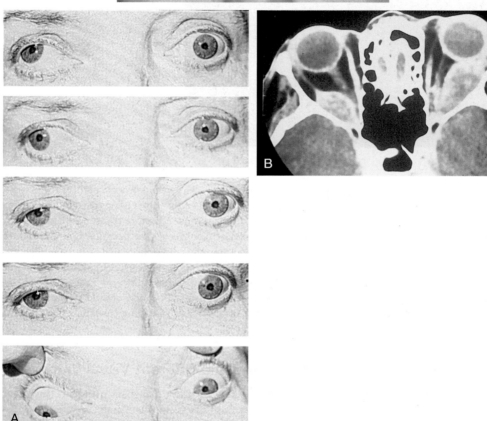

FIGURE 8.29 Orbital metastases. Top: Middle-aged woman with breast cancer metastasis to left orbit showing blepharoptosis of left upper eyelid and minimal proptosis. Bottom: A, There is exotropia in primary gaze (middle photograph) with globally decreased ductions. B, CT scan reveals masses in each orbit involving the lateral rectus muscles. (Top, From Shields JA, Shields CL. *Eyelid, Conjunctival, and Orbital Tumors: An Atlas and Textbook.* 3rd ed. Philadelphia, PA: Wolters Kluwer; 2015. A and B, From Savino P, Danesh-Meyer H. *Neuro-Ophthalmology.* 3rd ed. Philadelphia, PA: Wolters Kluwer; 2018.)

degeneration. Patients develop insidious onset loss of bilateral central vision over a period of months, along with dyschromatopsia, photopsias, light sensitivity, and impaired dark adaptation with nyctalopia. The retina often appears entirely normal on funduscopic examination though some cases may show retinal pigment epithelial disturbances or signs of intraocular inflammation (including anterior or posterior uveitis, cystoid macular edema, and retinal vasculitis). Multimodal retinal imaging is incredibly useful in diagnosis: optical coherence tomography reveals bilateral disruption of the outer retina with loss of photoreceptor inner-outer segments (**FIGURE 8.31**), and autofluorescent imaging shows a

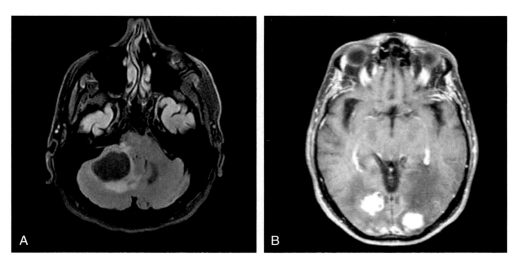

FIGURE 8.30 Cancer metastatic to the brain may present with visual symptoms. A, T2-weighted MRI of metastatic lung cancer to the right cerebellum with surrounding edema. A 64-year-old male with a history of NSCLC treated 1 year prior with carboplatin/taxol chemotherapy and radiation presented to the optometrist with blurry vision, double vision, and dizziness. Examination showed a right CN4 palsy and constant right-beating nystagmus worst on right gaze. Biopsy of the cerebellar mass demonstrated metastatic squamous carcinoma. B, MRI showing bilateral occipital lobe lesions from lung metastasis. A 67-year-old man complained of flashing lights lasting 15 minutes for 2 months. Visual fields showed a right homonymous defect with some involvement of the left homonymous field. (Figure credit: Rachel Druckenbrod, OD, VA Boston Healthcare System.)

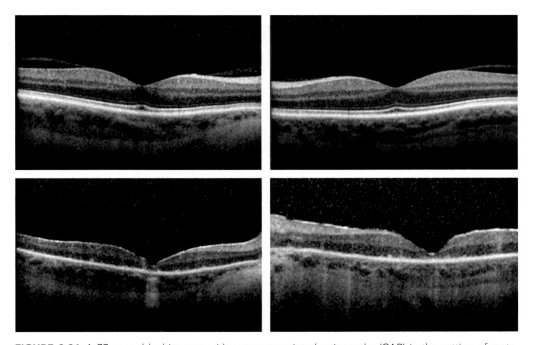

FIGURE 8.31 A 77-year-old white man with cancer-associated retinopathy (CAR) in the setting of metastatic anaplastic neuroendocrine tumor. The cancer diagnosis was made just days before death, several months after the onset of his visual symptoms. Vision declined from 20/25 to bare light perception OD and no light perception OS over a period of less than 6 months. Optical coherence tomography imaging of the maculae showed total absence of the photoreceptors bilaterally (bottom images) with normal anatomy on a routine scan several years earlier (top images). (Image credit: Dr Emily Carell, OD, VA Boston Healthcare System.)

ring of hyperautofluorescence involving the fovea. Electroretinogram testing shows global retinal dysfunction. A small majority (60%) of CAR patients will be seropositive for one or more autoantibodies against retinal proteins, including alpha-enolase (30%), recoverin (10%), transducin, and carbonic anhydrase II, among others. The diagnosis is otherwise one of exclusion and suspicion. Patients with suspected CAR should undergo an extensive investigation for cancer if a cancer diagnosis is not already present. Even when cancer is identified and treated, visual prognosis is guarded in CAR, though some evidence suggests benefit with immunosuppressive or immunomodulatory therapies such as systemic corticosteroids, azathioprine or mycophenolate mofetil, and rituximab.[73,74,112,113]

TALKING ABOUT CANCER

Discussions with patients about difficult topics such as cancer prognosis are challenging. Published studies as well as the author's (DS) own data confirm that these conversations occur too infrequently, leaving patients and families with limited advance notice regarding the risks and possible time frame for disease progression and death. Clear and forthright conversations about prognosis are critically important to help patients anticipate and plan around difficult times with advancing illness, progressive disability, and ultimately, death. Clinician education around initiating these difficult conversations is an important component of training and continuing education.

REFERENCES

1. Harris N. *The International Normalized Ratio: How Well Do We Understand This Measurement?* Washington, DC: AACC Scientific Shorts; 2012. https://www.aacc.org/community/aacc-academy/publications/scientific-shorts/2012/the-international-normalized-ratio-how-well-do-we-understand-this-measurement.

2. Camaschella C. Iron-deficiency anemia. *N Engl J Med.* 2015;372:1832-1843. doi:10.1056/NEJMra1401038.

3. https://ods.od.nih.gov/factsheets/VitaminB12-HealthProfessional/.

4. Stabler S. Vitamin B12 deficiency. *N Engl J Med* 2013;368:149-160. doi:10.1056/NEJMcp1113996.

5. Rodriguez NM, Shackelford KS. *Pernicious anemia.* In: *StatPearls.* Treasure Island, FL: StatPearls Publishing; 2019. https://www.ncbi.nlm.nih.gov/books/NBK540989/.

6. Vaggu SK, Bhogadi P. Bilateral macular hemorrhage due to megaloblastic anemia: a rare case report. *Indian J Ophthalmol.* 2016;64(2):157-159. doi:10.4103/0301-4738.179720.

7. Foulds WS, Chisholm IA, Stewart JB, Wilson TM. The optic neuropathy of pernicious anemia. *Arch Ophthalmol.* 1969;82(4):427-432. doi:10.1001/archopht.1969.00990020429001.

8. Chavala SH, Kosmorsky GS, Lee MK, Lee MS. Optic neuropathy in vitamin B12 deficiency. *Eur J Intern Med.* 2005;16(6):447-448.

9. Turkyilmaz K, Oner V, Turkyilmaz AK, et al. Evaluation of peripapillary retinal nerve fiber layer thickness in patients with vitamin B12 deficiency using spectral domain optical coherence tomography. *Curr Eye Res.* 2013;38(6):680-684.

10. Pineles SL, Bacler LJ. *Optic neuropathies.* In: *Liu, Volpe, and Galleta's Neuro-Ophthalmology.* 3rd ed. China: Elsevier; 2018:176-177.

11. Anand OP, Choudhary SK, Gupta S. Vitamin B12 deficiency induced optic neuropathy. *Digit J Ophthalmol.* 2019;29:125-126.

12. Piel FB, Steinberg MH, Rees DC. Sickle cell disease. *N Engl J Med.* 2017;376:1561-1573. doi:10.1056/NEJMra1510865.

13. Nelson DA, Deuster PA, Carter R, Hill OT, Wolcott VL, Kurina LM. Sickle cell trait, rhabdomyolysis, and mortality among U.S. Army soldiers. *N Engl J Med.* 2016;375:435-442. doi:10.1056/NEJMoa1516257.

14. Naik RP, Derebail VK, Grams ME, et al. Association of sickle cell trait with chronic kidney disease and albuminuria in African Americans. *J Am Med Assoc.* 2014;312(20):2115-2125. doi:10.1001/jama.2014.15063.

15. Hasan SP, Hashmi S, Alhassen M, Lawson W, Castro O. Depression in sickle cell disease. *J Natl Med Assoc.* 2003;95(7):533-537.

16. Vichinsky EP. Overview of the clinical manifestations of sickle cell disease. Debaum NR, Tirnauer JS, eds. *UpToDate.* Waltham, MA: UptoDate Inc. Accessed on December 22, 2019. https://www.uptodate.com.

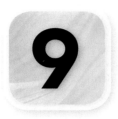

9

Infectious Diseases

David M. Shein and Rachel C. Druckenbrod

Infectious diseases have always been a threat to human health; with the approval of antibiotics in the 1940s, antivirals in the 1960s, and antifungals in the 1970s, effective therapies are now available for many infections. In addition to reductions in death from infectious diseases, advances in many other areas of medicine allow for longer life while contributing to a population with a higher burden of disease and risks for more serious infections. An understanding of infections that affect the eye, periocular structures, and the body as a whole will better position the optometrist to screen, diagnose, and manage a broad range of ocular and periocular diseases.

This chapter is divided into two sections: Section 1, Clinical Syndromes, explores important diagnoses and focuses on select pathogens. Section 2, Infectious Agents, focuses on important pathogens that often contribute to multisystem disease. Chapter 10 also covers many of these pathogens, but with a focus on manifestations and evaluation in the setting of HIV infection.

Clinical syndromes
   Pneumonia and pneumonitis
   Sinusitis
   Cellulitis
   Meningitis and encephalitis
   Hepatitis
   Sepsis
Pathogens
   Tuberculosis
   Herpes simplex virus type 1 and 2

Varicella-zoster virus
Cytomegalovirus
Human herpesvirus 8
Molluscum contagiosum
Toxoplasmosis
Candidiasis
Cat scratch disease
Rubella
Lyme disease
Syphilis

SECTION 1
CLINICAL SYNDROMES

By separating the diagnosis of a clinical syndrome from its cause, clinicians can avoid anchoring bias, which occurs when a diagnosis is made before adequate data are collected. For example, because conjunctivitis is often associated with infectious bacterial causes, many urgent care presentations with pink eye yield a topical antibiotic ointment prescription after a summary assessment without much data gathering. Because community-acquired infectious conjunctivitis is most often a self-limited viral infection (for which antibiotics offer no benefit), despite an incorrect diagnosis and ineffective treatment, the symptoms do resolve, and the outcome is unaffected. Clinicians thus continue to practice with the same anchoring bias, and occasionally, other important causes of conjunctivitis that need specific therapy may be overlooked. By considering the clinical syndrome apart from typical triggers, the clinician can conduct an appropriate history, examination, and data collection, apply advanced decision-making, and formulate a thorough differential diagnosis. This process will ultimately lead to a higher likelihood of arriving at the correct diagnosis. In this chapter, after considering common clinical syndromes and their differential diagnosis, common pathogens for the syndromes will be reviewed.

PNEUMONIA AND PNEUMONITIS

Inflammatory conditions involving the lungs may be infectious or triggered by other exposures. Although inflammation is most often the result of an infectious agent causing the clinical syndrome of *pneumonia*, a noninfectious *pneumonitis* can be caused by inhalation of chemicals such as chlorine gas. Aspiration of oral contents may result in a combination of chemical pneumonitis and bacterial pneumonia, often with oral anaerobic bacteria.

Patients with pneumonia develop inflammation of the lung parenchyma, which results in exudation of fluid and inflammatory cells into the alveoli, impairing gas exchange and resulting in pulmonary symptoms, most often cough, with shortness of breath or dyspnea in more severe cases, along with hypoxia. Pneumonia is usually accompanied by a clinical syndrome consistent with the systemic infection including fevers, chills, sweats, fatigue, and malaise.

Risk factors for pneumonia include impaired immunity as can occur with infections such as HIV (Chapter 10), with immunosuppression after organ transplants or cancer chemotherapy (Chapter 8). Diabetes (Chapter 5) and underlying lung diseases such as chronic obstructive pulmonary disease (COPD) (Chapter 14) are also risk factors for pneumonia. Impaired host mechanical defenses can occur with neurologic conditions; stroke, for example, may impair the gag reflex or swallowing function and increase the risk for aspiration of oral contents. Smoking and other toxic inhalations impair mucociliary clearance of inhaled pathogens and irritants. Impaired ventilation is also a risk, as can occur with chest wall injuries, after chest surgery, and in areas of the lung with localized airway obstruction from a lung mass. Bacterial pneumonia can also occur secondarily after other infections; this is a significant risk factor associated with influenza virus infection. Increasing age is also a risk factor for pneumonia.

Pneumonia can occur in several settings, and the potential pathogens and approach to treatment will differ. Community-acquired pneumonia describes pneumonia in a community-dwelling individual, whether they are healthy at baseline, or have a chronic illness. Nosocomial pneumonia is acquired in association with a current or recent stay in a healthcare setting, such as hospitals or nursing homes. Aspiration pneumonia occurs from inhaling oral contents; as described earlier, it occurs in patients with impaired swallowing in neurological diseases, impaired consciousness from intoxication or acute medical illness such as a seizure; or as a complication of anesthesia administration. Pneumonia in an immunocompromised host requires consideration of a wide array of pathogens and warrants an extended workup and broad-spectrum initial therapy.

The syndrome of bronchitis is commonly diagnosed but differs from pneumonia in several important ways. Bronchitis represents airway inflammation and irritation, and a lingering cough diagnosed as bronchitis may even be postinfectious. In contrast, pneumonia represents inflammation and infection of the lung parenchyma. Symptoms of bronchitis often overlap with pneumonia, especially cough; however, bronchitis is rarely accompanied by a high fever (low-grade elevation or normal temperature is typical), and while patients with bronchitis may develop mild malaise, they are

FIGURE 9.3 Schematic of sinuses. (Asset Provided by Anatomical Chart Co.)

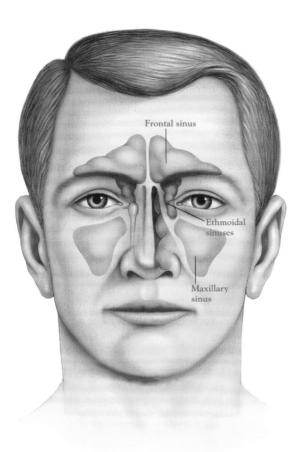

Frontal sinus

Ethmoidal sinuses

Maxillary sinus

On examination, the typical patient with sinusitis appears only minimally ill. Coryza may be present, with watery rhinitis, which is typically seen with viral and allergic triggers. Bacterial sinusitis may be accompanied by purulent nasal discharge. Tenderness over maxillary or facial sinus regions can be present with more significant inflammation. Rarely, facial erythema can be seen and may be an indication of a complication such as cellulitis. One feature that may help differentiate viral and allergic from bacterial causes (which may warrant treatment with antibiotics) is lateralizing symptoms. Bilateral symptoms are more typical of viral and allergic causes; unilateral facial pain or tenderness along with purulent nasal discharge is more suggestive of a bacterial cause.

The vast majority of acute, infectious rhinosinusitis episodes will be self-limited and resolve without specific therapy within 7 to 10 days. Most are caused by viral infections, for which antibacterial antibiotics are not useful. However, even for the subset of immunocompetent patients with acute rhinosinusitis triggered by pathogens that may be sensitive to antibacterial antibiotics, studies consistently demonstrate that the majority of these infectious will resolve on their own with time.[8-10] Unfortunately, in clinical practice antibiotics are commonly prescribed for conditions such as this in which they have no utility, exposing patients to the adverse effects without the opportunity for benefit, and contributing to the increase in antibiotic resistance.[11] Symptomatic management should include over-the-counter analgesia with acetaminophen or a low- to moderate-dose nonsteroidal anti-inflammatory drug (NSAID) (eg, naproxen 220 mg one or two times daily, ibuprofen 200-400 mg up to three times daily) and nasal saline irrigation. Topical nasal glucocorticoids such as fluticasone nasal spray can also be recommended for symptomatic relief. Intranasal decongestants such as oxymetazoline are sold over the counter and often used by patients. However, caution is advised because more than 3 days of use can trigger dependence and rebound nasal mucosal edema when the drug is stopped. The oral decongestant pseudoephedrine may also help with symptomatic relief, but as a stimulant, the systemic side effects limit their use in patients with hypertension, cardiovascular disease, tremors, and anxiety disorders. In addition, for some patients, they trigger urinary retention and should be avoided. The stimulant effect can impact sleep, and evening use is best avoided. Antihistamines have not been demonstrated to offer benefits in infectious sinusitis, although sedating first-generation antihistamines are often included in multisymptom cold and flu medications sold over the counter. Many physicians discourage the use of these mixed multisymptom medications, because the combination of medications increases the likelihood of side effects and drug interactions.

For subacute sinusitis, and for patients with bacterial rhinosinusitis symptoms that linger beyond 10 days, treatment for an underlying bacterial infection is considered, especially when accompanied by fevers, chills, or a so-called double sickening. This refers to initial clinical improvement from an upper respiratory viral illness (such as rhinosinusitis), followed by clinical worsening, often accompanied by a fever, suggesting a secondary bacterial infection. Patients with recurrent bacterial sinusitis may also benefit from earlier consideration of antibiotic treatment. Coverage is aimed at *Streptococcus* species, *Haemophilus influenzae,* and *Moraxella catarrhalis,* the most common pathogens.

Allergic sinusitis is often seasonal or may be related to indoor allergens or exposures at work or other settings (Chapter 14). Systemic nonsedating antihistamines and topical nasal glucocorticoids can be helpful in management. First-generation sedating antihistamines like diphenhydramine are best avoided due to the risk for sedation and impairment in motor function such as driving. When accompanied by asthma or other allergic symptoms, a more detailed evaluation and comprehensive treatment may be required.

Chronic rhinosinusitis is often related to an underlying chronic condition, and more detailed evaluation, including referral to an appropriate specialist, may be appropriate.

Complications of acute and subacute sinusitis are rare but can occur. Major complications include orbital cellulitis, preseptal cellulitis, and meningitis (all are discussed below).

CELLULITIS

Cellulitis is an infection of the dermis and subcutaneous fat. Although the appearance of a skin rash is typical, topical treatments are ineffective, and initial use can delay appropriate systemic treatment. Cellulitis can be invasive and may progress rapidly if untreated.

The most important risk factor for the development of cellulitis is impairment in the normal integumentary barrier. Intact skin plays a critical role in keeping bacteria out of the dermis. Although some episodes of cellulitis result from known, high-risk events such as animal bites or lacerations, cellulitis can also develop from skin breaks seen with underlying tinea pedis or small injuries such as splinters. Chronic dry and cracking skin can also result in bacterial entry and the development of cellulitis. Poor lymphatic drainage is also a risk factor, as might occur after axillary lymph node dissection as part of surgical treatment for breast cancer. Impaired host defenses also contribute to cellulitis development and progression. This includes mild impairment from diabetes, vascular disease with poor circulation, significant immune impairment with infections like HIV, and treatments like cancer chemotherapy, immune suppression after organ transplantation, and chronic glucocorticoid use for inflammatory diseases.

Symptoms typically develop over the course of several days, although infections with invasive pathogens may progress over just a few hours. Systemic symptoms such as fevers and chills require prompt evaluation and initiation of therapy.

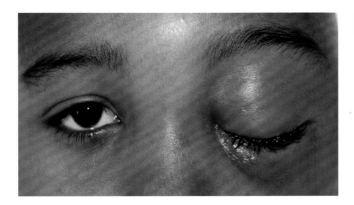

FIGURE 9.4 Orbital cellulitis. (Courtesy of Scott Goldstein, MD.)

The examination in patients with cellulitis is typically marked by skin erythema, increased warmth, and local swelling. Regional lymph nodes may also be enlarged and tender (for example, axillary nodes in upper extremity cellulitis or inguinal lymph nodes in lower extremity cellulitis). Proximal extension of the erythema along lymphatic channels, also sometimes called streaking erythema, is a very concerning finding and requires prompt initiation of antibiotic therapy when present.

Cellulitis most commonly occurs on the lower extremity, although any other region of the skin may be involved. Two specific syndromes that are especially relevant to the optometrist include preseptal and orbital cellulitis.

In preseptal cellulitis, the infection is superficial and there are no ocular symptoms or findings on examination. Systemic treatment and observation are appropriate, typically with oral antibiotics and outpatient follow-up.

In contrast, orbital cellulitis is a potentially serious deep infection and is both sight threatening and life threatening (**FIGURE 9.4**) (Chapter 15). Ocular symptoms may develop due to direct infection or compression due to adjacent inflammation. Orbital pain, extraocular muscle impairment resulting in diplopia, and vision impairment in more severe cases can be present. Management includes immediate initiation of intravenous antibiotics, and patients are often observed in a hospital setting initially. Imaging with CT or MRI may also be pursued to define the degree of anatomic involvement, assess for bone involvement with osteomyelitis, and exclude complications (such as abscess), comorbid conditions (such as a tumor), and monitor therapy.

Cellulitis is typically caused by common gram-positive skin colonizers including species of *Streptococcus* and *Staphylococcus*.[12] Specific risk factors such as occupational, lifestyle, or animal exposures can result in infection with other, less common pathogens. For example, cat and other animal bites often introduce the gram-negative *Pasteurella multocida*. Fishing and harvesting clams, for example, are associated with infection by *Vibrio*[13] species. Thus, a thorough history is important to guide assessment and treatment.

Staphylococci are gram-positive bacteria that grow in clusters (**FIGURE 9.5**); several species cause infections in humans, including *S. aureus* that produces a coagulase enzyme. Species that do not produce coagulase are grouped together as coagulase-negative staph; several of these species colonize the skin and may become pathogens, though typically only in patients with impaired immunity or foreign objects like long-term catheters or prosthetic joints. Antibiotic resistance among staphylococci is a serious public health problem, especially in patients previously exposed to antibiotics and those with recent encounters in healthcare settings, such as hospitalizations. However, community spread of resistant strains has been recognized, and this is becoming an increasingly serious problem with mounting antibiotic resistance.[14] Resistance to methicillin, an extended-spectrum penicillin with activity against susceptible staphylococci, has been recognized

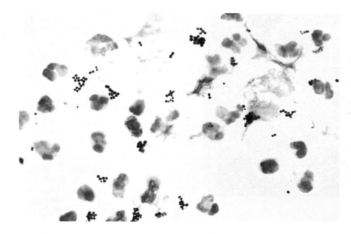

FIGURE 9.5 Clusters of *Staphylococcus* bacteria seen on tissue Gram stain. (Reprinted with permission from McClatchey KD. *Clinical Laboratory Medicine*. 2nd ed. Philadelphia, PA: Lippincott Williams & Wilkins; 2002.)

in association with hospital exposure and is commonly known as MRSA (methicillin-resistant *Staphylococcus aureus*). In cases of MRSA, vancomycin is often used; however, vancomycin resistance has been documented. Adherence to antibiotic prescribing guidelines is the most important tool to combat resistance. This includes avoiding antibiotics when unnecessary and using narrow-spectrum drugs whenever possible. This approach is also commonly cost-effective, because older, generic antibiotics are often less costly.

Treatment of cellulitis typically begins with empiric therapy once the infection is recognized. Clinical considerations including immune status, location of the infection, and recent exposures such as hospitalization, animal bites, dental procedures (especially those involving the upper teeth and superior alveolar ridge), occupation, hobbies, and travel. MRSA, *Pasteurella*, *Vibrio*, and other less common and potentially severe pathogens must be covered with initial therapy when a history compatible with significant exposure is present. Unless an abscess or other source of purulent drainage is present, or the infection is severe enough to warrant a biopsy, a culture of cellulitis typically will not yield a pathogen. Careful initial clinical assessment and ongoing monitoring in the management of severe or complicated cases (for example, orbital cellulitis) is necessary.

Cellulitis treatment requires systemic antibiotics. Most cases are mild and amenable to outpatient treatment with oral antibiotics, limb elevation, and medical follow-up. More severe cases, such as with streaking erythema, orbital cellulitis, and in some patients with immune compromise, intravenous therapy may be initiated with initial observation in the hospital to assess for clinical response. Very severe cases of cellulitis with progression to fasciitis can occur due to bacteria that produce toxins or gas that triggers swelling and circulatory impairment. Surgery may be necessary for drainage and debridement.

MENINGITIS AND ENCEPHALITIS

Two clinical syndromes that involve the central nervous system include meningitis and encephalitis. Although the two can be differentiated, there is also considerable overlap and patients are sometimes diagnosed with meningoencephalitis.

Meningitis reflects inflammation of the meninges, the tissues that surround the brain and spinal cord (**FIGURE 9.6**). Inflammation can occur due to a range of causes; infectious bacterial meningitis is probably considered most often; however, aseptic meningitis can occur due to viruses or drug reactions, and some cancers can cause carcinomatous meningitis.

Hallmark symptoms of meningitis are fever, headache, and nuchal rigidity (stiff neck). Although not all patients will have all three symptoms, many have at least two, and in the absence of any of

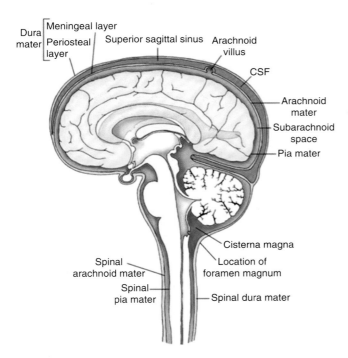

Dura mater {
Meningeal layer
Periosteal layer
}   Superior sagittal sinus   Arachnoid villus

CSF

Arachnoid mater

Subarachnoid space

Pia mater

Cisterna magna

Spinal arachnoid mater

Location of foramen magnum

Spinal pia mater

Spinal dura mater

FIGURE 9.6 Image of meninges, demonstrating the layers of the meninges and surrounding structures. The meninges surround the brain and spinal cord. *CSF*, cerebrospinal fluid. (From Gould DJ. *Lippincott's Pocket Neuroanatomy.* Philadelphia, PA: Wolters Kluwer; 2013.)

them, a diagnosis of meningitis is unlikely.[15] A change in mental statuses such as confusion, lethargy, or coma can also occur. With bacterial causes, rashes may also be present. Meningitis can be a community-acquired or a healthcare-associated infection.

In contrast to meningitis, encephalitis involves brain tissue inflammation and is accompanied by focal neurological deficits such as speech or motor impairment, ataxia, or seizure. Although meningitis also can impact mental status, these effects are usually related to sensorium, such as lethargy or coma, rather than the focal deficits of encephalitis. Seizures, however, can also occur with both encephalitis and meningitis. Encephalitis is more often viral as compared to meningitis, and viruses can cause both active infections as well as postinfectious syndromes with demyelination after the resolution of the active infection. Some cancers cause a paraneoplastic syndrome that manifests as encephalitis.

Patients presenting with meningitis are likely to be identified as having a significant illness. In addition to high fever, which is typical in infectious cases, the headache, which is generally diffuse, can be significant. A stiff neck with limited motion due to meningeal irritation can be assessed by having the patient flex the neck (chin to chest). Signs of other bacterial infection such as sinusitis or otitis media (middle ear infections) may be present, though these are uncommon triggers and the vast majority of sinusitis and otitis media do not result in severe complications such as meningitis. The presence of a rash is consistent with a bacterial cause, especially *Neisseria meningitidis* (see below). Seizures can occur in patients with acute meningitis from any cause.

Papilledema may occur from meningitis, encephalitis, and meningoencephalitis due to viral, bacterial, and other pathogens. The incidence ranges from 2% to 25%, with the lowest reported incidence among cases of viral/aseptic meningitis, and the highest incidence associated with tuberculosis meningitis.[16-18] Papilledema is uncommon with meningitis due to varicella, mumps, and rubella.[19] Papilledema in the setting of meningitis and encephalitis usually occurs secondary to diffuse cerebral edema. When intracranial pressure is normal, but the optic discs appear swollen, other infectious mechanisms are more likely, such as direct optic nerve infiltration or immune-mediated

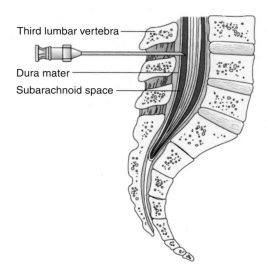

Third lumbar vertebra

Dura mater

Subarachnoid space

FIGURE 9.7 Lumbar puncture: A spinal needle is inserted between lumbar vertebrae to obtain a sample of cerebrospinal fluid (CSF) for clinical evaluation. Assessment of the opening pressure is done first in cases of suspected intracranial hypertension. (From Nath JL. *Short Course in Medical Terminology.* 4th ed. Philadelphia, PA: Wolters Kluwer; 2018.)

inflammation.[20] Papilledema in meningitis/encephalitis is often mild and transient, especially in aseptic cases, and resolves with resolution of cerebral edema. If optic atrophy occurs due to especially severe or prolonged papilledema, patients can develop permanent vision loss.

Lumbar puncture is the key diagnostic procedure for confirming the diagnosis and determining the cause (**FIGURE 9.7**). Leukocytes in the CSF, along with low glucose and elevated protein, are consistent with a bacterial cause. Gram stain and culture of the cerebrospinal fluid should be done to guide therapy. However, due to the severity of meningitis, treatment with empiric antibiotics should be initiated immediately. Viral meningitis or encephalitis will typically have fewer white blood cells in the CSF as compared to bacterial meningitis. Specific tests for viral pathogens can be performed in the laboratory if suspicion is high. In cases of encephalitis, brain imaging is typically performed to exclude tumor or infection and identify a pattern that may assist with the diagnosis. Aseptic meningitis related to medication use can be clarified by history, although a full evaluation for infectious causes should be initiated, and often empiric antibacterial antibiotic therapy is initiated as well, until a bacterial cause is excluded. Cancer cells in the CSF or other findings that are suspicious for the presence of malignancy should prompt an immediate consultation with a cancer specialist.

Rapid identification of meningitis is critical to the prompt initiation of effective treatment. Timely treatment should occur in parallel with appropriate diagnostics, most importantly lumbar puncture (LP). When there is evidence of increased intracranial pressure (for example, papilledema on examination), CT scanning may first be necessary to assess for imaging evidence of an intracranial lesion as the cause. Removing CSF via LP in the setting of increased intracranial pressure will lower spinal pressure resulting in downward pressure on the brain, resulting in a risk of herniation. When imaging and decision-making take up valuable time in the early assessment of a possible case of acute meningitis, there is consensus that initiation of treatment should not be delayed as this increases the risk of adverse outcomes.[21] Empiric therapy for meningitis includes broad-spectrum antibiotics until a cause can be identified; treatment is then completed with an appropriate narrow-spectrum drug. Viral causes of meningitis and encephalitis often cannot be treated directly, thus supportive measures are provided as necessary. Exceptions include herpes simplex encephalitis, which often involves the temporal lobe and imaging as well as diagnostic testing can assist in the diagnosis. HIV can cause encephalitis, although typically at a late stage of illness, and the diagnosis can only be confirmed after excluding a wide differential diagnosis of opportunistic infections and other causes (Chapter 10). In both of these situations, specific antiviral treatments should be initiated. Noninfectious triggers should be addressed with the removal of any drugs that may be a trigger; cancers are treated as appropriate for the tumor type and clinical stage in consultation with cancer specialists.

The prognosis for meningitis depends upon the cause, but given the severity of the clinical syndrome, the prognosis may be poor. Bacterial meningitis has a fatality rate of about 20% despite treatment, and much higher untreated.[10,15] Even for survivors, persistent neurological impairment can occur, most often hearing loss. For other infections, outcomes depend upon the underlying cause. For herpes encephalitis, the prognosis is poor despite appropriate therapy.[22] HIV encephalitis occurs less often today as antiretroviral treatments have improved, yet for patients who develop this complication, timely initiation of effective treatment has been reported to result in a favorable outcome.[23]

Most episodes of community-acquired bacterial meningitis are caused by *S. pneumoniae* or *N. meningitidis*.[10] A less common cause, but a condition worthy of consideration in specific cases is *Listeria monocytogenes*.

N. meningitidis is a gram-negative diplococcus for which humans are the only reservoir. People can carry *N. meningitidis* in the nasopharynx without being infected; however, nasopharyngeal carriage is associated with higher risks for infection. During *N. meningitidis* epidemics, the proportion of the population with asymptomatic nasopharyngeal carriage is increased. The bacterium is spread through close contact, including close living situations, kissing, and through respiratory secretions. In addition to meningitis, *N. meningitidis* can also cause bacteremia, either alone or with meningitis.

Community risk for *N. meningitidis* can be endemic or epidemic. In regions of endemic infection such as the United States, outbreaks can occur, for example, in college dorms. However, due to widespread vaccination against the more common infectious causes (including *S. pneumoniae* and *N. meningitidis*), the overall rate of bacterial meningitis in the United States has been on the decline.[24,25] Epidemic spread can result in population rates of infection as high as 1 per 10,000. In regions of sub-Saharan Africa where meningitis can be epidemic, approximately 30,000 people die annually from this disease.[26]

The risk of infection is associated with the following:

Nasopharyngeal carriage of the bacterium
Close contact with infected individuals (family members, roommates, intimate partners)
Close living situations (college dorms, military barracks)
Geographic risks (so-called meningitis belt in Africa[27]) (**FIGURE 9.8**)
Travel risks (Islamic Haaj in Mecca)
Immune deficiency (including complement deficiency)

Identification of individuals at risk is an important first step to prevention. Both pneumococcal and meningococcal vaccines are routinely recommended for children in the United States, and a review of vaccine status with appropriate updates to vaccination is typical before entry into college, military service, or high-risk travel. Cases of bacterial meningitis are evaluated by public health authorities in the United States, and antibiotic prophylaxis is recommended to contacts of cases when appropriate.

L. monocytogenes is a less frequent cause of both bacterial meningitis and encephalitis,[28] but due to its association with foodborne illness, it is an important public health consideration. *Listeria* are gram-positive rods and are found in decaying organic matter and in sewage. *Listeria* can survive refrigeration, and outbreaks have been reported in association with processed meat and unpasteurized dairy products. Commercial food outbreaks typically result in product recalls to limit additional exposures. Clinical symptoms can include gastroenteritis and meningoencephalitis. Pregnant women are at higher risk for complications including fetal loss if exposed to *Listeria*. The common advice to avoid unpasteurized milk during pregnancy is in part to minimize the risk of *Listeria* exposure. People with immune disorders are also at risk.

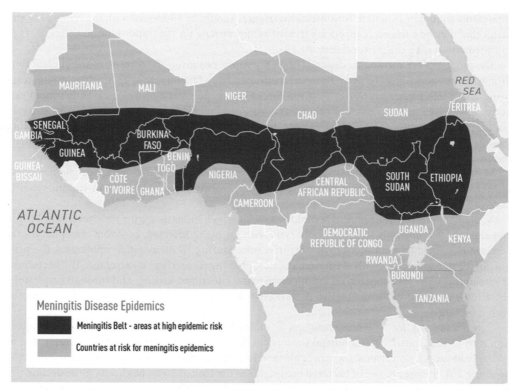

FIGURE 9.8 Meningitis Belt and region of high meningitis risk in central Africa. (Centers for Disease Control and Prevention. *CDC Yellow Book 2020: Health Information for International Travel.* New York: Oxford University Press; 2017. Centers for Disease Control and Prevention. CDC Yellow Book 2020: Health Information for International Travel. New York: Oxford University Press; 2017.)

Cryptococcus neoformans and *Cryptococcus gatii are* opportunistic yeast found in pigeon or chicken dropping as well as rotting vegetation and soil. As a pathogen, *Cryptococcus* species affect people with cell-mediated immune impairment. Since the 1980s, clinical infections have been seen most commonly in people with advanced HIV (Chapter 10). Patients on immunosuppressive medications, particularly after solid organ transplants, are also at risk.

In addition to meningitis, *Cryptococcus* can also cause ocular, dermatological, and pulmonary disease. Visual dysfunction is an unfortunate but relatively frequent occurrence with cryptococcal infection especially in the setting of HIV, reported to occur in as many as 47% of patients with meningitis.[22] Ocular signs and symptoms with *Cryptococcus* include papilledema from raised intracranial pressure (most commonly); ophthalmoplegia/diplopia due to cranial neuropathy of cranial nerves 3, 4, or 6; uveitis and retinochoroiditis caused by endogenous endophthalmitis; and/or optic neuropathy or chiasmopathy due to direct fungal invasion or immune-mediated mechanisms. Visual prognosis can be very poor, and ophthalmic involvement is often a sign of disseminated disease, with poor prognosis overall.

Pulmonary cryptococcus can cause pneumonia, and dermatological involvement results in a rash, often accompanied by fever. Dermatologic presentations vary, from lesions that appear like cellulitis, to raised skin lesions including nodules.[29] *Cryptococcus* is an important consideration in the differential diagnosis for skin lesions in immunosuppressed patients, especially when fevers are present.

Criteria have been defined to identify patients with sepsis and deliver timely, comprehensive care. The quickest assessment is the qSOFA (quick sequential organ failure assessment) that assesses three areas in patients with a serious infection that may have progressed to sepsis.

- Respiratory rate >22
- Impairment in mental state
- Systolic blood pressure <100 mm Hg

Patients meeting two or all three criteria are at risk for having sepsis and require further clinical assessment.

A thorough clinical examination is necessary, including assessment of brain perfusion with mental status assessment, along with attention to possible sites of infection including lungs, skin, central nervous system, heart valves, GI system, urinary, and genital tracts. Laboratory assessment includes complete blood count, kidney and liver function, electrolyte and lactate levels, cultures from regions of potential infection, and a chest x-ray. Other tests and imaging studies are performed as guided by the patient's history and clinical findings. Treatment of sepsis varies depending upon the trigger and severity, and includes prompt treatment of the inciting infection and initiation of intravenous fluids to counter hypotension. Care for patients with sepsis is often delivered in bundles to assure a comprehensive approach to the complex and often very ill patient with sepsis.

Although the prognosis for patients with sepsis has improved over the past few decades, mortality, especially from severe sepsis remains high; thus, prompt diagnosis and aggressive treatments are critical for survival.

SECTION 2
PATHOGENS

LEARNING OBJECTIVES

This section will focus on important bacterial, fungal, and viral pathogens in human disease. The spectrum of clinical disease for each of these includes ocular infection, making these pathogens important for the optometrist to consider in the differential diagnosis when appropriate.

TUBERCULOSIS

Mycobacterium tuberculosis (MTB) is an aerobic, rod-shaped bacterial pathogen. Tuberculosis (TB) primarily infects humans, and infected people are responsible for ongoing transmission. TB can exist in latent and active forms. In contrast to active TB, patients with latent TB infection are asymptomatic and have no evidence of active disease. Latent TB is not infectious; however, it can reactivate later in life or with immunocompromise. The World Health Organization estimates that one-third of the world population is infected with latent tuberculosis. Tuberculosis is one of the ten most common causes of death worldwide, responsible for an estimated 10 million deaths annually. Fortunately, that statistic is falling, with a drop of about 40% in deaths over the past 2 decades. In contrast, multidrug resistance is a growing problem, and the burden of TB in HIV-infected individuals remains a challenging public health concern[40] (Chapter 10). Tuberculosis rates vary in different regions of the globe, with the highest rates seen in southern Africa, India, and Southeast Asia.[41] In the United States, there are about 9000 active cases of TB reported annually while about 13 million people are living with the disease.[42] Most cases of active TB in the United States are imported, as the individual acquired the infection overseas and the disease activated while in the United States. Homelessness and incarceration are also risk factors for TB.

The cell wall of organisms in the *Mycobacterium* genus stains variably with Gram stain and thus is not generally characterized as either gram negative or positive. The cell wall is resistant to dye removal during the acidic or ethanolic wash with gram staining; hence, different stains are used when mycobacteria are suspected. The most common of these acid-fast stains include Ziehl-Neelsen or auramine. Auramine staining has higher sensitivity but requires access to fluorescence microscopy. Both will identify mycobacterial species, and this characteristic confers the alternate name acid-fast bacillus, or AFB. As a slow-growing bacterium, it may take weeks for the pathogen to be diagnosed on routine culture media. Newer techniques for culture and identification, such as liquid media and nucleic acid amplification via polymerase chain reaction (PCR), can expedite the confirmation of the tuberculosis diagnosis when present. As an aerobic bacterium, MTB has a propensity to cause pulmonary infections (**FIGURE 9.9**).

On tissue biopsy, tuberculosis and other mycobacterial infections are characterized by granuloma formation. As sarcoidosis frequently affects the lungs and also forms granulomas, identification of *M. tuberculosis* in the specimen or on culture is critical for making a correct diagnosis when mycobacterial infection is present. Distinction between the granulomas of tuberculosis and those of sarcoid can often be made based on the fact that the granulomas of TB usually exhibit caseation necrosis at their core, whereas the granulomas of sarcoid are noncaseating.

Pulmonary TB, which represents more than half of cases, results in cough, which aerosolizes the bacteria; inhalation is the dominant mode of transmission. Exposure of a healthy individual to a person infected with pulmonary TB results in an approximately 25% risk of infection. After transmission, primary infection can occur with a full-blown infection at the time of the initial exposure.

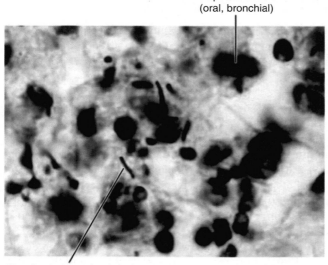

Sputum cells
(oral, bronchial)

Mycobacterium tuberculosis

FIGURE 9.9 Sputum specimen with bronchial cells and a gram-positive staining *Mycobacterium tuberculosis* bacterium. (Reprinted with permission from Creason C. *Stedman's Medical Terminology*. Philadelphia, PA: Wolters Kluwer; 2010.)

Patients with HIV are at higher risk of developing active disease with the primary infection. However, in most cases, there is successful control of the acute infection, although not all organisms are cleared, and the patient enters a latent phase.

As previously noted, in its latent form, TB is not transmissible, but it does pose a risk for future reactivation. It is reactivation that often results in transmission. Reactivation occurs at the highest rates within the first 2 years after infection and then decades later, as individuals age. The risk of reactivation in the short- and very long-term time frames are each about 5%, resulting in a 10% overall risk of lifetime reactivation in immunocompetent individuals. In immunocompromised individuals, TB reactivates at a higher rate, and nonpulmonary TB appears more often and may be especially difficult to diagnose in the setting of HIV coinfection.[43] Immunosuppressive therapies, particularly the biologic agents that inhibit tumor necrosis factor to treat autoimmune conditions, such as inflammatory bowel disease, rheumatoid arthritis, and multiple sclerosis among others, should be preceded by a TB test so patients with the latent disease can be identified and treated to decrease the risk of reactivation during the immunosuppressive therapy.

Active TB causes both systemic and organ-specific symptoms, depending upon the location of the reactivation. As noted, the pulmonary disease is most common. The initial focus of pulmonary TB in primary infection is termed a tubercle. When the tubercle is seen on x-ray, it is described as the Ghon focus. As the organism spreads to regional lymph nodes, this finding on x-ray is described as a Ghon complex. A successful immune response may control the infection at this point. Absent a successful immune response, tuberculosis proliferates. The result is the destruction of lung tissue, creating cavities filled with the acid-fast bacteria that become aerosolized with coughing, spreading the pathogen. However, TB can occur in almost any organ, and involvement of the kidney, spine, and adrenal gland are some of the more common extrapulmonary TB sites. The diffuse spread of TB to multiple organs is known as military TB and is often fatal.

Systemic symptoms of TB include fever, fatigue, and weight loss. Organ-specific symptoms typically occur based upon the site of infection, such as cough and pleuritic chest pain (worse with breathing) for pulmonary TB, back pain with spinal TB, and adrenal insufficiency with adrenal TB (Chapter 10 for discussion of TB infection in HIV).

Ocular TB affects structures of both the anterior and posterior segments of the eye, either by direct infection or by an immune response to TB antigens. Incidence of ocular involvement in TB infection ranges from 1% to 4% in nonendemic areas (such as the United States) and up to 26% in highly endemic areas[44] and is more likely in an immunocompromised host. The disease usually results from the dissemination of systemic TB rather than a primary ocular inoculation, though the latter is possible. Ocular findings mimic other disease processes, and thus, the diagnosis of TB-related eye disease can be challenging; standard TB testing (including chest x-ray, PPD, sputum culture, and microscopic examination, discussed below), as well as biopsy of superficial/localized eye lesions with PCR analysis, can help with the diagnosis. Anterior segment findings in TB most commonly manifest as a chronic granulomatous anterior uveitis (with "mutton-fat" keratic precipitates and iris nodules), which may or may not accompany posterior inflammation. TB can also cause immune keratitis in the form of phlyctenular keratoconjunctivitis or interstitial keratitis (neither of which is specific to TB). Phlyctenular keratoconjunctivitis presents as a limbal or bulbar conjunctival nodule with associated neovascularization that encroaches on the cornea, creating symptoms of photophobia, irritation, and tearing (**FIGURE 9.10**). Interstitial keratitis creates a stromal haze that may reduce vision and may be associated with scleritis or uveitis. Isolated episcleritis or scleritis due to TB is uncommon. Also uncommonly, primary tubercles of the conjunctiva or cornea may occur.[45]

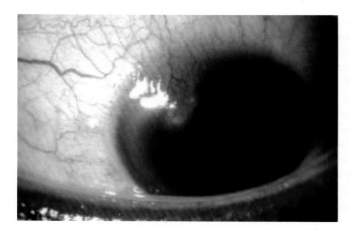

FIGURE 9.10 Corneal phlyctenule. (From Gerstenblith AT. *Wills Eye Manual*. 6th ed. Philadelphia, PA: Wolters Kluwer; 2012.)

Posterior segment involvement includes the formation of choroidal granuloma and/or inflammation with one or more findings of chorioretinitis, vasculitis, vitritis, and optic disc edema[46] (**FIGURE 9.11**). Choroidal tubercles appear as one or more ill-defined, yellow-white or gray nodules in the posterior pole that may lead to exudative retinal detachment. A "serpiginous" chorioretinopathy may occur in TB with plaque-like, ameboid choroidal inflammation. Orbital granuloma in TB is possible but uncommon. TB-related eye disease is primarily treated with systemic disease management. Adjunctive standard treatments for anterior uveitis and keratitis are appropriate, and some evidence exists for a role for laser photocoagulation in choroidal granuloma due to TB.[47]

Screening for latent TB in countries with a low disease prevalence such as the United States is performed in several settings, including the following:

- Exposure risk (eg, healthcare providers, high-risk travel)
- Contacts of active pulmonary TB cases
- Patients newly diagnosed with HIV
- Patients initiating immunosuppressive drug treatments

The typical approach to screening for latent infection is with the TB skin test (TST). A fixed-dose of MTB purified protein derivative (PPD—an alternate name for the skin test) is injected intradermally. In individuals sensitized to TB due to prior exposure, a skin reaction is identified upon examination of the injection site at 48 to 72 hours with induration (a raised reaction), caused by infiltration of the skin with responding immune cells. Merely detecting erythema (redness) at the injection site is not indicative of latent TB. A similar immune response evaluation can be performed on a blood sample tested in vivo with an interferon-γ release assay (IGRA). Though more convenient because a second visit within a specific time-window for the skin examination is not required, IGRA testing is not used as often because it is more expensive and does not have the same performance characteristics (reliability of positive and negative results) as the time-tested TST that has been used to define clinical practice and public health standards for decades.

In an individual with a positive TST or IGRA, assessment for risk of active disease must take place as latent TB and active disease are vastly different clinical scenarios. Generally, the patient with a positive test for latent TB is questioned about systemic and pulmonary symptoms, along with the performance of a chest x-ray to exclude a cavitary lesion or other evidence of pulmonary TB. If both symptom assessment and chest x-ray are normal, then latent TB can be diagnosed.

Bacille Calmette-Guérin (BCG) is an attenuated mycobacterial strain that was developed for the purposes of vaccination against TB. The BCG vaccine remains an important treatment that is administered worldwide in regions of high TB prevalence, as BCG administration has been associated with decreased childhood mortality. In contrast, BCG vaccination is not given in regions of low overall TB transmission risk such as the United States. For several years after BCG administration, the TST may remain positive due to reaction with BCG antigens, although most adults given BCG in infancy will no longer react. Thus, in North American clinical practice, the administration of BCG in infancy should not be a factor in interpreting the tuberculin skin test in an adult. However, the IGRA is more specific for *Mycobacterium tuberculosis* and will remain negative in a BCG recipient.

When a patient presents with a history and symptoms suggestive of pulmonary tuberculosis, the evaluation must take place along with isolation to limit potential transmission. Chest x-ray in pulmonary TB has a characteristic appearance, described as the cavitary lung lesion (**FIGURE 9.12**). Culture and acid-fast or auramine staining of sputum can be useful for diagnosis with pulmonary TB; occasionally bronchoscopy is required to obtain this specimen. With extrapulmonary TB, a biopsy is often necessary to make the diagnosis and direct treatment. Active TB is a reportable disease in all 50 US states, and it is the responsibility of the provider to report the diagnosis to the appropriate public health authority. Cases are investigated by regional public health authorities to identify exposure risks in the community for testing and follow-up. Overall rates are tracked nationally.

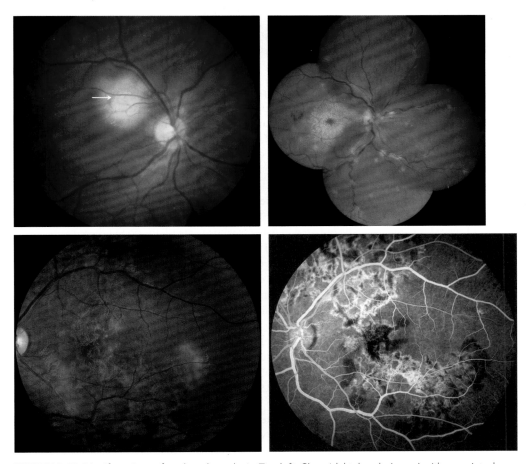

FIGURE 9.11 Manifestations of ocular tuberculosis. Top-left: Choroidal tubercle (arrow) with associated exudative retinal detachment. Top-right: Retinal vasculitis, choroiditis, and optic disc edema with macular exudate (neuroretinitis). Bottom-left: Serpiginous chorioretinopathy with pigmented scarring from old inflammation and yellow-white areas of active inflammation. Bottom-right: Early-phase fluorescein angiogram of the eye in bottom-left image. (Top-left and right, From Garg SJ. *Uveitis.* 2nd ed. Philadelphia, PA: Wolters Kluwer; 2018. Bottom left and right, Courtesy of Sunir J. Garg, MD.)

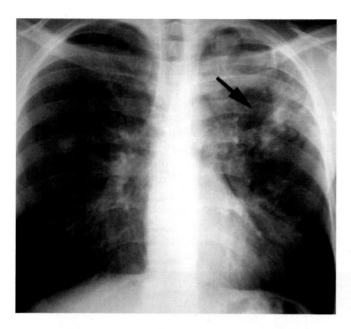

FIGURE 9.12 Chest x-ray with evidence of cavitary tuberculosis (TB) (arrow, left upper lobe). (From Daffner RH. *Clinical Radiology.* 3rd ed. Philadelphia, PA: Wolters Kluwer; 2007.)

Active TB is usually treated with an initial three-drug regimen, followed by ongoing two-drug treatment to complete a 6-month course of therapy. Shorter courses increase the risk of incomplete treatment and recurrence of active disease. Resistance testing should be conducted, and when resistance is present, the regimen should be modified as appropriate. Patients living in regions of high resistance, or those believed to have acquired the disease from an individual with a resistant strain, should begin treatment with a multidrug regimen designed around the predicted resistance until specific testing can be done on the bacteria isolated from the case patient.[48] Resistance is a substantial problem in some parts of the world. It typically develops in association with incomplete treatment, including single-drug therapy and poor medication adherence. Monitoring of therapy, including directly observed treatment, can be initiated in patients who are at risk for poor adherence.

Important considerations in the treatment of TB include the long duration of therapy with multiple drugs. This results in a substantial risk for drug adverse effects, occurring in over 10% of individuals treated with standard regimens. Rates are even higher when second-line agents are used for drug-resistant infections.[5] In sensitive strains, isoniazid and rifampin are commonly used together. Both can cause hepatitis, and liver test monitoring is necessary. In addition, isoniazid can cause peripheral neuropathy, which can be prevented by taking vitamin B6 (pyridoxine) during the course of therapy. Rifampin is secreted into saliva and tears that can result in orange discoloration of soft contact lenses during treatment. Ethambutol is often added to initial treatment until drug sensitivity is known. Ethambutol may cause an optic neuropathy in about 1% of patients and is dose dependent, with the greatest risk occurring at doses above 15 mg/kg/day.[49] All patients should be monitored regularly during therapy with visual acuity, color vision, and Amsler grid testing (at a minimum); comprehensive eye examination with visual field testing and optical coherence tomography imaging is indicated when patients are symptomatic with visual acuity loss, visual field loss, or color vision disturbances. Streptomycin, which is only available as an injected drug, is reserved for use in cases of highly resistant TB. Permanent hearing loss and vestibular dysfunction are unfortunate but common adverse effects, even at therapeutic doses.

Latent TB, in contrast, can be treated with a single drug, usually isoniazid, for 6 to 9 months or a drug combination for a shorter period. Therapy for latent TB therapy decreases the risk of reactivation by 90% or more.

The rash in a typical untreated course of zoster lasts 7 to 10 days. Until all lesions have scabbed, active viral replication and shedding is taking place and VZV may be transmitted to anyone who is susceptible to the virus, meaning they have not had the primary infection with varicella or received the vaccination. Infants (who are too young for vaccination) and susceptible vaccine-age children and adults (who have not had natural infection or vaccination) are at risk for viral infection and development of the primary disease, and thus contact precautions are indicated.

For most patients, the rash and acute pain resolve within a few days; however, a subset of patients with zoster, particularly older patients, will develop the chronic, persistent pain of PHN. PHN usually persists as a continuum of pain at the site of the original rash. Typically PHN is diagnosed when pain persists more than 90 days after the acute infection, but even within that 90-day window significant distress and disability can result from the pain of zoster, often interrupting sleep and contributing to decreased appetite. In elderly patients, PHN can contribute to a significant overall decline in health.

Ophthalmic zoster results when the virus reactivates along the ophthalmic division of the trigeminal nerve (V1), termed herpes zoster ophthalmicus (HZO). HZO represents only 7% to 20% of zoster cases but carries a risk for significant ocular morbidity and a chronic disease course, especially for elderly patients.[62,63] Like zoster affecting other dermatomes, it may begin with a prodrome of pain several days before the appearance of the rash, with globe involvement usually several days after the rash (though sometimes simultaneously). The eyelids may be edematous due to the surrounding skin inflammation/edema, sometimes to the point of complete mechanical ptosis, and there is risk for eyelid scarring, entropion, ectropion, or eyelid necrosis in severe cases. Globe involvement in HZO occurs in roughly 50% of cases and is more likely in the presence of Hutchinson sign (vesicular rash involving the side and/or tip of the nose, due to involvement of the nasociliary nerve) and in patients older than 50 years.[64,65] There may be papillary conjunctivitis, mild scleritis, and mild epithelial punctate keratitis in early stages. Some patients develop a pseudodendritic keratitis early on resembling the dendrite of HSV keratitis, but without terminal end bulbs and with central rather than edge-heaping of the devitalized epithelium (**FIGURE 9.16**). Stromal edema is common in the presence of epithelial disease or may occur in isolation, often initially as focal areas of small round or ill-defined anterior stromal haze (nummular keratitis). A deeper, focal endotheliitis or disciform keratitis may occur along with keratic precipitates and uveitis with elevated intraocular pressure (**FIGURE 9.17**); this deeper inflammation can be a latent complication several months after initial symptoms, and it is unclear whether it represents a direct infectious process or an immune-mediated response. Chronic HZO-related inflammation results in interstitial keratitis with permanent corneal scarring, neovascularization/fibrosis, and significant vision loss (**FIGURE 9.17**). Patients with HZO keratitis often develop corneal anesthesia, and this can be a helpful diagnostic sign in cases of unclear diagnosis presenting after the resolution of the skin rash,

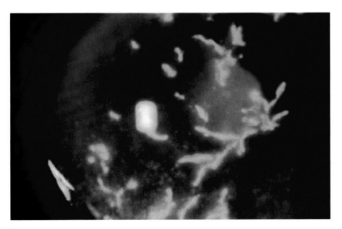

FIGURE 9.16 Pseudodendritic keratitis due to herpes zoster. Note the lack of a classic "tree branch" pattern, elevated edges, and terminal end bulbs that are typical for herpes simplex dendritic keratitis. (From Rapuano CJ. *Wills Eye Institute - Cornea.* 2nd ed. Philadelphia, PA: Wolters Kluwer; 2011.)

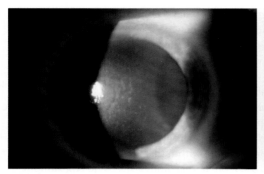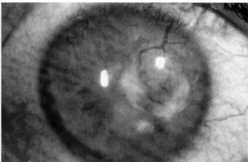

FIGURE 9.17 Deep stromal involvement in herpes zoster keratitis can lead to permanent corneal scarring. Left: Herpes zoster disciform keratitis with associated keratic precipitates. Right: Significant corneal neovascularization and scarring with lipid deposition after an episode of herpes zoster ophthalmicus 8 years prior. (From Rapuano CJ. *Cornea*. 3rd ed. Philadelphia, PA: Wolters Kluwer; 2018.)

particularly in cases of isolated HZO-related iritis, which can also feature significant patchy iris stromal and sphincter atrophy and poor pupil reactivity. Neurotrophic keratitis after HZO results from loss of epithelial trophic support in the anesthetic cornea and can lead to ulceration corneal perforation. Treatment of HZO-related anterior segment eye disease is focused on quieting the ocular inflammation to minimize permanent corneal scarring and inflammatory complications such as uveitic glaucoma. Though many ocular manifestations of HZO are felt to be immune-based and not due to direct viral infection, most clinicians treat active HZO-related eye disease with oral antiviral coverage in addition to topical ophthalmic treatment, which may include a combination of mydriatic drops, corticosteroids, intraocular pressure-lowering therapy, and ophthalmic lubricants.

Posterior segment ocular complications of VZV are uncommon and similar to those that occur in HSV eye disease (see that discussion above); retinal vasculitis with or without optic neuritis and necrotizing chorioretinitis (ARN and PORN) are all possible and more likely to occur in VZV infection than in HSV infection. A nonnecrotizing form of chorioretinitis felt related to occlusive retinal vasculitis ("herpes zoster chorioretinopathy") rarely occurs in zoster, is often delayed in onset, and may be associated with ischemic anterior segment signs (such as iris atrophy and poor pupil reactivity).[66] Ischemic oculomotor palsy (with or without symptomatic diplopia) has long been described in association with zoster and is also associated with ischemic anterior segment ocular signs.[67] The neuroophthalmologic complications of VZV are increasingly recognized as part of an entity known as varicella zoster virus vasculopathy (VZVV), which occurs when VZV infects cerebral and extracranial arteries. This classically results in contralateral hemiparesis though a spectrum of neurological signs and symptoms is now recognized, including ophthalmoplegia and ischemic optic neuropathy.[68,69] VZVV with neuroophthalmic complications occurring in older adults can mimic the systemic vasculitis giant cell arteritis (Chapters 11 and 12).[70] Detection of VZV in CSF aids in diagnosis.

Treatment with the nucleoside analogues that are active against herpes virus infections (acyclovir, valacyclovir, famciclovir) is indicated for primary varicella and specific cases of zoster. Treatment should be initiated as soon as possible, ideally within 72 hours for zoster. Once 72 hours have elapsed in cases of uncomplicated zoster or in patients without significant risk factors for complications, as long as no new vesicles are forming, there is limited benefit to initiating treatment. With early initiation of antiviral therapy in uncomplicated zoster, the course is shortened, viral shedding is decreased, and acute pain is diminished.[8] Antiviral therapy has not, however, been shown to reliably decrease the risk of postherpetic neuralgia.[60] Zoster complications are addressed on a case-by-case basis, with antiviral therapy a mainstay of management.

Prevention with vaccination is important for both primary chickenpox infection in children and to prevent zoster and PHN in older adults. Vaccination guidelines have evolved over time; current guidelines recommend a two-vaccine series for both varicella[71] and zoster prevention.[72]

Cytomegalovirus (CMV) is a common virus reflected by seropositivity in most US adults. Higher rates of seropositivity are seen with aging and with lower socioeconomic factors, including higher rates in developing countries. Transmission occurs with close casual content (such as household family members, daycare settings), sexual contact, vertically (mother to baby), and with organ transplants. CMV rarely causes disease in immunocompetent adults, but in the setting of immune compromise, critical illness,[73] pregnancy, and childbirth, it can cause systemic illness, congenital abnormalities, and sight-threatening infections. As with the other herpesviruses, after the initial exposure, latent infection results, and many clinical syndromes represent reactivation of latent infection.

In immunocompetent individuals, CMV can cause mononucleosis syndrome. Although Epstein-Barr virus (EBV), another member of the herpesvirus family, is the most common cause of the mononucleosis syndrome, CMV is a well-described cause and should be considered when EBV testing is negative. As the most common cause of neonatal infections in the United States, CMV is a significant cause of permanent hearing loss from birth.[74]

In immunocompromised individuals, CMV can infect many organs, with CMV retinitis representing the most common cause of ocular infection in HIV before the availability of highly active antiretroviral therapy (HAART)[75] (Chapter 10). CMV can also cause esophagitis, colitis, hepatitis, pneumonitis, encephalitis, and myocarditis.

Treatment with antiviral agents ganciclovir, valganciclovir, foscarnet, and cidofovir can be used for CMV therapy. Ganciclovir and valganciclovir are also used most commonly for the prevention of CMV reactivation in immunocompromised patients with positive CMV antibodies.

Human herpesvirus 8 (HHV 8) is the causative agent of Kaposi sarcoma (KS). Before the HIV epidemic in the 1980s, this vascular-associated malignancy was seen uncommonly, and generally only in several discrete populations. They included older men living in the Mediterranean region (as described by the eponymous Dr. Kaposi) and certain regions of Africa, as well as in transplant recipients. As cases of this uncommon malignancy were increasingly seen in the population with AIDS during the early 1980s, the associations with immunocompromise and sexual transmission became evident (Chapter 10).

Clinical findings are often dermatological, with violaceous (purple-colored) lesions occurring in the skin and mucous membranes, including the eyelids, conjunctiva (**FIGURE 9.18**), and rarely the orbit. Ocular KS mimics other adnexal vascular lesions (such as hemangioma), subconjunctival hemorrhage, or atypical chalazion and most commonly occurs in the setting of HIV/immunosuppression, though cases also occur in immunocompetent patients.[76-78] HIV testing is indicated in all patients without a past history of testing or preexisting HIV diagnosis. Tissue biopsy with immunohistochemistry for HHV8 markers is definitive for diagnosis, and treatment of focal ocular lesions is successful with local surgical resection, radiation, cryotherapy, or intralesional chemotherapy. Ocular KS lesions associated with HIV respond to HAART. Pulmonary involvement can also be seen in HIV, presenting with hemoptysis and shortness of breath. Pulmonary evaluation in the setting of KS reveals abnormal imaging on chest x-ray and CT scan. The presence of simultaneous mucocutaneous lesions can be an important key to making the correct diagnosis. In the era of HAART, the frequency of KS has decreased substantially in treated individuals.[79]

To treat KS in immunosuppressed patients with HIV, initiating HAART if not already prescribed is critical. Radiation and cancer chemotherapy are also options for refractory lesions.

Other Pathogens

Molluscum contagiosum is a human poxvirus, from the same family as the smallpox virus. Individual lesions are called mollusca, and true to the name, they are contagious with person-to-person contact, as well as contact with infected fomites such as towels and toys. Children are affected most commonly with lesions often on the face, extremities, and torso. Sexual contact with an infected partner can result in the spread of molluscum to the genital region.

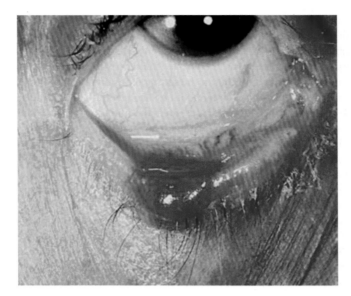

FIGURE 9.18 Kaposi sarcoma. Kaposi sarcoma appears as an elevated, red tumor on the lid margin in a patient with AIDS. (Courtesy of Robert Penne, MD.)

Molluscum lesions are raised and flesh-colored papules, with a small central depression, often described as umbilicated. In immunocompetent individuals, a limited number of small lesions are typically present, and the infection is self-limited, resolving on its own within a few months. Patients may also develop a variant of molluscum that occurs at the lid margin as a solitary nodule that does not disrupt the continuity of the lash line. In these cases, a persistent viral conjunctivitis is often present as the shedding of virus reinoculates the conjunctival cul-de-sac (**FIGURE 9.19**).

Immunocompromised patients can suffer from large lesions and clusters of lesions, involving the face and eyelids, much of the torso and extremities (**FIGURE 9.20**).

Many immunocompetent patients with limited, nongenital infections choose not to be treated, as this self-limited infection resolves without scarring, typically within weeks or a few months. Covering the lesions and attention to personal hygiene are important to limit spread. Genital infections and more extensive involvement may warrant local treatments to remove the lesions. Once the lesions resolve, an individual is no longer infectious.[80] The optometrist should be alert to the possibility of molluscum in the differential diagnosis for facial and eyelid lesions.

Toxoplasma gondii is a protozoan parasite and the causative agent of toxoplasmosis. Host organisms are primarily mammals and birds, with cats serving as the definitive host and a major vector of transmission. Cat feces and undercooked meat are the primary modes of transmission to humans. Toxoplasmosis is asymptomatic in most immunocompetent hosts, and an estimated 11% of Americans have been infected, most of them without any symptoms.[81] Tissue cysts in muscle, brain, and other organs develop, yet remain asymptomatic in the setting of normal immune function. However, toxoplasmosis does pose significant risks in association with immunosuppression and pregnancy. As with many of the other pathogens covered here, toxoplasmosis occurs as both a primary infection and reactivation.

In pregnancy, primary infection (and not reactivation) results in congenital toxoplasmosis. Presentations range from miscarriage to asymptomatic infection. The typical syndrome of congenital toxoplasmosis is marked by retinochoroiditis (**FIGURE 9.21**), hydrocephalus, and brain calcifications. However, a wide range of symptoms can be seen including microphthalmia and microcephaly. Neonates who are asymptomatic at birth may develop late manifestations including ocular infection, intellectual disabilities, hearing loss, and seizures. To avoid primary infection

association with candidemia is less certain. Patients with *Candida* chorioretinitis are usually asymptomatic and visual prognosis at this stage is good. In a minority of cases, fungal organisms seed the vitreous and lead to endophthalmitis, with risk for devastating vision loss. This appears as a diffuse or localized vitritis within the posterior pole, often with multiple white, fluffy, "snowballs" representing vitreal fungal abscesses (**FIGURE 9.24**). Fungal endogenous endophthalmitis is much more common than bacterial endophthalmitis. Prompt initiation of systemic antifungal treatment, detection of early chorioretinitis with surveillance dilated eye examinations, and continuation of systemic therapy until ocular lesions and candidemia fully resolve are effective for minimizing endophthalmitis risk. Some patients will demonstrate delayed-onset chorioretinitis for up to 14 days after initiation of systemic treatment, so fundoscopy should be performed at 1-week and 2-weeks to maximize detection. Patients with endophthalmitis may benefit from intravitreal antifungals in addition to systemic therapy.

Mucocutaneous candidiasis is often diagnosed with a surface scraping examined under the microscope for the presence of budding yeast with hyphae. When systemic infection is a concern, cultures and biopsy can also be obtained. The presence of yeast on blood culture or organ biopsy confirms the diagnosis of systemic infection.

Treatment with a topical or brief course of an oral antifungal agent is effective for most mucocutaneous infections; underlying factors should be addressed whenever possible to aid in treatment and prevent a recurrence. This includes improved glucose management in poorly controlled diabetes, rinsing the mouth after inhaled corticosteroids, or counseling on personal hygiene factors in recurrent genital infections. Systemic infections in severely ill and immunocompromised patients require longer term systemic therapy and often involves consultation with an infectious disease specialist.

While current medical practice can identify and treat many clinical manifestations of *Candida* infections, there remain nontraditional approaches to defining, diagnosing, and treating *Candida* syndromes. As *Candida* species are common human colonizers, merely finding *Candida* on a culture from a patient with nonspecific symptoms does not reliably establish its role as a pathogen. Conditions such as *Candida* hypersensitivity syndrome and chronic candidiasis have been described in the medical literature, and in some cases, traditional scientific methods have found them to be "speculative and unproved."[86] Yet patients so diagnosed often suffer with a range of symptoms that have otherwise defied diagnosis and treatment. In addition to remaining empathic to the patient's symptoms that may go unvalidated without a formal diagnosis, clinicians should keep in mind that

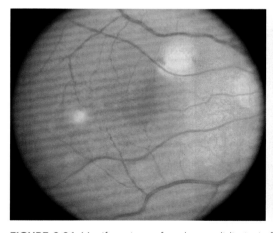
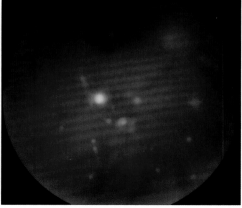

FIGURE 9.24 Manifestations of ocular candidiasis. Left: *Candida* chorioretinitis. Right: *Candida* endophthalmitis. There are many small vitreous abscesses in the case of fungal endophthalmitis caused by *Candida albicans*. (Left, Reprinted with permission from Hartnett ME. *Pediatric Retina*. 2nd ed. Philadelphia, PA: Wolters Kluwer; 2013. Right, Courtesy of MidAtlantic Retina, the Retina Service of Wills Eye Hospital.)

first do no harm is a useful frame of reference in these situations. Unproven treatments may bring limited benefit in exchange for the exposure to their potential adverse effects and often high financial cost that may not be covered by health insurance.

Bartonella henselae is a gram-negative bacterium and the etiologic agent in cat scratch fever. True to its name, human scratches from infected cats will transmit this bacterial pathogen. Kittens are more often associated with this infection, which can also be caused by cat bites and flea bites. The disease is transmitted to cats via infected fleas; thus, flea-infested cats are at the highest risk for infection and transmission to humans. Cats are often asymptomatic despite harboring the bacteria in their blood and saliva. Cases have been reported in all regions of North America as well as many other parts of the globe.

Most cases of cat scratch fever are diagnosed in children and are self-limited, localized infections that resolve without intervention. At the site of infection, patients may develop a vesicular lesion followed by regional lymphadenopathy. Occasionally, a lymph node may drain. The lymphadenopathy may persist for months, but will often resolve without treatment. Low-grade fever can occur, and occasionally, cat scratch fever has been a cause for prolonged, undiagnosed fevers. About 10% of patients will experience systemic symptoms including myalgia or arthralgia. Cat ownership and history of a scratch or bite are useful components of the history in the evaluation of patients with unexplained unilateral lymphadenopathy. Diagnosis is typically made by history along with serology to detect the presence of *Bartonella* antibodies. Observation is the typical course of management for most cases of lymphadenopathy in otherwise healthy patients.

While cat scratch fever is usually an uncomplicated and self-limited clinical syndrome, ocular complications such as Parinaud oculoglandular syndrome and neuroretinitis may occur (discussed below). Patients with immune compromise are at higher risk for developing other uncommon, but severe, systemic complications including encephalitis, the liver infection peliosis hepatitis, and a systemic infection known as bacillary angiomatosis characterized by the formation of tumor-like vascular masses in the skin and organs. Complicated cases or disease that occurs in patients at risk for complications is often treated with one or more oral antibiotics including azithromycin and doxycycline. Immunocompromised patients are generally treated as well.[87]

The ocular complications in cat scratch disease include Parinaud oculoglandular syndrome (an anterior segment complication) and neuroretinitis (a posterior segment complication). Parinaud oculoglandular syndrome occurs in 5% of patients and constitutes a triad of head and neck lymphadenopathy, unilateral follicular conjunctivitis, and fever (**FIGURE 9.25**). Enlarged nodes can be found in the preauricular, cervical, or submandibular regions. Regional exposure to cat saliva or

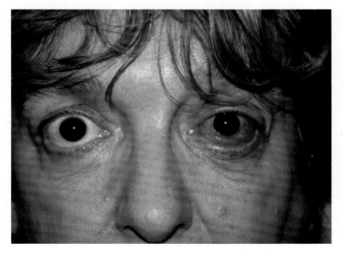

FIGURE 9.25 Parinaud oculoglandular syndrome. The left eye has a conjunctival injection with epiphora. The left preauricular node is enlarged. (Reprinted from Garg SJ. *Uveitis.* 2nd ed. Philadelphia, PA: Wolters Kluwer; 2018.)

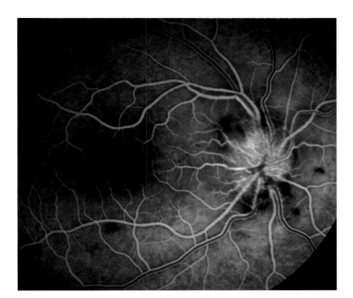

FIGURE 9.26 Neuroretinitis due to cat scratch disease. (From Garg SJ. *Uveitis.* 2nd ed. Philadelphia, PA: Wolters Kluwer; 2018.)

a scratch is often the trigger, and patients will demonstrate positive serologic titers to *B. henselae* (note that tularemia, infection with the bacterium *Francisella tularensis*, is another common cause of Parinaud oculoglandular syndrome, and a number of other infections can also infrequently cause the syndrome). Neuroretinitis is an uncommon ocular complication of *Bartonella* infection, seen in about 1% to 2% of patients.[88] This is characterized by unilateral optic disc edema and macular edema with the formation of a "macular star" composed of stellate lipid exudate over several days to weeks (**FIGURE 9.26**). Some patients also have an associated vitritis and retinitis. It is important to note that *B. henselae* is not the only cause of neuroretintis, as other infectious and inflammatory etiologies (including syphilis and sarcoidosis) may cause a similar presentation. While visual acuity may be significantly reduced during the acute stages of the disease due to extensive macular edema and disc swelling, the visual prognosis is excellent, even without treatment.[89] There is no standardized treatment for the ocular complications of *Bartonella* and the natural history suggests that observation may be appropriate, though some reports also suggest benefit with a variety of oral antibiotics such as rifampin, doxycycline, ciprofloxacin, erythromycin, and trimethoprim-sulfamethoxazole.[90]

Rubella, commonly known as German measles, is a viral pathogen that causes a common childhood infection in the absence of vaccination. A vaccine was licensed in 1969, and in 2004 rubella was declared eliminated in the United States.[91] A small number of imported cases from overseas transmission continue to occur each year. While young children are the most commonly infected, nonimmune adults can also be infected, and the congenital rubella syndrome is an especially serious infection that can result from maternal infection during pregnancy. It is estimated that the congenital rubella syndrome affects about 100,000 neonates every year across the world.[92]

The hallmark clinical finding in acute rubella is a maculopapular rash with lymphadenopathy. The rash typically begins on the face, spreads to the torso, and then becomes generalized over a 24-hour period. The median duration of rash is 3 days, although it may last up to 5 days. Patients can be contagious for up to 7 days before and after the rash appears. Infection is spread via droplets with coughing and sneezing. Adults with rubella frequently develop arthralgia (70%), which can persist for weeks.[21] With neck lymphadenopathy, conjunctivitis and low-grade fever may occur. Encephalitis due to rubella has been reported, though it is a rare complication (estimated 1 in 5000) and is associated with a poor prognosis.[93]

The most common serious complications of rubella infection involve children who are infected in utero. The first trimester of pregnancy is the period of highest fetal risk from maternal infection as rubella can infect the placenta and the fetus, impacting organogenesis at this critical stage. The offspring of 90% of mothers infected at this early time experience complications of fetal infection including stillbirth, preterm birth, and severe congenital birth defects that constitute the congenital rubella syndrome (CRS).[94] CRS most commonly involves the eyes,[95] inner ear, heart, and central nervous system (CNS); when CRS is suspected, ocular, cardiovascular, and audiology examinations are important components of the evaluation. Over 50% of children with CRS have bilateral deafness and CRS remains a leading cause of neonatal sensorineural hearing loss in regions without vaccination. About 50% of infants born with CRS have congenital heart defects (including pulmonary artery stenosis, patent ductus arteriosus, and ventricular septal defect) and 25% have congenital cataracts (see ocular complications below).[96] It can also cause microcephaly, developmental delay, and autism. Children with congenital rubella are also at increased risk for renovascular hypertension and endocrine disorders, including diabetes and thyroid disease, later in life.[97]

Ocular manifestations of rubella are common after congenital infection. A long-term epidemiological study of 125 patients with congenital rubella followed for over 32 years at the Mayo Clinic found that ocular complications were highly prevalent (78%) and significantly associated with hearing loss, cardiac abnormalities, and cognitive impairment.[98] The most common finding was pigmentary retinopathy (60%) (**FIGURE 9.27**) followed by bilateral cataracts (27%), nystagmus (25%), strabismus (24%), microphthalmia (23%), amblyopia (16%), and glaucoma (9%). Less frequently reported ocular complications included optic atrophy, iris coloboma, and corneal haze. Ophthalmic complications are usually bilateral. A notable unilateral, later-onset ocular condition associated with rubella is Fuch heterochromic iridocyclitis. Patients have chronic, asymptomatic anterior uveitis in one eye characterized by low-grade cells and flare with diffusely distributed stellate keratic precipitates and a notable absence of ocular injection, often also with associated heterochromia (lighter pigmentation on the affected side). There is an increased risk for glaucoma in the affected eye. Rubella recently emerged as a causative agent for Fuch heterochromic iridocyclitis after several studies reported the detection of intraocular antibodies against rubella virus in 100% of tested patients. Epidemiological evidence of declining incidence of Fuch heterocyclitis after the widespread implementation of the MMR vaccine in the United States is also suggestive.[99]

Spirochetes

Spirochetes are spiral-shaped bacteria and include the causative agents of syphilis and Lyme disease. Common features of the clinical presentations include multiple stages of the disease

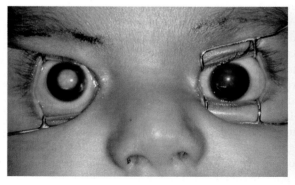
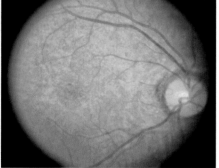

FIGURE 9.27 Ocular findings in congenital rubella. Left: Mature cataract in the right eye and early cataract in the left eye in a child with congenital rubella. Right: Pigmentary retinopathy in congenital rubella. (Left, Reprinted from Garg, SJ. *Uveitis*. 2nd ed. Philadelphia, PA: Wolters Klluwer; 2018. Right, Reprinted with permission from Hartnett, ME. *Pediatric Retina*. 2nd ed. Philadelphia, PA: Wolters Kluwer; 2013.)

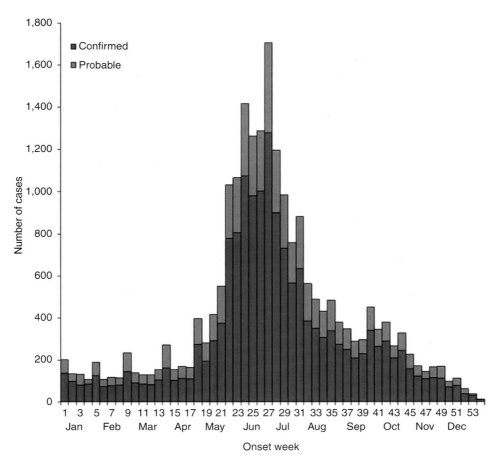

FIGURE 9.28 Lyme disease—Reported confirmed and probable cases by week of disease onset, United States, 2018. (Content source: Centers for Disease Control and Prevention. *National Center for Emerging and Zoonotic Infectious Diseases (NCEZID), Division of Vector-Borne Diseases (DVBD).* Accessed November 22, 2019. https://www.cdc.gov/other/imagereuse.html.)

(including early and late stages) as well as initial dermatological manifestations and CNS involvement. The extent of ocular involvement, however, differs between the two infections; ocular findings in syphilis are myriad, while significant ocular manifestations are less common in Lyme disease.

Lyme disease is a tick-borne illness. In the United States, *Borrelia bergdorferi* is the spirochete responsible for most of these infections, and Lyme disease itself is responsible for 82% of all reported tick-borne illness.[100] Typically, hard-bodied ticks in the *Ixodes* genus transmit Lyme disease, including the black-legged tick *Ixodes scapularis* on the east coast and midwest, while *Ixodes pacificus* is endemic on the west coast. The most concentrated reports of Lyme disease cases in the United States by region include the mid-Atlantic, northeast, and upper midwest.[101] Cases are also reported in Europe and Asia.

The lifecycle of the *Ixodes* tick, responsible for disease transmission in the eponymous region (Lyme, Connecticut) includes the white-footed mouse and white-tailed deer. The ticks ultimately reside on tall grasses and latch on to people and animals passing by. The ticks die off in the winter; thus, Lyme disease is only transmitted during temperate weather, with the highest risk in the summer months of June through September in the temperate regions of the US Documented changes in global temperature patterns over the past decades, including the later onset of freezing temperatures and warmer winter weather, are associated with ongoing Lyme transmission well into the autumn and even into the winter, as well as with geographic spread of the infection.

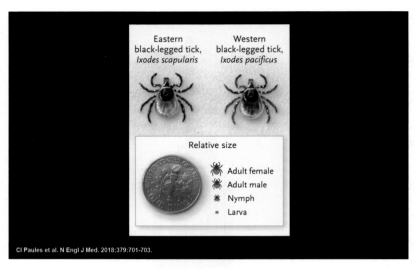

CI Paules et al. N Engl J Med. 2018;379:701-703.

FIGURE 9.29 Common ticks associated with Lyme disease in North America. (Paules CI, Marston HD, Bloom ME, Fauci AS. Tickborne diseases – Confronting a growing threat .*N Engl J Med.* 2018;379:701-703.)

When the tick attaches to a human, it often moves to a warm region of the body including axilla, waist, or groin, where it attaches. Burrowing into the skin and extracting blood from the host for nutrition, the tick simultaneously transmits the spirochete directly to the host.

Management of tick exposure is a common scenario in settings such as primary care and urgent care during summer and early autumn months. The first step in management is to obtain a history, including likely timing of tick attachment, frequency of tick exposure risk, and the presence of possible tick-borne illness symptoms. Patients with frequent exposure risks (eg, hikers, suburban landscapers) require assessment for the current episode along with the possibility of prior Lyme exposure. Patients with rare exposure risks can often pinpoint a time frame for tick attachment (eg, a city dweller who went for a one-time walk in a wooded area). The next step is to assess the tick. When the tick can be evaluated at the visit (still attached, or brought in by the patient after removal at home), assessment of the tick appearance will help determine if the arthropod is an *Ixodes* tick (responsible for transmitting Lyme disease), or a larger dog tick that does not transmit Lyme disease. When the tick is not evaluable, using a photograph of tick sizes to show the patient may help clarify the likelihood of an *Ixodes* tick (vs. a larger dog tick) and, thus, the risk of Lyme transmission.

Proper removal of an embedded tick requires tweezers to grab the insect as close to the skin as possible. With the tweezers, pull firmly away from the skin without twisting (**FIGURE 9.30**).

How to remove a tick.[101]

1. Use fine-tipped tweezers to grasp the tick as close to the skin's surface as possible.
2. Pull upward with steady, even pressure. Don't twist or jerk the tick; this can cause the mouth-parts to break off and remain in the skin. If this happens, remove the mouthparts with tweezers. If you are unable to remove the mouth easily with clean tweezers, leave it alone and let the skin heal.
3. After removing the tick, thoroughly clean the bite area and your hands with rubbing alcohol or soap and water.
4. Never crush a tick with your fingers.

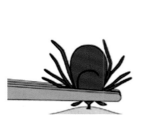
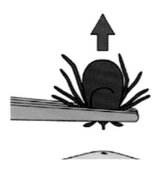

FIGURE 9.30 How to remove a tick. (Content source: Centers for Disease Control and Prevention. *National Center for Emerging and Zoonotic Infectious Diseases (NCEZID), Division of Vector-Borne Diseases (DVBD).* Accessed November 22, 2019. https://www.cdc.gov/other/imagereuse.html.)

Ticks attached for less than 72 hours do not pose a significant risk of Lyme transmission.[102] Since most ticks are identified and removed within 48 hours, the overall risk of Lyme transmission from a single tick exposure is low. Thus, a narrow time frame between the exposure and removal of an unengorged tick can help make the determination of a very low-risk exposure. An uncertain duration between attachment and removal, or the finding of an engorged *Ixodes* tick, raises the risk. In this situation, consideration should be given to the options of empiric treatment versus confirmatory antibody testing, which typically requires several weeks to allow for sufficient antibody production by the host. Some laboratories are able to test the tick itself, and in this setting, a risk assessment can be made based upon the infectious status in the tick. The highest risk for Lyme transmission occurs with nymphal tick attachment, a developmental stage in the tick life cycle between the immature larval stage and the adult stage. Because the nymphal tick is tiny (see **FIGURE 9.30** above), many infected individuals are unaware of the tick exposure.

Erythema migrans (EM) may be the first symptom of Lyme disease infection. This rash, typical of acute Lyme disease, usually develops in warm regions of the body such as the groin, axilla, waist, and thighs. A single lesion often develops in the region of exposure to the *Borrelia* spirochete; however, the initial infection may disseminate early resulting in multiple regions of EM rash. EM is often a flat erythematous lesion and is often asymptomatic, though pruritus and occasionally pain may occur. The rash is typically round, and untreated it expands and may develop central clearing with the frequent description of a bulls-eye rash (**FIGURE 9.31**). However, the bulls-eye appearance may not always be present, and the center of the legion may have enhanced erythema or vesicles. Some patients may not be aware of an EM rash, for example, if it occurs on the back or posterior thigh. While many people with the EM rash have no other symptoms, others will develop systemic

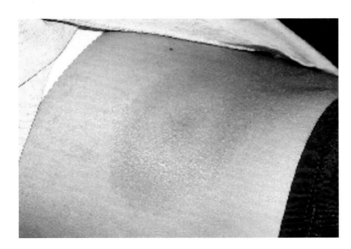

FIGURE 9.31 Erythema migrans rash of Lyme disease. (From Kline-Tifford AM, Haut C. *Lippincott Certification Review: Pediatric Acute Care Nurse Practitioner.* Philadelphia, PA: Wolters Kluwer; 2015.)

symptoms including myalgia, arthralgia, headache, and fatigue. Conjunctivitis and fever can also develop with the initial infection, but this presentation occurs infrequently.

Disseminated Lyme disease causes cardiac, neurological, and joint manifestations. Carditis (often presenting with heart block), peripheral facial nerve palsy, and meningitis can occur within weeks of the initial infection. Peripheral facial palsy, in particular, is associated with Lyme disease, and Lyme should be considered in all cases before diagnosing an idiopathic Bell palsy Lyme arthritis is a later stage symptom, typically developing weeks to several months after infection. It most commonly involves large joints (knee, ankle) as migratory, inflammatory arthritis, moving from joint to joint. An illustrative case presented to one of the authors (DS) in a patient with difficulty driving a manual shift car (requiring both feet to drive) because of swelling that migrated from one knee to the other.

Ocular symptoms in Lyme disease are uncommon, and symptoms such as mild conjunctivitis are minor, self-limited, and often go unnoticed. Indeed, many physicians are unaware of the association, and a number of general medicine reviews on Lyme disease reviewed by the editors do not include mention of ocular symptoms or findings. Acute Lyme can present with follicular conjunctivitis, reported to occur in up to 10% of individuals. Because the conjunctivitis is limited in duration and can be a part of the initial presentation of the disease, it may be the only clue that enables early diagnosis of Lyme disease. A history to assess for Lyme disease risks such as exposure to long grass or wooded areas, or a known tick bite, plus examination for EM should be a part of the general evaluation of conjunctivitis when season and geography are compatible with potential *Ixodes* tick exposure. Keeping Lyme disease in mind when evaluating follicular conjunctivitis is especially important because up to 20% of patients with Lyme disease will not develop the typical EM rash, potentially leaving conjunctivitis as one of the sole indicators of early disease. Because the conjunctivitis is self-limited, the window for early recognition and definitive treatment of Lyme disease may be lost if Lyme is not considered, even in the absence of EM. Laboratory investigation for *B. burgdorferi* antibodies is not warranted in all cases of conjunctivitis; testing should be reserved for situations when history and examination are compatible with this diagnosis. It is useful to remind patients and parents of young patients presenting in summer months in Northern climates of the signs and symptoms of ocular Lyme disease and the importance of seeking treatment if these symptoms develop.

Disseminated Lyme disease can be accompanied by a range of inflammatory ocular conditions including keratitis, vitritis, and uveitis. Reported cases of neuroretinitis, optic atrophy, and disc edema have also been associated with Lyme disease. Though overall not a common cause of intraocular inflammation, Lyme testing should be included as part of the standard workup for these patients. Generally responding to treatment, it is making the diagnosis that may be most challenging. A vitreous tap may be necessary in cases without a clinical diagnosis.[103,104]

As noted above, the diagnosis of early Lyme is made when the clinical finding of an EM rash is present along with a compatible history. Patients presenting without the typical rash, or with later stages of disseminated disease require additional evaluation, as the differential diagnosis for the range of symptoms that can occur in Lyme disease is broad. Testing for Lyme disease is a two-stage process, starting with an ELISA (enzyme-linked immunosorbent assay) test. If negative, the result is reported as such. If equivocal or positive, a Western blot is done to confirm, and this result is then reported.

There are situations when the antibody tests will not be definitive or timely in the assessment. A very recent tick exposure with an early EM rash may not yet be met with a detectable host antibody response, and clinical assessment alone often guides treatment in the setting of acute Lyme disease. In a patient with a prior positive Lyme antibody test who has been treated, antibodies often remain positive, and the diagnosis of a recurrent infection can only be made on clinical grounds. Empiric Lyme treatment is often initiated in patients presenting with acute symptoms such as facial nerve palsy, meningitis, or heart block when geography, along with occupational and/or leisure activities, puts them at risk for Lyme disease. Follow-up assessment can be done when antibody blood test results are available—typically within a few days.

Treatment for a recent high-risk exposure without symptoms can be done with a single high dose of doxycycline. An alternative approach is clinical monitoring and follow-up antibody testing several weeks later, with treatment only prescribed for positive test results or if typical symptoms develop (eg, EM rash) in the interim. An initial test is often done as well so that if a previously transmitted infection is present, prompt treatment can be initiated. In patients with a low-to-moderate risk of *Borellia* infection, this testing approach can help minimize antibiotic exposure while still providing timely treatment for an infection. There is no indication that a delay of a few weeks (typically, 6-8) to await seroconversion for antibody confirmation will impact long-term outcomes. Thus, treatment can be safely deferred for a few weeks when the clinical presentation is not definitive.

The EM rash of early Lyme disease is often treated with a 2-week outpatient course of appropriate antibiotics—usually doxycycline or amoxicillin. Facial nerve palsy is also treated orally, often with 3 weeks of therapy. Meningitis, carditis, and ocular inflammatory disease may require an intravenous third-generation cephalosporin, and treatment recommendations in more complicated cases such as these are usually guided by consultation with an infectious disease specialist.

The prognosis for Lyme disease eradication is excellent with early identification and treatment. Later disease identification and treatment are also effective, but in some cases, outcomes are more variable. Some patients experience lingering symptoms, and there remains uncertainty as to whether so-called chronic Lyme represents persistent infection, immunologic or other sequelae from a fully treated infection, or something else entirely when an overlap of nonspecific and otherwise undiagnosed symptoms coincidentally occur in a patient with a history of Lyme disease. Long-term use of antibiotics without a confirmed ongoing infection has been studied; this approach has not offered meaningful improvement in clinical outcomes,[105] and the risks, including bacterial resistance, are a concern.

Prevention of tick exposure can reduce Lyme disease risk. Appropriate clothing before outdoor activities that entail a risk of tick exposure (long sleeves and pants tucked into socks or boots) and use of insect repellent are important. Avoiding high-risk areas (such as staying on hiking paths and avoiding walking into tall grasses) should also be reinforced in endemic regions. Checking for and removing ticks and/or showering to dislodge ticks after potential exposures can remove the arthropods before they latch on and transmit disease.

Treponema pallidum is the pathogen responsible for syphilis; humans are the only known host. With documented outbreaks in Europe as early as the 1490s, syphilis has been recognized as a sexually transmitted disease for centuries. It was also the subject of an egregious case of racially motivated scientific misconduct in the Tuskegee Project for several decades through the 1900s, prompting a formal apology from US President Clinton. The incidence of syphilis in the United States has been increasing over the past 2 decades. Having achieved a nadir around the turn of the millennium, cases have increased nearly fivefold in the United States since 2001, with most cases occurring in men who have sex with men. However, heterosexual transmission continues to occur, posing an ongoing risk for congenital syphilis.

Any sexually transmitted bacterial infection will increase the risk of cotransmission of HIV. Underlying HIV infection also impacts the progression of other sexually transmitted diseases such as syphilis; for example, ocular findings are more common in patients with HIV coinfection. Any patient being screened for a sexually transmitted bacterial infection should also have HIV testing. Conversely, anyone diagnosed with syphilis or another sexually transmitted disease should be screened for HIV infection (Chapter 10).

Syphilis is transmitted sexually and vertically (mother to fetus). The infection progresses through stages of the disease if untreated, from primary to secondary (early stages of syphilis) to latent and tertiary (late-stage syphilis). Ocular inflammation is a manifestation of the later stages of syphilis and is an important consideration in the differential diagnosis for ocular inflammation, particularly when occurring together with other neurological findings. The astute clinician will both consider

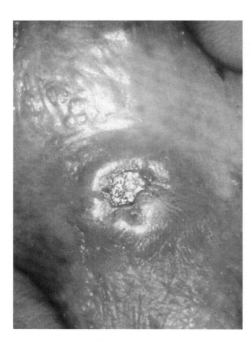

FIGURE 9.32 Cutaneous chancre of primary syphilis. (From Sweet RL, Gibbs RS. *Atlas of Infectious Diseases of the Female Genital Tract.* Philadelphia, PA: Lippincott Williams & Wilkins; 2005.)

syphilis when appropriate and initiate a sensitive discussion to review the differential diagnosis with the patient, encouraging syphilis testing with information for referral when necessary. Ocular syphilis is discussed further below.

Primary syphilis commonly begins with a chancre or sore at the site of inoculation and spirochete invasion, typically the genitals (penis or labia), anorectal region, or mouth. The lesion is ulcerative, well-demarcated, and nontender (**FIGURE 9.32**) and heals spontaneously over several weeks. Regional lymph nodes may also be enlarged and tender. Identification at this point is important, as early treatment can be initiated to prevent the progression of the disease and further transmission. Primary syphilis is highly contagious to sexual partners. The initial infection also begins the approximately 4-year period during which an infected woman harbors active infection (if untreated), and pregnancy can result in congenital syphilis.[106] Untreated, the chancre will resolve and syphilis will progress to subsequent stages of the disease.

Secondary syphilis develops about 8 weeks after primary infection. One of the most prominent features of secondary syphilis is rash; however, many organs can be involved with a variety of signs, and systemic symptoms including fever, headache, and joint pain can also occur. The rash of secondary syphilis commonly involves the palms and soles but can affect other regions as well including the torso, legs, and arms. The typical rash is copper-colored and may be confluent or maculopapular (with both flat and raised regions) (**FIGURE 9.33**). Patchy alopecia (hair loss) can develop on the scalp, and condylomata lata can also appear at this stage (**FIGURE 9.34** below). These soft, raised regions develop near the site of inoculation and contain the active spirochetal infection, making them highly infectious. Early neurosyphilis may develop as part of the secondary stage, along with uveitis.[107] While early neurosyphilis is often asymptomatic, the presence of inflammatory cells on the CSF confirms this diagnosis.

Like primary syphilis, most signs and symptoms of secondary syphilis will resolve spontaneously over time without treatment, though some untreated patients will experience relapses of secondary syphilis for as long as 5 years after the initial episode.[108] Relapse as primary syphilis is infrequent.

After 2 to 4 years of infection, syphilis becomes latent. At this stage, patients are asymptomatic but will still demonstrate infection with *T. pallidum* by serologic testing. The risk of transmission decreases and this stage, especially with an increasing duration of time since active signs or symptoms were present. Congenital syphilis remains a risk relatively early on (within 4 years of active disease).

Between 15% and 40% of people progress to late or tertiary syphilis. The onset of this stage can occur anywhere from 1 to 30 years after primary infection.[109] Neurological, ocular, cardiovascular, dermatological, and bone involvement are common manifestations. Syndromes of neurosyphilis include

- Meningitis, with headache and neck stiffness; the presentation can include cerebral arterial inflammation leading to stroke symptoms
- Tabes dorsales, often manifesting with damage to the posterior spinal columns resulting in loss of position sense and a flat-footed gait
- Argyll-Robertson pupil (discussed below)
- Paresis, a syndrome with memory loss and impaired judgment that often leads to dementia; psychiatric symptoms such as depression, mania, and psychosis can occur

The involvement of the aortic valve and ascending aorta, likely from infiltration of the vaso vasorum (small arteries that supply the aorta itself), results in aortic aneurysm and aortic valve damage. Gummas, granulomatous lesions that can develop on the skin and in the GI tract, bones, or other organs, are rare but characteristic findings in late syphilis.

Ocular syphilis usually presents as a form of neurosyphilis, occurring in the secondary or tertiary disease stages. Rarely, eyelid or conjunctival chancre may be a presentation of primary syphilis. Ocular involvement is infrequent overall but can serve as an important diagnostic marker, especially for tertiary syphilis, as proper diagnosis with treatment initiation can prevent further serious complications. Ophthalmic manifestations are more likely to occur in the setting of HIV infection with an incidence as high as 10% in this population (Chapter 10). The advent of HAART has improved the prognosis for ocular syphilis in the setting of HIV, though delay in diagnosis beyond 28 days has been associated with less favorable outcomes.[110] The diagnosis of ocular syphilis can be challenging since virtually any ocular tissue can be affected and the signs and symptoms mimic other diseases; thus, a high degree of suspicion is necessary for prompt diagnosis, and syphilis should be included in the differential for ocular inflammation of unknown cause. Occasionally, patients present with ocular manifestations of secondary syphilis, which mainly involve anterior segment inflammation such as interstitial keratitis, iridocyclitis, episcleritis, and scleritis. Anterior uveitis due to syphilis is more common in HIV-infected patients.[111] Posterior segment inflammation is also possible in late secondary syphilis; acute syphilitic posterior placoid chorioretinitis is a rare but characteristic manifestation featuring one or more yellowish, placoid outer retinal lesions with faded center and

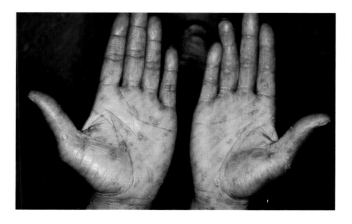

FIGURE 9.33 Typical rash of the palms in secondary syphilis. (Courtesy of Arthur Eisen, MD, Division of Dermatology, Washington University School of Medicine.)

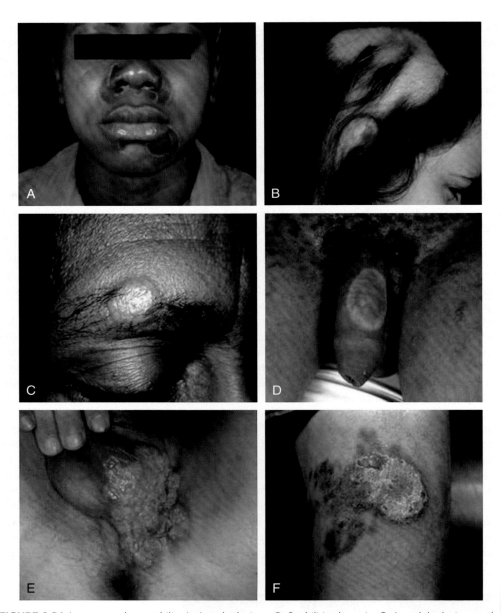

FIGURE 9.34 Late secondary syphilis. A, Annular lesions. B, Syphilitic alopecia. C, A nodular lesion on the eyebrow. D, An annular lesion on the penis. E, Condylomata lata in the groin area. F, Psoriatic-type syphilitic lesion on the leg. (From Hall BJ, Hall JC. *Sauer's Manual of Skin Diseases*. 11th ed. Philadelphia, PA: Wolters Kluwer; 2017.)

with adjacent RPE disturbance (**FIGURE 9.35**). Most commonly, ocular syphilis occurs as a complication of tertiary syphilis and patients present due to symptoms of blurry vision or light sensitivity. Examination reveals panuveitis with a characteristic multifocal retinochoroiditis described as having the appearance of "ground glass," from aggregation of discrete, yellow-white retinal lesions overlying deeper, white-gray, placoid areas of inflammation, usually also with some degree of vitritis[110] (**FIGURE 9.36**). Necrotizing chorioretintis, cystoid macular edema, serous retinal detachment due to syphilitic infiltration, occlusive retinal vasculitis, and optic neuropathies including neuroretinitis, optic atrophy, inflammatory optic neuritis, and gummatous optic nerve infiltration are also possible

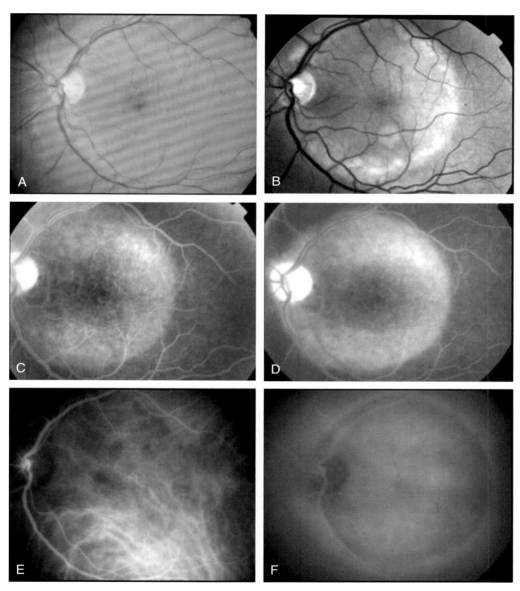

FIGURE 9.35 Color fundus photograph (A), red-free photograph (B), fluorescein angiogram (C and D), and indocyanine green angiography (E and F) of an acute syphilitic posterior placoid chorioretinitis, often seen in patients with HIV. (Reprinted from Garg SJ. *Uveitis*. 2nd ed. Philadelphia, PA: Wolters Kluwer; 2018.)

ocular manifestations of syphilis infection. Neuroophthalmic manifestations of syphilis are always a component of neurosyphilis and result from stroke (due to CNS arteritis) or gumma formation within the meninges or brain parenchyma. Virtually any neuroophthalmic abnormality is possible, including eye movement abnormalities, pupillary abnormalities, and visual field loss. The Argyll-Robertson pupil is a classic pupillary abnormality associated with neurosyphilis (**FIGURE 9.37**). Pupils are bilaterally irregular, miotic, and nonreactive to light, with intact near response (light-near dissociation). The etiology is thought to be interrupted signaling along the efferent pupillary light pathway, between the Edinger-Westphal nuclei and the pretectal nuclei.

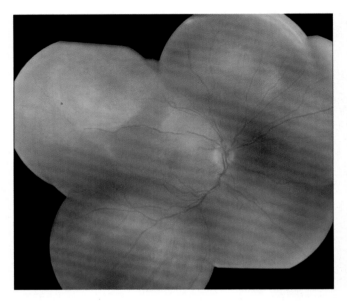

FIGURE 9.36 A 44-year-old man presented with bilateral decreased vision. He had a recent skin rash that was diagnosed as mononucleosis. His vision was 20/80 OD and 20/800 OS. Color fundus photograph of the right eye showing large, patchy, multifocal yellow areas in the outer retina/choroid. (Courtesy of Paul Baker, MD.)

Congenital ocular syphilis involves inflammatory eye disease as in acquired cases, and may be diagnosed in infancy (after the 18th week) or later in life depending on the severity and particular manifestations. Early cataract formation is also a complication of congenital syphilis with risk for amblyopia is children who are not diagnosed early in life. Before the advent of antibiotics, congenital syphilis was a leading cause of interstitial keratitis and corneal blindness, which is now surpassed by herpes simplex virus.[112] Patients with a history of chorioretinitis due to congenital syphilis typically demonstrate a characteristic "salt and pepper" RPE mottling throughout the posterior poles of both eyes later in life, representing quiescent retinal scarring from past chorioretinitis (**FIGURE 9.38**).[113]

The visual prognosis in ocular syphilis declines with delay in treatment and in the presence of HIV. Permanent visual loss can occur from amblyopia due to unrecognized congenital cataracts, retinal scarring, or neuroophthalmic manifestations such as optic atrophy and stroke. Inflammatory eye disease that is promptly identified and treated has a generally good visual prognosis. All eye disease is treated with the same regimen as neurosyphilis (regardless of results of a CSF analysis); the current recommendation is intravenous penicillin G 18 to 24 million units per day for 10 to 14 days. There can be transient worsening of eye disease due to a phenomenon known as the Jarisch-Herxheimer reaction, which is an immune-mediated inflammatory reaction to the dying spirochete, and which

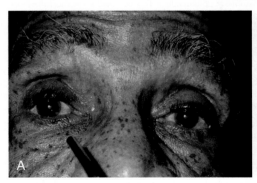
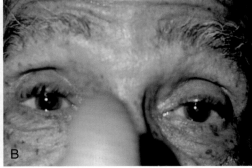

FIGURE 9.37 Argyll Robertson pupils: The pupils react poorly to direct light (A) but become more miotic on near testing (B). (From Savino P, Danesh-Meyer H. *Neuro-Ophthalmology*. 3rd ed. Philadelphia, PA: Wolters Kluwer; 2018.)

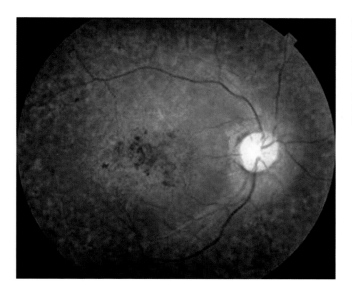

FIGURE 9.38 Patient with congenital syphilis with diffuse pigmentary retinopathy with optic disc pallor, retinal vascular attenuation resembles retinitis pigmentosa. (From Huang JJ, Gaudio PA. *Ocular Inflammatory Disease and Uveitis Manual.* Philadelphia, PA: Wolters Kluwer; 2010.)

can also cause systemic reactions such as fever, headache, myalgias, and malaise.[114] This reaction is not an indication to stop treatment, and IV methylprednisolone may be used in conjunction with penicillin to minimize the reaction in some cases.

Diagnostic laboratory testing for syphilis typically employs two-stage blood testing: the initial reactive plasma reagin screening test is confirmed, when positive, with a subsequent antitreponemal test. The RPR (rapid plasma reagin) test measures nonprotective antibodies; the level is used to determine the current level of disease activity and to titrate treatment. Antitreponemal tests (TPPA or FTA-Abs) determine whether the patient has ever had the disease and, in exposed patients, will remain positive for life. The antitreponemal tests may be reported as negative (nonreactive) if testing is done at a very early stage, before antibodies have developed. Darkfield microscopy and silver stain can be used to examine specimens and scrapings. Syphilis remains sensitive to penicillin, which is the preferred therapy for all stages.[115]

Prevention of transmission is an important public health goal. The use of a barrier method, chiefly condoms during sexual encounters, is a very effective way to prevent sexual transmission of syphilis and many other sexually transmitted infections.

REFERENCES

1. Metlay JP, Waterer GW, Long AC, et al. Diagnosis and treatment of adults with community-acquired pneumonia. An official clinical practice guideline of the American thoracic society and infectious diseases society of America. *Am J Respir Crit Care Med.* 2019;200(7):e45-e67. doi:10.1164/rccm.201908-1581ST.

2. JainS, Self WH, Wunderink RG, et al; CDC EPIC Study Team. Community-acquired pneumonia requiring hospitalization among U.S. Adults. *N Engl J Med.* 2015;373(5):415-427.

3. Zivich PN, Grabenstein JD, Becker-Dreps SI, Weber DJ. Streptococcus pneumoniae outbreaks and implications for transmission and control: a systematic review. *Pneumonia (Nathan).* 2018;10:11. doi:10.1186/s41479-018-0055-4.

4. Matanock A, Lee G, Gierke R, Kobayashi M, Leidner A, Pilishvili T. Use of 13-valent pneumococcal conjugate vaccine and 23-valent pneumococcal polysaccharide vaccine among adults aged ≥65 years: updated recommendations of the advisory committee on immunization practices. *MMWR Morb Mortal Wkly Rep.* 2019;68:1069-1075. doi:10.15585/mmwr.mm6846a5.

5. Truong J, Ashurst JV. *Pneumocystis (Carinii) Jiroveci Pneumonia.* [Updated 2019 February 22]. In: *StatPearls [Internet].* Treasure Island, FL: StatPearls Publishing; 2019. https://www.ncbi.nlm.nih.gov/books/NBK482370/.

6. https://www.cdc.gov/fungal/diseases/pneumocystis-pneumonia/index.html.

7. Perry JT, Chen WS. Acute mycoplasma pneumoniae infection presenting with unilateral anterior uveitis and perineuritis. *J AAPOS*. 2016;20(2):178-180. doi:10.1016/j.jaapos.2015.12.003.

8. Young J, De Sutter A, Merenstein D, et al. Antibiotics for adults with clinically diagnosed acute rhinosinusitis: a meta-analysis of individual patient data. *Lancet*. 2008;371:908.

9. Lindbaek M, Butler CC. Antibiotics for sinusitis-like symptoms in primary care. *Lancet*. 2008;371:874.

10. Williamson IG, Rumsby K, Benge S, et al. Antibiotics and topical nasal steroid for treatment of acute maxillary sinusitis: a randomized controlled trial. *J Am Med Assoc*. 2007;298:2487.

11. Rosenfeld RM, Piccirillo JF, Chandrasekhar SS, et al. Clinical practice guideline (update): adult sinusitis executive summary. *Otolaryngol Head Neck Surg*. 2015;152(4):598-609. doi:10.1177/0194599815574247.

12. Jeng A, Beheshti M, Li J, Nathan R. The role of β-hemolytic streptococci in causing diffuse, nonculturable cellulitis: a prospective investigation. *Medicine (Baltimore)*. 2010;89:217-226.

13. King M, Rose L, Fraimow H, Nagori M, Danish M, Doktor K. *Vibrio vulnificus* infections from a previously non-endemic area. *Ann Intern Med*. 2019;171:520-521. doi:10.7326/L19-0133.

14. Fridkin SK, Hageman JC, Morrison M, et al. Methicillin-resistant *Staphylococcus aureus* disease in three communities. *N Engl J Med*. 2005;352:1436-1444.

15. van de Beek D, de Gans J, Spanjaard L, Weisfelt M, Reitsma JB, Vermeulen M. Clinical features and prognostic factors in adults with bacterial meningitis. *N Engl J Med*. 2004;351(18):1849.

16. Hanna LS, Girgis NI, Yassin MW, et al. Incidence of papilloedema and optic atrophy in meningitis. *Jpn J Ophthalmol*. 1981;25:69-73.

17. Drake RL. Ocular syphilis. III. Review of the literature and report of a case of acute syphilitic meningitis and meningoencephalitis with special reference to papilledema. *Arch Ophthalmol*. 1933;9:234-243.

18. Pedersen E. Papilledema in encephalitis. *Arch Neurol*. 1965;13:403-408.

19. Friedman DI. Papilledema. Miller NR, Newman NJ, Biousse V, Kerrison JB, eds. *Walsh and Hoyt's Clinical Neuro-Ophthalmology*. 6th ed. Philadelphia, PA: Lippincott Williams & Wilkins; 2005:237-291.

20. Silverstein A. Papilledema with acute viral infections of the brain. *Mt Sinai J Med*. 1974;41:435-443.

21. Tunkel AR, Hartman BJ, Kaplan SL, et al. Practice guidelines for the management of bacterial meningitis. *Clin Infect Dis*. 2004;39(9):1267-1284. doi:10.1086/42536.

22. Atherton RR, Ellis J, Cresswell FV, Rhein J, Boulware DR. Ophthalmic signs in Ugandan adults with HIV-associated cryptococcal meningitis: a nested analysis of the ASTRO-CM cohort. *Wellcome Open Res*. 2018;3:80.

23. Shah P, Paul R, Gold R, Tashima K, Flanigan T. Treating HIV encephalopathy with antiretroviral therapy: a clinical case demonstrating the success of HAART. *Clin Infect Dis*. 2004;39(10):1545-1547. doi:10.1086/425119.

24. Pellegrino P, Carnovale C, Perrone V, et al. Epidemiological analysis on two decades of hospitalisations for meningitis in the United States. *Eur J Clin Microbiol Infect Dis*. 2014;33:1519-1524. doi:10.1007/s10096-014-2102-2.

25. Hsu HE, Shutt KA, Moore MR, et al. Effect of pneumococcal conjugate vaccine on pneumococcal meningitis. *N Engl J Med*. 2009;360:244-256.

26. *WHO Fact Sheet: Meningococcal Meningitis*. 2018. Accessed October 27, 2019. https://www.who.int/news-room/fact-sheets/detail/meningococcal-meningitis.

27. Centers for Disease Control and Prevention. *CDC Yellow Book 2020: Health Information for International Travel*. New York: Oxford University Press; 2019.

28. Mailles A, Stahl JP; Steering Committee and Investigators Group. Infectious encephalitis in France in 2007: a national prospective study. *Clin Infect Dis*. 2009;49(12):1838-1847. doi:10.1086/648419.

29. Hayashida MZ, Seque CA, Pasin VP, Enokihara MMSES, Porro AM. Disseminated cryptococcosis with skin lesions: report of a case series. *An Bras Dermatol*. 2017;92(5 suppl 1):69-72. doi:10.1590/abd1806-4841.20176343.

30. Sloan DJ, Parris V. Cryptococcal meningitis: epidemiology and therapeutic options. *Clin Epidemiol*. 2014;6:169-182. doi:10.2147/CLEP.S38850.

31. https://www.who.int/news-room/fact-sheets/detail/hepatitis-a.

32. Ryder SD, Beckingham IJ. ABC of diseases of liver, pancreas, and biliary system: acute hepatitis. *Br Med J*. 2001;322(7279):151-153. doi:10.1136/bmj.322.7279.151.

33. Centers for Disease Control and Prevention. In: Hamborsky J, Kroger A, Wolfe S, eds. *Epidemiology and Prevention of Vaccine-Preventable Diseases*. 13th ed. Washington, D.C: Public Health Foundation; 2015.

34. https://www.who.int/news-room/fact-sheets/detail/hepatitis-b.

35. Centers for Disease Control and Prevention (CDC). Updated U.S. Public health service guidelines for the management of occupational exposures to HBV, HCV, and HIV and recommendations for postexposure prophylaxis. *MMWR Recomm Rep*. 2001;50:1-42.

36. https://www.who.int/news-room/fact-sheets/detail/hepatitis-c.

37. Moyer VA; U.S. Preventive Services Task Force. Screening for hepatitis C virus infection in adults: U.S. Preventive services Task Force recommendation statement. *Ann Intern Med.* 2013;159:349-357.

38. https://www.who.int/news-room/fact-sheets/detail/hepatitis-e.

39. Seymour CW, Liu VX, Iwashyna TJ, et al. Assessment of clinical criteria for sepsis: for the third international consensus definitions for sepsis and septic shock (Sepsis-3). *J Am Med Assoc.* 2016;315(8):762-774. doi:10.1001/jama.2016.0288.

40. World Health Organization *Global Tuberculosis Report 2019.* https://www.who.int/tb/publications/factsheet_global.pdf?ua=1. Accessed November 29, 2019.

41. Zumla A, Raviglione M, Hafner R, von Reyn CF. Tuberculosis. *N Engl J Med.* 2013;368:745-755.

42. https://www.cdc.gov/tb/statistics/default.htm.

43. Small PM, Fujiwara PI. Management of tuberculosis in the United States. *N Engl J Med.* 2001;345:189-200.

44. Abu El-Asrar AM, Abouammoh M, Al-Mezaine HS. Tuberculous uveitis. *Int Ophthalmol Clin.* 2010;50:19-39.

45. Tabbara KF. Ocular tuberculosis: anterior segment. *Int Ophthalmol Clin.* 2005;45(2):57-69.

46. Demirci H, Shields CL, Shields JA, Eagle RC. Ocular tuberculosis masquerading as ocular tumors. *Surv Ophthalmol.* 2004;49(1):78-89.

47. Thompson MJ, Albert DM. Ocular tuberculosis. *Arch Ophthalmol.* 2005;123(6):844-849.

48. Horsburgh CR, Barry CE, Lange C. Treatment of tuberculosis. *N Engl J Med.* 2015;373:2149-2160.

49. Chamberlain PD, Sadaka A, Berry S, lee AG. Ethambutol optic neuropathy. *Curr Opin Ophthalmol.* 2017;28(6):545-551.

50. Prober C. Sixth disease and the ubiquity of human herpesviruses. *N Engl J Med.* 2005;352:753-755.

51. Gnann JW, Whitley RJ. Genital herpes. *N Engl J Med.* 2016;375(7):666-674.

52. Liesegang TJ. Herpes simplex virus epidemiology and ocular importance. *Cornea.* 2001;20(1):1-13.

53. Herpetic EyeDisease Study Group. Predictors of recurrent herpes simplex virus keratitis. Herpetic Eye Disease Study Group. *Cornea.* 2001;20:123-128.

54. Collum LMT, McGettrick P, Akhtar J, Lavin J, Rees PJ. Oral acyclovir (Zovirax) in herpes simplex dendriticcorneal ulceration. *Br J Ophthalmol.* 1986;70:435-438.

55. Sozen E, Avunduk AM, Akyol N. Comparison of efficacy of oral valacyclovir and topical acyclovir in the treatment of herpes simplex keratitis: a randomized clinical trial. *Chemotherapy.* 2006;52(1):29-31.

56. Wilhemlus KR. The treatment of herpes simplex virus epithelial keratitis. *Tr Am Ophth Soc.* 2000;98:505-532.

57. Goldstein DA, Li A, Palestine A, et al. Necrotizing herpetic retinitis. In: Larochelle M, ed. *American Academy of Ophthalmology, EyeWiki;* 2019. Accessed March 7, 2020. https://eyewiki.aao.org/Necrotizing_Herpetic_Retinitis.

58. Bodaghi B, Rozenberg F, Cassoux N, Fardeau C, LeHoang P. Nonnecrotizing herpetic retinopathies masquerading as severe posterior uveitis. *Ophthalmology.* 2003;110(9):1737-1743.

59. Corey L, Wald A, Patel R, et al. Once-daily valacyclovir to reduce the risk of transmission of genital herpes. *N Engl J Med.* 2004;350(1):11-20.

60. Cohen JI. Herpes zoster. *N Engl J Med.* 2013;369(3):255-263. doi:10.1056/NEJMcp1302674.

61. Breuer J, Fifer H. Chickenpox. *BMJ Clin Evid.* 2011;2011:0912.

62. Liesang TJ. Herpes zoster ophthalmicus. Natural history, risk factors, clinical presentation, and morbidity. *Ophthalmology.* 2008;115(2):S3-S12.

63. Brazis PW, Miller NR. Viruses (except retroviruses) and viral diseases. In: Miller NR, Newman NJ, eds. *Walsh & Hoyt's Clinical Neuro-Ophthalmology.* 6th ed. Philadelphia, PA: Lippincott Williams & Wilkins; 2005.

64. Amaki S, Suzuki S, Shinbo R, et al. A statistical study of ocular complications of herpes zoster ophthalmicus and its prolongation factors. *Nippon Ganka Gakkai Zasshi.* 1995;3:289-295.

65. Zaal MJ, Volker-Dieben HJ, D'Amaro J. Prognostic value of Hutchinson's sign in acute herpes zoster ophthalmicus. *Graefe's Arch Clin Exp Ophthalmol.* 2003;241:187-191.

66. Roberts TV, Francis IC, Kappagoda MB, Dick AD. Herpes zoster chorioretinopathy. *Eye.* 1995;9:594-598.

67. Marsh RJ, Dulley B, Kelly V. External ocular motor palsies in ophthalmic zoster: a review. *Br J Ophthalmol.* 1977;61:677-682.

68. Hilt DC, Buchholz D, Krumholz A, et al. Herpes zoster ophthalmicus and delayed contralateral hemiparesis caused by cerebral angiitis: diagnosis and management approaches. *Ann Neurol.* 1983;14:543-553.

69. Nagel MA, Jones D, Wyborny A. Varicella zoster virus vasculopathy: the expanding clinical spectrum and pathogenesis. *J Neuroimmunol.* 2017;308:112-117.

70. Nagel MA, Bennett JL, Khmeleva N, et al. Multifocal VZV vasculopathy with temporal artery infection mimics giant cell arteritis. *Neurology.* 2013;80:2017-2021.

71. Centers for Disease Control. Prevention of varicella: recommendations of the advisory committee on immunization practices (ACIP). *MMWR Recomm Rep.* 2007;56(RR-4):1-40.

72. Dooling KL, Guo A, Patel M, et al. Recommendations of the advisory committee on immunization practices for use of herpes zoster vaccines. *MMWR Morb Mortal Wkly Rep.* 2018;67:103-108. doi:10.15585/mmwr.mm6703a5.

73. Limaye AP, Kirby KA, Rubenfeld GD, et al. Cytomegalovirus reactivation in critically ill immunocompetent patients. *J Am Med Assoc.* 2008;300(4):413-422. doi:10.1001/jama.300.4.413.

74. Bale JF. Screening newborns for congenital cytomegalovirus infection. *J Am Med Assoc.* 2010;303(14):1425-1426. doi:10.1001/jama.2010.424.

75. Whitcup SM. Cytomegalovirus retinitis in the era of highly active antiretroviral therapy. *J Am Med Assoc.* 2000;283(5):653-657. doi:10.1001/jama.283.5.653.

76. Sousa Neves F, Braga J, Cardoso da Costa J, Sequeira J, Prazeres S. Kaposi's sarcoma of the conjunctiva and the eyelid leads to the diagnosis of human immunodeficiency virus infection – A case report. *BMC Cancer.* 2018;18(1):708.

77. Abalo-Lojo JM, Abdulkader-Nallib I, Pérez LM, Gonzalez F. Eyelid Kaposi sarcoma in an HIV-negative patient. *Indian J Ophthalmol.* 2018;66(6):854-855.

78. Coblentz J, Park JY, Discepola G, Arthurs B, Burnier M. Conjunctival Kaposi's sarcoma with orbital extension in an HIV-negative man. *Can J Ophthalmol.* 2018;53(3):e111-e113. doi:10.1016/j.jcjo.2017.09.014.

79. Nwabudike SM, Hemmings S, Paul Y, et al. Pulmonary Kaposi sarcoma: an uncommon cause of respiratory failure in the era of highly active antiretroviral therapy – Case report and review of the literature. *Case Rep Infect Dis.* 2016;2016:9354136. doi:10.1155/2016/9354136.

80. Centers for Disease Control and Prevention. *National Center for Emerging and Zoonotic Infectious Diseases (NCEZID), Division of High-Consequence Pathogens and Pathology (DHCPP).* Accessed December 2, 2019. https://www.cdc.gov/ncezid/dhcpp/poxvirus_rabies/index.html.

81. Centers for Disease Control and Prevention, *Global Health, Division of Parasitic Diseases.* Accessed December 3, 2019. https://www.cdc.gov/parasites/toxoplasmosis/epi.html.

82. Petersen E, Kijlstra A, Stanford M. Epidemiology of ocular toxoplasmosis. *Ocul Immunol Inflamm.* 2012;20(2):68-75.

83. Butler NJ, Furtado JM, Winthrop KL, Smith JR. Ocular toxoplasmosis II: clinical features, pathology and management. *Clin Exp Ophthalmol.* 2013;41(1):95-108.

84. Oude Lashof AM, Rothova A, Sobel JD, et al. Ocular manifestations of candidemia. *Clin Infect Dis.* 2011;53(3):262-268.

85. Vaziri K, Pershing S, Albini TA, Moshfeghi DM, Moshfeghi AA. Risk factors predictive of endogenous endophthalmitis among hospitalized patients with hematogenous infections in the United States. *Am J Ophthalmol.* 2015;159:498-504.

86. Anderson JA, Chai H, Clemon HN, et al. Candidiasis hypersensitivity syndrome [Position statement]. *J Allergy Clin Immunol.* 1986;78:271-273.

87. Klotz SA, Ianas V, Elliott SP. Cat scratch disease. *Am Fam Physician.* 2011;83(2):152-155.

88. Reed JB, Scales DK, Wong MT, Lattuada CP Jr, Dolan MJ, Schwab IR. Bartonella henselae neuroretinitis in cat scratch disease. Diagnosis, management, and sequelae. *Ophthalmology.* 1998;105(3):459.

89. Subramanian P. Bacteria and bacterial diseases. In: Miller JR, Newman NJ. *Walsh and Hoyt's Clinical Neuro-Ophthalmology.* 6th ed. Philadelphia, PA: Lippincott Williams & Wilkins; 2005:2647-2773.

90. Rosen BS, Barry CJ, Nicoll AM, Constable IJ. Conservative management of documented neuroretinitis in cat scratch disease associated with Bartonella henselae infection. *Aust N Z J Ophthalmol.* 1999;27(2):153-156.

91. *Content source: National Center for Immunization and Respiratory Diseases (NCIRD), Division of Viral Diseases.* Accessed December 17, 2019. https://www.cdc.gov/rubella/hcp.html.

92. Lambert N, Strebel P, Orenstein W, Icenogle J, Poland GA. Rubella. *Lancet.* 2015;385(9984):2297-2307. doi:10.1016/S0140-6736(14)60539-0.

93. Sherman FE, Michaels RH, Kenny FM. Acute encephalopathy (encephalitis) complicating rubella: report of cases with virologic studies, cortisol-production determinations, and observations at autopsy. *J Am Med Assoc.* 1965;192(8):675-681. doi:10.1001/jama.1965.03080210019005.

94. World Health Organization Fact Sheets: *Rubella.* Accessed October 4, 2019. https://www.who.int/news-room/fact-sheets/detail/rubella.

95. Matalia J, Shirke S. Congenital Rubella. *N Engl J Med* 2016;375:1468. doi:10.1056/NEJMicm1501815.

96. Reef SE, Plotkin S, Cordero JF, et al. Preparing for elimination of congenital Rubella syndrome (CRS): summary of a workshop on CRS elimination in the United States. *Clin Infect Dis*. 2000;31(1):85-95.

97. Sever JL, South MA, Shaver KA. Delayed manifestations of congenital rubella. *Rev Infect Dis*. 1985;7(suppl 1):S164.

98. Givens KT, Lee DA, Jones T, Ilstrup DM. Congenital rubella syndrome: ophthalmic manifestations and associated systemic disorders. *Br J Ophthalmol*. 1993;77(6):358-363.

99. Liu Y, Takusagawa HL, Chen TC, Pasquale LR. Fuchs heterochromic iridocyclitis and the rubella virus. *Int Ophthalmol Clin*. 2011;51(4):1-12.

100. Paules CI, Marston HD, Bloom ME, Fauci AS. Tickborne diseases – Confronting a growing threat .*N Engl J Med*. 2018;379:701-703.

101. Centers for Disease Control and Prevention. *National Center for Emerging and Zoonotic Infectious Diseases (NCEZID), Division of Vector-Borne Diseases (DVBD)*. Accessed December 9, 2019. Page last reviewed: November 22, 2019. https://www.cdc.gov/lyme/datasurveillance/maps-recent.html.

102. Nadelman RB, Nowakowski J, Fish D, et al. Prophylaxis with single-dose doxycycline for the prevention of Lyme disease after an Ixodes scapularis tick bite. *N Engl J Med*. 2001;345:79-84.

103. Weinberg RS. Ocular involvement in Lyme disease. *Am Acad Ophthalmol News*. 2008. Accessed November 5, 2008. https://www.aao.org/current-insight/ocular-involvement-in-lyme-disease#references.

104. Lesser RL. Ocular manifestations of Lyme disease. *Am J Med*. 1995;98(4A):60S-62S.

105. Klempner MS, Hu LT, Evans J, et al. Two controlled trials of antibiotic treatment in patients with persistent symptoms and a history of Lyme disease. *New Engl J Med*. 2001;345(2):85-92.

106. Peeling RW, Mabey D, Kamb ML, Chen XS, Radolf JD, Benzaken AS. Syphilis. *Nat Rev Dis Primers*. 2017;3:17073. doi:10.1038/nrdp.2017.73.

107. O'Byrne P, MacPherson P. Syphilis. *Br Med J*. 2019;365:l4159.

108. Clark EG, Danbolt N. The Oslo study of the natural course of untreated syphilis: an epidemiologic investigation based on a re-study of the Boeck-Bruusgaard material. *Med Clin North Am*. 1964;48:613.

109. Rosahn PD. *Autopsy Studies in Syphilis. 649 Information Supplement #21, J Venereal Disease*. Washington, DC: U.S. Public Health Service Venereal Disease Division; 1947.

110. Dutta Majumder P, Chen EJ, Shah J, Ching Wen Ho D. Ocular syphilis: an update. *Ocul Immunol Inflamm*. 2019;27(1):117-125.

111. Moradi A, Salek S, Daniel E, Gangaputra S. Clinical features and incidence rates of ocular complications in patients with ocular syphilis. *Am J Ophthalmol*. 2015;159(2):334-343.

112. Aldave AJ, King JA, Cunningham ET Jr. Ocular syphilis. *Curr Opin Ophthalmol*. 2001;12(6):433-441.

113. Boot JM, Oranje AP, de Groot R, Tan G, Stolz E. Congenital syphilis. *Int J STD AIDS*. 1992;3(3):161-167.

114. Fathilah J. The jarisch-herxheimer reaction in ocular syphilis. *Med J Malaysia*. 2003;58(3).

115. Workowski KA, Bolan GA; Centers for Disease Control and Prevention. Sexually transmitted diseases treatment guidelines, 2015. *MMWR Recomm Rep*. 2015;64(RR-03):1.

116. Barron BA, Gee L, Hauck WW, et al. Herpetic Eye Disease study. A controlled trial of oral acyclovir for herpes simplex stromal keratitis. *Ophthalmol*. 1994;101:1871-1882.

117. Wilhelmus KR, Gee L, Hauck WW, et al. Herpetic Eye Disease study. A controlled trial of topical corticosteroids for herpes simplex stromal keratitis. *Ophthalmol*. 1994;101:1883-1896.

118. The Herpetic Eye Disease Study Group. A controlled trial of oral acyclovir for iridocyclitis caused by herpes simplex virus. *Arch Ophthalmol*. 1996;114:1065-1072.

119. The Herpetic Eye Disease Study Group. The Epithelial Keratitis Trial. A controlled trial of oral acyclovir for the prevention of stromal keratitis or iritis in patients with herpes simplex virus epithelial keratitis. *Arch Ophthalmol*. 1997;115(6):703-712.

120. The Herpetic Eye Disease Study Group. Acyclovir for the prevention of recurrent herpes simplex virus eye disease. *N Engl J Med*. 1998;339:300-306.

HIV Infection

Richard Serrao

LEARNING OBJECTIVES

This chapter will review the natural history of HIV infection from acute HIV to AIDS, opportunistic infections, and comorbidities that occur as a result of HIV infection and preventative and treatment strategies.

KEY CONCEPTS

Section 1: Epidemiology and diagnosis
  Definitions and history
  Modes of transmission, risk behaviors, and statistics
  Diagnostic testing
Section 2: Symptoms and stages of HIV infection
  The relationship between HIV viral load and CD4 counts
  Acute HIV infection
  Chronic HIV infection
Section 3: AIDS
  Endogenous and exogenous organisms: from normal flora to pathogens
  How diseases behave in HIV-positive persons

  CD4 count and associated diseases, prevention, and treatments
  AIDS-associated infections
  HIV-related malignancies
Section 4: HIV-associated diseases
  HIV-related diseases affecting the eye and vision
Section 5: Vaccinations, screening, and primary care of the HIV-infected patient
Section 6: Treatment and prevention of HIV
  Antiretroviral therapy
  Adherence and resistance
    Timing of ART and potential complications: IRIS
  PEP and PREP
  HIV vaccines and cure strategies

SECTION 1: EPIDEMIOLOGY AND DIAGNOSIS
DEFINITIONS AND HISTORY

The **human immunodeficiency virus** (HIV) is a retrovirus, replicating by using host (human) DNA to reverse-transcribe its own genetic code (**FIGURE 10.1**). It is the causative agent of AIDS, the acquired immunodeficiency syndrome: *acquired* predominantly by sexual activity that causes a *deficiency* of the CD4+ T lymphocytes (CD4 cells or T-cells) that are crucial in achieving a regulated and effective immune response to pathogens.

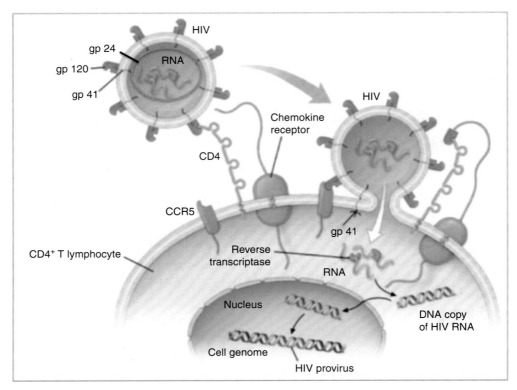

FIGURE 10.1 Schematic diagram of the HIV infection of helper CD4+ T-cell. Human immunodeficiency virus (HIV) is an RNA virus that contains the enzyme reverse transcriptase. The HIV capsid is form by the p24 protein which surrounds the viral genetic material. The envelope of the HIV virus contains the glycoprotein gp120, which bind to the CD4 molecules on helper T-cells. This results in formation of the CD4-gp120 complex, initiating a process that anchors virus to the helper T-cell lymphocyte's cell membrane. The C-C chemokine receptor type 5 (CCR5), is a major co-receptor for this process. The viral envelope then fuses with the T-cell membrane, allowing the virus to inject its genetic information (viral RNA with reverse transcriptase) into the T-cell cytoplasm. Reverse transcriptase produces a double-stranded DNA copy of a single-stranded viral RNA. The newly synthetized viral DNA is then transported into the T-cell nucleus. The viral enzyme integrase incorporates the viral DNA into the cell genome, at which point it is referred to as a "provirus." Viral RNA in the T-cell cytoplasm is translated by the cell, resulting in the synthesis of new viral proteins. (From Pawlina W, Ross MH. *Histology: A Text and Atlas*. 8th ed. Philadelphia, PA: Wolters Kluwer; 2018.)

Via phylogenetic analyses of stored human blood, HIV arose in the 1920s via cross-species zoonotic transmission of simian immunodeficiency virus from consumption and cross contamination of blood in the slaughter of nonhuman primates along trade routes in sub-Saharan Africa.[1] On June 4, 1981, the *MMWR* published the first case report of a cluster of unusual infections among five men who have sex with men (MSM) in Los Angeles that included oropharyngeal candidiasis (thrush), *Pneumocystis carinii* (now *Pneumocystis jirovecii*) pneumonia ("PCP"), and cytomegalovirus (CMV) infection, marking this the first description of a burgeoning new syndrome to be named.[2] Coincident case reports substantiated these stories: a wasting syndrome characterized by profound weight loss and diarrhea labeled "slim disease" was found among a "heterosexually promiscuous population" in rural Uganda. Some cases were associated with Kaposi sarcoma (KS) and some clinical features resembled an enteropathic acquired immunodeficiency syndrome being identified concurrently in Zaire.[3]

The unifying etiology for these mysterious immunocompromised conditions was ultimately deemed to be one and the same: HIV. In successive years, two distinct types (HIV-1 and HIV-2) and several groups of HIV have been identified worldwide. The cases found in the 1980s were just the tip of the proverbial iceberg of the pandemic that was to come. In this chapter, we will focus predominantly on the nature, pathogenesis, treatment, and prevention of disease of the most common type: HIV-1.

MODES OF TRANSMISSION, RISK BEHAVIORS, AND STATISTICS

HIV is predominantly a sexually transmitted infection (STI), yet it can be spread perinatally (during pregnancy or at delivery), through breast milk, and through exposure to infected blood such as from the sharing of contaminated needles. HIV cannot be transmitted through saliva, kissing, tears, or touching, unless body fluids like blood, semen, or vaginal secretions enter broken skin or mucus membranes. Currently, blood products and organ transplantation rarely, if ever, transmit HIV.

Politics aside, risk *groups* have been reclassified as risk *behaviors*. *Anyone* can become infected with HIV based on the probability of acquisition per *risk factor*. For example, there is an approximate 1 in 300 chance of acquiring HIV per high-risk exposure such as from a needle stick exposure to HIV-infected blood,[4] yet there is a 2000-fold higher relative risk for infection in unprotected receptive anal intercourse than there is in insertive oral sex.[5] Most infections are transmitted from someone newly infected when the amount of virus in the circulation (viremia) is at its highest,[6] and the rest are mainly from those who are not aware they are HIV positive—an estimated 8.1 million worldwide[7]—or not fully suppressed.[8] HIV transmissibility is heightened when other active STIs exist such as a chancre (painless ulcer) from syphilis, or an inflamed cervix from gonorrhea because of disruption of the mucosal barrier.[9] Those who are on treatment and can fully suppress their virus are generally not able to transmit it to their sexual partners.[10]

Worldwide as of 2018, rates of new infections and deaths are decreasing, yet United Nations AIDS data estimate that 37.9 million people were living with HIV; 770,000 died from AIDS-related ill and 1.7 million people became newly infected predominantly in Eastern Europe, Central Asia, Middle East, and North Africa at a rate of 5000 infections per day.[7] Eastern and southern Africa continue to bear the brunt of global infections with 20.6 million people, the majority of these afflicting young women from heterosexual transmission.[11] Among resource-rich settings like the United States, where an average of 40,000 infections continue to occur yearly and where there are just over one million persons currently HIV positive, a resurgence of new infections has impacted MSM populations.[12] Other sexual minorities, women, and people of color are overrepresented[13] (**FIGURE 10.2**). Although HIV has historically been a young person's disease, one in six new infections in the United States are in those aged 50 years or older.[14]

DIAGNOSTIC TESTING

HIV can be diagnosed as early as 15 days after infection using very sensitive fourth-generation immunoassay blood tests that detect both antibodies and glycoprotein p24 antigens that form the capsid of HIV 1 and 2 (**FIGURE 10.1**). Positive tests are confirmed by a differentiation immunoassay. If indeterminate (or even negative), which can sometimes be seen during the early "window period" of infection when antibodies are not fully formed or in false-positives, testing for the virus itself via the ultrasensitive polymerase chain reaction (PCR) confirms the diagnosis as early as 5 days after infection. The PCR quantifies the amount of virus circulating in the blood and is reported as a "viral load."

Testing has increased through verbal rather than written consent, home kits, and an "opt out" approach where testing "will be included as part of your care, unless you decline" rather than "would you like to be tested?"

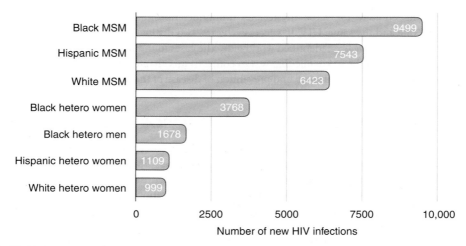

FIGURE 10.2 New HIV diagnoses in the United States and dependent areas for most affected subpopulations, 2018. (Image credit Richard Serrao, MD.)

SECTION 2: SYMPTOMS AND STAGES OF HIV INFECTION

HIV infection has three major stages: acute infection, chronic infection, and AIDS. In order to understand these stages, it is important to first appreciate the interaction between the two most important factors in disease progression and symptoms: HIV viral load and CD4 count.

THE RELATIONSHIP BETWEEN HIV VIRAL LOAD AND CD4 COUNTS

The HIV **viral load** (the number of viral particles per cubic milliliter of blood: copies/mL^3) and **CD4 cell count** (the number of cells per cubic milliliter of blood: cells/mL^3) correlate inversely (**FIGURE 10.3**): the higher the viral load, the higher the infectiousness, the faster the rate of CD4 decline, and consequently, the faster progression to AIDS. Of note, an undetectable viral load while on therapy reflects effective control of viral reproduction.

Normal CD4 counts range between 800 and 1400 cells/mL^3. Uncontrolled viral replication itself can lead to wasting and cachexia (loss of muscle and fat tissue leading to a skeletal appearance) akin to that described in "slim disease," yet it is the progressive immunologic decline and the consequent diseases that account for the predominant mortality in persons with HIV in those not receiving specific HIV medications. This process takes an average of 10 years from initial infection but can vary depending on several factors, mainly through the interplay between the host's immune makeup and the viral strain (**FIGURE 10.4**).

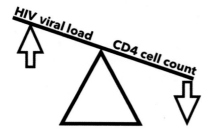

FIGURE 10.3 The inverse relationship between viral load rise and CD4 count drop. (Image credit Richard Serrao, MD.)

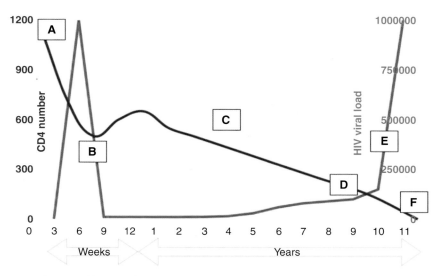

FIGURE 10.4 The natural history of HIV/AIDS: A, primary infection; B, acute HIV infection, wide dissemination of virus, seeding of lymphoid organs; C, clinical latency; D, constitutional symptoms; E, opportunistic diseases; F, death. (Image credit Richard Serrao, MD.)

At two ends of the spectrum, some HIV-positive individuals are "elite controllers" who are able to natively control viral replication and others are "rapid progressors," individuals who are unable to naturally control HIV leading to a more accelerated course to AIDS. At one extreme, a small percentage of the world's population carries the genetic profile that results in a lack of the CCR5 or CXCR4 coreceptors on macrophages or T-cells that make these persons functionally resistant to HIV, provided the strain of HIV they are exposed to requires those receptors to gain cell entry.[15] The viral load in these individuals can be as low as a few hundred copies or not detectable at all since viral replication is inefficient. As a result, CD4 counts are generally unmoved and the patient does not progress to AIDS. This scenario is the exception.

For most chronically infected HIV-positive individuals not on treatment, the HIV viral load settles to around the tens of thousands, which leads to the typical *gradual* decline in CD4 count over years. In contrast, those with the most symptoms during the acute HIV syndrome can manifest a viral load in the millions, and CD4 counts can acutely plummet in some. In those on treatment, mortality is best predicted by viral load rather than by CD4.[16]

ACUTE HIV INFECTION

Acute HIV is the initial syndrome experienced by 40% of people, on average 2 weeks after infection, and is characterized predominantly by a prolonged fever, pharyngitis, and diffuse lymphadenopathy due to significant viremia. Up to 50% of individuals can manifest a morbilliform (measles-like) rash (**FIGURE 10.5**). These symptoms mimic infectious mononucleosis caused by the Epstein-Barr virus (EBV) and to a lesser extent other viruses like CMV or herpes simplex viruses (HSVs). Given the similarities in presentation, acute HIV must be considered in all cases of mononucleosis.

Acute HIV is suspected on clinical grounds and diagnosed by patterns in antibody/antigen/viral load tests that characterize the aforementioned "window period": namely negative or early and evolving antibody patterns with positive viral loads. Identifying this syndrome is valuable because early treatment, especially in those with a profoundly symptomatic acute phase, preserves cellular immunity and minimizes transmission risk to others. Delays in diagnosis yield poorer results overall in reconstituting an HIV-positive patient's immunity.[17]

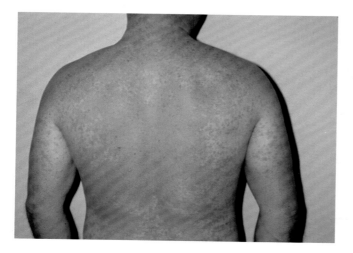

FIGURE 10.5 Characteristic morbilliform rash of acute HIV. (From Goodheart HP. *Goodheart's Photoguide of Common Skin Disorders.* 2nd ed. Philadelphia, PA: Lippincott Williams & Wilkins; 2003.)

Chronic HIV Infection

After acute infection, most patients' symptoms subside, and they enter the chronic phase of HIV that for most lasts many years. This period is spent predominantly in clinical *latency* where patients remain asymptomatic, although some can experience a variety of constitutional findings that could be suggestive of, yet not specific to, HIV. These include fatigue, fever, night sweats, weight loss, diarrhea, lymphoepithelial parotid cysts, and persistent generalized lymphadenopathy. The latter two present with fullness in the face and diffusely enlarged lymph nodes throughout the body, respectively. These findings typically correlate with high viral loads and when seen can be a harbinger for a faster progression to AIDS. It is not until CD4 cells decline substantially that a patient is at risk for what are called AIDS-defining conditions.

SECTION 3: AIDS

AIDS is defined as a CD4 count of <200 cells/mL^3 or the presence of AIDS-defining conditions (TABLE 10.1) in an HIV-positive individual, irrespective of their CD4 count.[18] HIV *itself* can create AIDS-defining conditions, which include HIV-related encephalopathy and wasting syndrome. HIV encephalopathy, also categorized as HIV-associated neurocognitive disorder (HAND), can manifest a range of symptoms from mild cognitive impairment and apathy to movement disorders to frank dementia. Progression of HAND can correlate with prolonged poor peripheral viremic control, yet can paradoxically occur in those who maintain robust peripheral CD4 counts and undetectable viral loads. Those most at risk for HAND progression are an AIDS diagnosis, male sex, lower educational level, and hepatitis B co-infection according to one study.[19]

As the name implies, HIV wasting refers to progressive weight loss and cachexia in the absence of an alternative disease process. HIV wasting tends to only occur in patients not on therapy.

ENDOGENOUS AND EXOGENOUS ORGANISMS: FROM NORMAL FLORA TO PATHOGENS

The concepts of *normal flora, colonization, virulence, pathogenicity, infection, disease,* and *reactivation* are salient with respect to *endogenous* and *exogenous* organisms in patients with AIDS.

The human body harbors more organisms than the number of cells that make up the entire body. These *endogenous* organisms are comprised mainly of bacteria and yeasts such as staphylococci,

TABLE 10.1   **AIDS-Defining Diagnoses in Order of Progressive Prevalence as CD4 Cells Decline. Some Infections/Diseases can Occur at Higher or Lower CD4 Counts**
Candidiasis of bronchi, trachea, lungs, or esophagus
Recurrent pneumonia** and/or multiple/recurrent bacterial infections*
Recurrent *Salmonella* septicemia
Chronic ulcers (>1-mo duration), bronchitis, pneumonitis, or esophagitis due to herpes simplex***
Pneumocystis jirovecii pneumonia ("PCP")
Invasive cervical cancer**
Disseminated or extrapulmonary histoplasmosis
Burkitt, immunoblastic, or primary central nervous system lymphoma
Intestinal cryptosporidiosis or isosporiasis of >1-mo duration
Cerebral toxoplasmosis***
Disseminated or extrapulmonary coccidioidomycosis
Extrapulmonary cryptococcosis
Disseminated or extrapulmonary *Mycobacterium tuberculosis***, Mycobacterium avium* complex (MAC), *Mycobacterium kansasii,* or other species
Kaposi sarcoma
Cytomegalovirus disease (other than liver, spleen, or nodes)*** or of retina with vision loss
HIV encephalopathy
Wasting syndrome attributed to HIV
Progressive multifocal leukoencephalopathy (PML)

*Age < 6 y, **Age ≥ 6 y, ***Age > 1 mo.

streptococci, enterococci, corynebacteria, lactobacilli, and candida coating the upper airway, gastrointestinal (GI) tract, skin, and urogenital system. In the absence of disease, endogenous organisms exist in homeostasis—a balance between each other and our body that has evolved to contribute to the physiologic functioning of the whole. When serving predominantly in this capacity, organisms are considered commensals, or *normal flora*. A swab of anyone's arm will always grow *Staphylococcus epidermidis* on culture media because this organism is considered normal flora of all human skin.

Exogenous organisms are organisms that are not part of our normal flora and are acquired through inhalation, ingestions, abrasions, contact, and insect bites, for example. These are usually *pathogens* because they create disease. Some examples and their respective diseases and routes of acquisition include the viruses rhinovirus and influenza causing the common cold and the flu through the air; the bacterium *Salmonella typhi* and the virus hepatitis A causing typhoid fever and liver failure from consumption of contaminated food or water; the parasite *Malaria malariae* and the spirochete *Borrelia burgdorferi* causing malaria and Lyme disease from bites from insect vectors like the *Anopheles* mosquitoes and *Ixodes scapularis* ticks; and *Treponema pallidum* (syphilis), *Neisseria gonorrhoeae* (gonorrhea), *Chlamydia trachomatis* (chlamydia), and HIV causing their respective infections from sexual activity.

Some endogenous and exogenous organisms inhabit niches they typically do not, and can briefly be reclassified as *colonizers* of those spaces. They may reach homeostasis within that environment but can shift from colonizers to *pathogens* based on the conditions of the environment they populate or their inherent capacity to create disease, also known as their *virulence*. For example, *Staphylococcus aureus*, a relatively virulent endogenous bacteria, can be found in many individuals inhabiting the skin of the groin, axillae, or inside the nose. However, when it asymptomatically colonizes the upper airway, it has a higher probability of causing pneumonia if aspirated into the lungs from this novel location.

The endogenous normal flora *Candida albicans* transforms into a pathogen when it creates "yeast infections." Candida is relatively avirulent, yet in areas of the body that have become favorable due to moisture, or disruption of normal flora from the use of antibiotics (which do not kill yeast), or when a patient has poorly controlled diabetes or HIV, for example, candidiasis appears as scattered patches of white overlying an inflamed mucous membrane. Common areas include the female genital tract (*vulvovaginal candidiasis*) or intertriginous areas such as under a breast or fold of tissue in the groin in men or women.

The exogenous fungus, *P. jirovecii*, which we will explore later, is an example of an exogenous organism that colonizes the lungs in many people. It is not remarkably virulent, until it can be.

HOW DISEASES BEHAVE IN HIV-POSITIVE PERSONS

Indirectly, most of the harm from HIV comes from its effects on T-cells, of which CD4+ cells are a subset. Among their many roles, these T-helper cells modulate the activity of B-cells, which in turn produce antibodies (*humoral immunity*) that principally combat bacterial infections. The T-cells chiefly provide *cell-mediated immunity*, which aims to sequester infectious agents that multiply intracellularly like mycobacteria, viruses, some bacteria, certain fungi, and protozoa. Since these infections are uncommon in hosts with normal immune function, HIV must always be considered when these are suspected or diagnosed.

Diseases of these kinds can also be found in other circumstances that affect cell-mediated immunity. These include antirejection medications in recipients of solid organ transplants, the use of monoclonal antibody drugs such as infliximab or tumor necrosis factor blockers like etanercept for the control of rheumatologic conditions such as rheumatoid arthritis, and disorders of the hematopoietic system like leukemias and their associated treatments.

Many of the organisms that can affect the HIV-positive patient have been addressed in Chapter 9, yet it is important to see how many of these behave within the context of progressive immunosuppression. Most diseases with which HIV associates are diseases that, through the destruction of the immune system, are *allowed to occur*. These are called *opportunistic infections* ("OIs"), infections that take the *opportunity* to create diseases when the immune system is incapable of controlling them when acquired anew (eg, bacterial pneumonia or *Salmonella* sepsis), permitting it to grow into a pathogen from a colonizer (eg, thrush or PCP), or preventing it from *reactivating* (eg, previously acquired tuberculosis, many chronic viruses, or fungi).

Most exogenous organisms invade, create disease, and are then eliminated by our immune system with or without sequelae or medications, resulting in a self-limited illness. Many infections, like HIV, persist for life. For those pathogens that are not fully eradicated, the term *infection* still applies, even though *disease* may not currently be present. Latent, or dormant, organisms can *reactivate* within the tissues of the body if the conditions to do so are favorable.

Latency within this context is distinct from the latent phases of HIV in that HIV is always replicating to some extent throughout the course of its natural history. On the other hand, clinically latent infections that reactivate due to HIV (or other immunocompromising disorders like diabetes, chronic kidney disease, or active malignancies) are not actively replicating until they can. Because of the nature of latency, a person's prior residences, food choices, occupations and sexual activities are as or more important than more recent exposures in determining the potential etiologies of infections in the HIV+ individual.

To clearly illustrate the concept of reactivation, *Mycobacterium tuberculosis* (MTB) serves as a good example. Tuberculosis as a *disease* can be characterized as a progressive destructive ("cavitary") pneumonia with prolonged fevers, night sweats, weight loss, and hemoptysis.

Only 5% to 10% of infected people will experience tuberculosis disease as a *primary* symptomatic infection after exposure. However, most tuberculosis infections are in a *latent* stage: though the immune system contains it during primary infection, it fails to fully eliminate it in approximately 90% of individuals.[20] Residual hardy organisms that survive are sequestered, and lay dormant within macrophages in lung tissue for life. This condition is called latent tuberculosis infection (LTBI) and, in contrast to active tuberculosis disease, has no symptoms. Diagnosis of LTBI is made within the appropriate epidemiologic context by transdermal skin testing or blood immune gamma release assays and, simultaneously, by confirming that there is no active disease with lung imaging, usually by chest x-ray.

A healthy 40-year-old California native with evidence of LTBI, no evidence for active disease, and no accumulation of any other immunocompromising conditions of significance in her lifetime can expect a cumulative risk of developing reactivation tuberculosis of about 4% to 10% simply due to the natural waning of her immunity as she ages toward 80. If that same individual is diagnosed with AIDS, however, her lifetime risk reaches 100%.[21] Not surprisingly, the global distribution of tuberculosis closely matches that of untreated HIV because untreated HIV contributes to tuberculosis disease activity.[22] More than 60% of those with tuberculosis in South Africa, for example, also have HIV.[23]

The behavior of the closely related viruses CMV, HSV, EBV (mononucleosis), and VZV (*varicella-zoster* virus: chicken pox, shingles) can further illustrate this concept. After initial infection, all four of these viruses remain clinically latent and remain dormant within tissues like lymph nodes or nerve roots. In the absence of risk factors for complications, most healthy individuals recuperate fully after primary infection.

The most likely of these to reactivate is herpes, a virus that lays inert within sensory nerves. In many people, herpes periodically breaks out during a person's lifetime as the characteristic vesicular (blister-like) eruption ("cold sore") on the lips (**FIGURE 10.6**) and genitalia. Much less commonly, ocular involvement is seen as herpetic keratitis with or without uveitis (see below).

One need not be immunocompromised to manifest these breakouts. The threshold for herpes to reactivate is already low. For instance, simple stressors such as cold air, sunlight, chapped lips, or another concurrent taxing event to the body can facilitate viral escape. On the other hand, CMV has a higher threshold to reactivate, and the immune system must be weaker before it has a chance to create disease (see below).

VZV, the etiologic agent for primary *varicella*, or "chicken pox," is a self-limited illness characterized by fever, malaise, and a generalized vesicular rash commonly affecting children (**FIGURE 10.7**). When it reactivates, it appears as the painful rash called *herpes zoster*, an eruption like the vesicles of chicken pox but confined to a *dermatome*, the sensory root distribution where it had laid dormant. This condition is known colloquially as shingles (**FIGURE 10.8**). The most common reason for shingles to present is advancing age. Cancer chemotherapy, poorly controlled diabetes, corticosteroid use, and HIV also increase the risk for shingles dramatically.

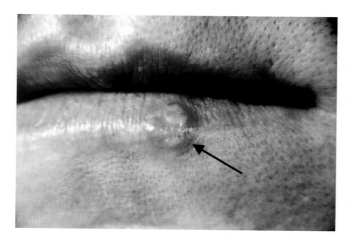

FIGURE 10.6 A crop of herpes simplex vesicles on the lower lip. (Public Health Image Library http://phil.cdc.gov/Phil/default.asp. PHIL ID# 1573.)

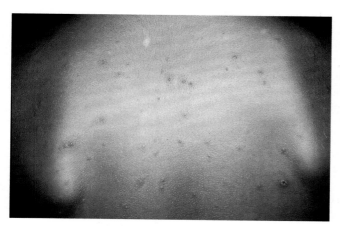

FIGURE 10.7 Chicken pox in a child caused by varicella-zoster infection. Vesicles are distributed across the body. (Reprinted from Goodheart HP. *Goodheart's Photoguide of Common Skin Disorders.* 2nd ed. Philadelphia, PA: Wolters Kluwer; 2003.)

FIGURE 10.8 Herpes zoster (shingles) in an adult. Vesicles are distributed in a band-like manner along a dermatome. (Reprinted from Edwards L, Lynch P. *Genital Dermatology Atlas and Manual.* 3rd ed. Philadelphia, PA: Wolters Kluwer; 2017.)

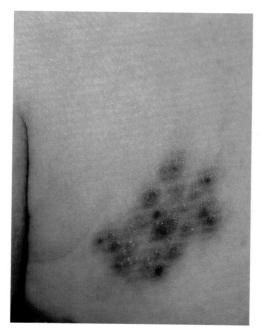

CD4 Count and Associated Diseases, Prevention, and Treatments

TABLE 10.2 lists some of the most prevalent OIs relative to specific CD4 counts. These breakpoints are not rigid, yet certain pivotal thresholds must generally be met before these diseases can become manifest. Conversely, when CD4 counts are well within the normal range, AIDS-defining diagnoses are not likely.

This listing is not all-inclusive because the epidemiology of OIs differs around the world. TABLE 10.2 relates predominantly to the OIs encountered in the United States. However, *Talaromyces marneffei*, a dimorphic fungus that behaves similarly to some fungi we will explore later in this chapter, affects individuals at CD4 counts ≤100 but is not listed in TABLE 10.2 because it is endemic only to Asia. Similarly, *Pneumocystis* is less, and tuberculosis is more prevalent in Africa than these diseases are in America.[24]

It should be emphasized up front that the centerpiece for management of all the OIs reviewed in this section is through the use of potent antiretroviral therapy (ART) as a preventative and treatment strategy (see section on antiretroviral therapy).

AIDS-ASSOCIATED INFECTIONS

When OIs occur in a setting of low and even lower CD4 counts, they are generally *more* symptomatic (many times in different ways), *more* aggressive, and *more* life-threatening than at the time of initial acquisition (provided that the individual infected is not immunocompromised at that time). They also can strike virtually every organ, including the eyes.

Any CD4

M. tuberculosis reactivates at any CD4 count and is inclined to spread beyond the lungs (ie, becoming *extrapulmonary*) at mostly lower CD4 numbers. TB can destabilize the spine as in Pott disease, seed the peritoneum, and obstruct the flow of cerebrospinal fluid (CSF) or the movement of the extraocular muscles by compressing the cranial nerves via the formation of granulomas at the base of the skull. Four drug regimens of rifampin, isoniazid, pyrazinamide and ethambutol are necessary to initially treat active tuberculosis infection.

TABLE 10.2	Prototypical Opportunistic Infections Relative to CD4 Count Thresholds
CD4	**Opportunistic Infection**
Any	*Mycobacterium tuberculosis*
≤500	Shingles, thrush, recurrent harpes/vulvovaginal candidiasis/pneumonia
≤250	Coccidioidomycosis
≤200	Pneumocystis
≤150	Histoplasmosis
≤100	Toxoplasmosis, cryptococcosis, primary central nervous system lymphoma, PML, KS
≤50	*Mycobacterium avium* complex (MAC), CMV, cryptosporidiosis, isosporiasis

CMV, cytomegalovirus; KS, Kaposi sarcoma; PML, progressive multifocal leukoencephalopathy.

In the absence of active tuberculosis, patients are offered *prophylaxis* for LTBI to prevent progression with once daily isoniazid for 6 to 9 months or longer, depending on the incidence of tuberculosis in the region acquired. Alternatively, shorter durations with the rifamycin class of anti-tuberculars (like rifampin alone or rifapentene in combination with isoniazid) can be used if there are no drug interactions with HIV-specific medications.

A thorough search for active tuberculosis disease is necessary in any HIV+ patient with positive TB skin or blood testing and/or TB epidemiologic risk factors like homelessness, incarceration, and prior residence or visitation to tuberculosis-endemic regions of the world, even when the only presenting symptom is a persistent fever. Because tissue destruction is partly mediated by the immune response to the pathogen, tuberculosis in advanced AIDS patients can paradoxically present without classic findings and evade detection.

CD4 ≤ 500

Appearing at around a CD4 count of 500 and below, recurrent vulvovaginal candidiasis, shingles, recurrent herpes, and recurrent pneumonias are all possible when CD4 cells relinquish control over these organisms.

Oropharyngeal candidiasis, also known as thrush, is the most common OI in patients with HIV (see **FIGURE 10.9**).

Because it is inherently difficult for candida to grow on the mucous membranes of the mouth where chewing and swallowing mechanically prevents it from doing so, the finding of thrush is strongly indicative of immunodeficiency. At even lower CD4 counts, the same process that results in thrush can spread down the alimentary tract causing esophageal candidiasis resulting in odynophagia (pain with swallowing). Candida can invade the bloodstream and attach to cardiac valves (fungal endocarditis) or the vitreous and/or aqueous humors of the eyes (candidal endophthalmitis) (**FIGURE 10.10**).

Candidal infections respond to topical agents depending on the extent of disease. For localized disease, nystatin, which binds to and increases the permeability of fungal walls, can be swished and swallowed to treat both oropharyngeal and esophageal infections. With repeated treatments,

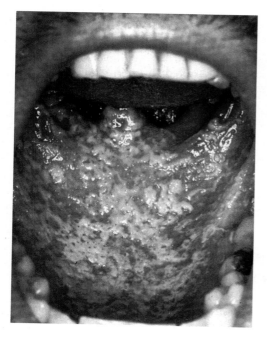

FIGURE 10.9 Oropharyngeal candidiasis (thrush). (Reprinted with permission from Harvey RA, Cornelissen CN. *Lippincott Illustrated Reviews: Microbiology.* 3rd ed. Philadelphia, PA: Wolters Kluwer; 2012.)

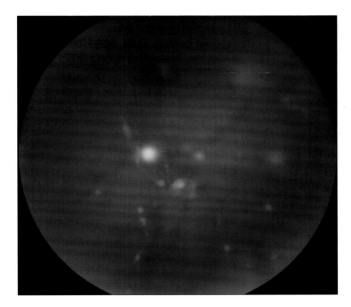

FIGURE 10.10 Endogenous fungal endophthalmitis. There are many small vitreous abscesses in a case of fungal endophthalmitis caused by *Candida albicans*. (Courtesy of MidAtlantic Retina, the Retina Service of Wills Eye Hospital.)

unfortunately, candida can become refractory to first-line agents. This requires escalation from the azole class of fluconazole or itraconazole to the later generation azole derivatives such as voriconazole or posaconazole. Intravenous therapy with the echinocandin class (eg, caspofungin, micafungin) and amphotericin is reserved for difficult-to-eradicate infections.

Herpes, typically localized to a small cluster of vesicles on the lips or genitalia at a CD4 count of 450, can markedly ulcerate and can spread to the eyes, GI tract, and brain when the CD4 count is 50. At this level of immunosuppression, herpes can affect the eyes as peripheral outer retinal necrosis (**FIGURE 10.11**), esophagus as ulcerations resulting in odynophagia, and brain as herpes *encephalitis* manifesting as hemorrhagic necrosis (bleeding and cell death) of the temporal lobes with concomitant seizures and coma.

Shingles in the patient with advanced AIDS not only is more common but has a higher potential to become *extradermatomal*. This scenario can resemble primary varicella (chickenpox) with the possibilities for coexistent varicella pneumonia or varicella encephalitis, resulting in altered mental status, altered motor function or sensation, and/or seizures.

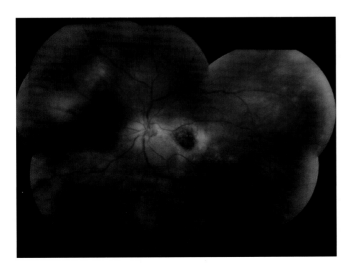

FIGURE 10.11 Progressive outer retinal necrosis, with large areas of outer retinal whitening involving the macula. Note the lack of vitritis and vasculitis. (Reprinted from Garg SJ. *Uveitis*. 2nd ed. Philadelphia, PA: Wolters Kluwer; 2018.)

Recurrent herpes and shingles are treated similarly. Episodic or suppressive use of inhibitors of herpes viral DNA polymerase (acyclovir, famciclovir, or valacyclovir) can abort or suppress herpes, and intravenous acyclovir is first-line therapy for disseminated zoster. HSV and VZV are prone to resistance in the HIV population due to frequent or prolonged use of these agents. More toxic therapies like foscarnet or cidofovir may become necessary.

Recurrent pneumonias are prevented via vaccination for vaccine preventable pathogens, such as *Streptococcus pneumoniae* and *Haemophilus influenzae*, as well as seasonal influenza vaccine and are treated with empiric or targeted antimicrobials (penicillins, cephalosporins, or macrolide antibiotics) or antivirals if applicable (eg, neuraminidase inhibitors like oseltamivir for influenza).

CD4 ≤ 250

The etiologic agent for "Valley fever," *Coccidioides immitis*, is a fungus endemic to the southwest United States (predominantly regions of California and Arizona), Central and South America. With progressive immunocompromise, coccidioidomycosis ("cocci") becomes possible. When acquired as a primary infection via the inhalation of arthroconidia (spores) that disseminate through the air during farming, construction, or windy periods, greater than 60% of infected people have no symptoms or experience a mild self-limited respiratory infection. As a result, very few people seek medical attention.

Cocci can remain in a dormant state predominantly in lung tissue and reactivate at a CD4 <250. Because of this latency, as with other reactivation diseases, clinicians must take a thorough travel and occupational history to increase the index of suspicion. It is not unusual for an advanced AIDS patient who had lived in the San Joaquin Valley of California as a child to present with reactivation cocci in New York many years later.

Coccidioidomycosis is typically extrapulmonary and can affect the skin, bone, joints, lymph nodes, and meninges in AIDS. It is treated with fluconazole or itraconazole except in severe cases (such as rapid progression or central nervous system [CNS] disease) with liposomal amphotericin B. There is no vaccine for coccidioides. In those who test positive for exposure to cocci via serologic testing and have a CD4 count <250, preemptive fluconazole can be used to suppress or eradicate residual cocci before it can create disease and can be stopped when CD4 counts rise above the level of risk via ART.

CD4 ≤ 200

The archetypal AIDS-defining diagnosis is PCP. It is still a threat to those with CD4 counts below 200 and is a significant cause of life-threatening pneumonia in HIV patients. A fungal colonizer of the lungs, *P. jirovecii* (reclassified from *P. carinii* to more accurately reflect the species affecting humans but keeping the PCP name) presents as an indolent nonproductive cough, fever, and progressive shortness of breath. PCP is typically more acute and aggressive in non-HIV at-risk populations with immunodeficiencies.

Securing a diagnosis of PCP requires a combination of high clinical suspicion, staining for fungi (eg, Gomori methenamine silver) or PCR on respiratory specimens, and supportive radiographic and laboratory findings. Because the pathogenesis of this disease occurs predominantly within the interstitial spaces (like scaffolding) of the lungs rather than the alveoli themselves, the chest x-ray may appear normal despite significant disease. Clues to more severe disease lie in assessment of arterial blood gas measurements and quantitation of serum lactate dehydrogenase levels which can demonstrate significant defects in gas exchange (abnormal alveolar-arterial gradient) and tissue damage, respectively. Testing for the presence of serum beta-D-glucan, a cell wall component of many fungi, can be supportive. Extrapulmonary disease is uncommon but can be subclinical (found mainly at autopsy) or cause progressive multisystem disease.

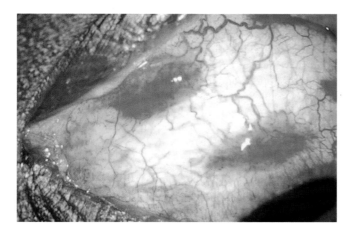

FIGURE 10.15 Fleshy vascular lesions on the conjunctiva in an AIDS patient with Kaposi sarcoma. (Reprinted from Chern KC, Saidel MA. *Ophthalmology Review Manual.* 2nd ed. Philadelphia, PA: Wolters Kluwer; 2011.)

explored and revealed that those who are seropositive for HHV-8 are more likely to develop the disease than those who are not. Their appearance can mimic bacillary angiomatosis, a systemic infection from *Bartonella* bacterial species transmitted from cat scratches or body lice. KS can involve the visceral structures such as the gums, oral cavity, GI tract, or lungs. Lesions localized to those areas can impede chewing, swallowing, digesting, or breathing. KS can also affect the conjunctiva, where it is generally asymptomatic and is reported as an area of "redness" (FIGURE 10.15).

KS lesions are stratified as cutaneous or visceral to establish the potential for complications and the treatment implemented. If KS involves just the skin, particularly if obstructing lymphatic flow, lesions have traditionally been treated with intralesional chemotherapy and radiation therapy. KS involving the viscera can be treated with systemic chemotherapy. These distinctions are presently less important because ART is most effective in treating both, "melting away" lesions with time (FIGURE 10.16).

Because of the immunologic control that ART affords, the prevalence (the number of cases present in a population at a given time) of malignancies resulting from these infections is decreasing, while the prevalence of non–AIDS-defining cancers is increasing.[32,33] Non–AIDS-defining cancers like lung, breast, and skin are rising because ART offers a longer lifespan that results in ample time to accumulate traditional environmental or genetic factors such as smoking and lung cancer, ultraviolet rays and skin cancer, and genetic markers for breast cancer. Using traditional screening tools,

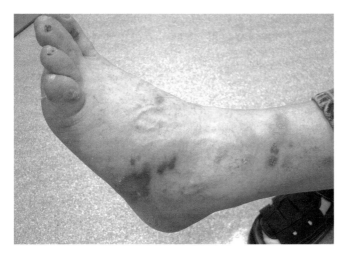

FIGURE 10.16 Classic violaceous papules on the skin of a patient with Kaposi sarcoma. (Photo credit to the author: Richard Serrao, MD.)

age-appropriate screening for all cancers is performed with mammographies for breast cancer, colonoscopies for colon cancer, Pap smears for cervical cancer, etc, as with the general population.

HIV+ patients who are co-infected with oncogenic strains of human papilloma virus or have chronic hepatitis B or C are assessed and surveilled for curative intent (eg, colposcopy or confocal microscopy of cervical or anal tissue; drugs to suppress or cure hepatitis B/C). These diseases are all preventable (through vaccines), modifiable (through behavioral changes), and curable (hepatitis C).

SECTION 4: HIV-ASSOCIATED DISEASES

In addition to OIs and malignancies, those who are HIV+ can experience a unique set of secondary medical issues directly related to HIV infection and/or its treatments (see section on treatment). Other infections that can come bundled with the same psychosocial risk factors that contributed to HIV acquisition (eg, unprotected sexual activity, intravenous drug use, neuropsychiatric diseases, psychosocial marginalization) are hepatitis B or C infection, tuberculosis, and STIs. An increased burden of general medical issues like accelerated aging; osteopenia; cardiovascular disease; metabolic syndromes; and chronic liver, lung, and kidney diseases also occur.[34] An estimated 20% of HIV-infected persons in the United States do not know their diagnosis[35] and are therefore more apt to present late to care in their disease course. Consequently, HIV itself can exploit and weaken the bone marrow, resulting in a reduction of all cell lines that include white blood cells, red blood cells, and platelets, resulting in pancytopenia. This increases their risk for infection, generalized weakness, malaise, and bleeding. HIV can preferentially destroy platelets causing idiopathic thrombocytopenic purpura which can result in spontaneous bleeding. With time, irrespective of CD4 decline, uncontrolled HIV viremia can establish an immune complex–mediated kidney disease known as HIV-associated nephropathy. Prior to more stringent use of early ART, many patients progressed to end-stage kidney disease directly related to HIV[36]; post-ART, patients' requirements for renal replacement therapy (ie, hemodialysis) are from HIV-related and non–HIV-related reasons as the population ages.[37]

Traditional risk factors like hypertension, smoking, diabetes, and hyperlipidemia in HIV-infected adults contribute predominantly to cardiovascular risk, although untreated HIV is directly myocardiotoxic and OIs like tuberculosis or pneumococcus can potentially fill the pericardial space with pus, restricting the pumping of the heart. HIV itself can occasionally alter the structure of the pulmonary circulation, leading to pulmonary hypertension, a condition that creates dyspnea on exertion, exertional chest pain, and fluid retention.

Principally through the accelerated progression to cirrhosis from chronic active hepatitis C or B infection and alcohol use, HIV+ patients can manifest a range of liver abnormalities, from mild fatty liver changes to advanced liver disease, including AIDS cholangiopathy, an infiltrative disease of the biliary tract resulting in strictures and obstruction of the flow of bile in those with CD4 counts less than 100.

In addition to the cutaneous manifestations of the many OIs discussed earlier materializing on the skin like cryptococcus, MAC, KS lesions, or HPV papillomas (warts), HIV-induced immunosuppression predisposes the patient to seborrheic dermatitis, a condition that is most commonly appreciated as dandruff, yet in HIV patients it also occurs on the face. It is presumed to be caused by the *Malassezia* yeast; it is treated with topical ketoconazole and regresses with ART. Eosinophilic folliculitis, a more diffuse dermatologic condition that as its name implies is an inflammatory condition of the hair follicles, is an intensely pruritic (itchy) condition that may be autoimmune or triggered by mites, bacteria, or yeast. It is also effectively treated with ART and can benefit from topical corticosteroids.

Finally, HIV is in many ways very much a psychosocial diagnosis as it is as a medical one. To this day, despite a clearer understanding of the epidemiology of HIV, many patients experience isolation and stigma that governs disclosure which inevitably impacts disease transmission, relationships, and adherence to treatment plans. There is a significant burden of neurocognitive diagnoses, especially as the population ages.[38] In the United States, nearly half of HIV-positive adults have substance use disorders.[39] Major depression is common following an HIV diagnosis and can be the result of subcortical brain damage caused by untreated HIV itself (see HAND, above). Posttraumatic stress disorder (PTSD), a condition where echoes of a significant psychosocial event are reexperienced, is common in HIV+ patients and can come from being given an HIV diagnosis or the circumstances that predated it. PTSD alone can contribute to behaviors that increase one's risk for acquisition. It also imparts physiologic changes in the body through elevation in biomarkers for immune reactivation and inflammation despite optimal virologic control.[40]

HIV-RELATED DISEASES AFFECTING THE EYE AND VISION

Anatomy of the Eye and Some Representative Pathogens Affecting Patients With HIV

All the structures necessary for optimal vision, from the eyelids to the visual cortex of the occipital lobes of the brain, can be affected by HIV, its comorbidities, and medications used to treat both (**FIGURE 10.17**). Acute changes in vision, pain, redness, photophobia, floaters, or flashes typically require urgent evaluation, especially in those with lower CD4 counts. Clinicians must attend not only to the eye and its adnexal structures but also to the *patterns* of vision changes and constitutional symptoms that can coexist.

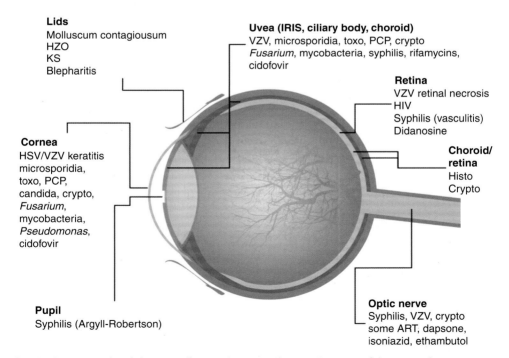

FIGURE 10.17 HIV-related diseases affecting the eye and vision. Anatomy of the eye and some representative pathogens affecting patients with HIV. HSV, herpes simplex virus; HZO, herpes zoster ophthalmicus; IRIS, immune reconstitution inflammatory syndrome; KS, Kaposi sarcoma; PCP, *Pneumocystis jirovecii* pneumonia; VZV, varicella-zoster virus. (Image credit: Richard Serrao, MD.)

To illustrate, a patient who notes binocular vision loss in a *hemianopsic* pattern, a pattern where *both* eyes appreciate a loss of vision in the same or mirrored visual fields, has a different differential and different portions of the visual pathway are implicated than a patient who has monocular pain and no loss of vision. The "omas" (crypto, toxo, lymphoma) and other encephalitic pathogens (like CMV, PML) previously discussed can compromise the optic tracts and/or the visual cortex producing hemianopsia that points to a neuro-ophthalmic origin rather than within the eye itself. Keratitis (corneal inflammation) in a patient with fevers, olfactory hallucinations, and seizures can implicate a pathogen potentially affecting both the globe(s) and the brain, like herpes, and a stroke in a patient who tests positive for syphilis and is not on ART could have syphilitic or HIV-mediated cerebrovascular disease as causes. When certain cranial nerves involved in the movement of the extraocular muscles are dysfunctional either in isolation or in conjunction with other nerves and symptoms like fever and headache are coexistent, basilar granulomatous meningitis from pathogens like tuberculosis or cryptococcosis is possible.

Molluscum contagiosum is a poxvirus that is for the most part asymptomatic when it occurs in children, though it can also spread with sexual exposure. Manifesting as clusters of painless umbilicated papules (raised flesh-colored lesions with a central dimple), it appears around the eyes and face when seen in children, or genitals when transmitted sexually. Many times, eye specialists may be the first to encounter these lesions. When involving the face, molluscum contagiosum lesions, like the lesions of KS, are typically of cosmetic significance, although both can affect vision when they impact mobility of the eyelids, conjunctiva, and potentially deeper structures. Molluscum contagiosum papules in most cases regress with ART from improvements in CD4 cells (**FIGURE 10.18**).

VZV is the causative agent of herpes zoster ophthalmicus (HZO), so-called when shingles arises from the ophthalmic (V1) distribution of the fifth cranial nerve. Given the disruption of intact skin from the rupturing of hemorrhagic vesicles, HZO puts the patient at risk for staphylococcal or streptococcal cellulitis or impetigo from normal flora. Prognosis is generally good if the cellulitis remains periorbital/preseptal and can be managed on an outpatient basis. The eye could be obscured by the intense edema of the lids making it a challenge, albeit compulsory, to examine. If the examination reveals ophthalmoplegia, anisocoria, proptosis, or chemosis, the structures deeper to the orbital septum are likely involved which raises concern for orbital cellulitis or suppurative cavernous sinus thrombosis, diagnoses requiring emergent imaging, surgical consultation, and intravenous antibiotics.

When HZO affects the nasociliary branch of V1 that provides sensation to the cornea responsible in large part for the blinking reflex, VZV can result in ipsilateral blepharoconjunctivitis, episcleritis, and scleritis, and threatens vision when it directly damages the cornea (keratitis).[41] In addition, VZV-mediated uveitis, acute retinal necrosis, progressive outer retinal necrosis, optic neuritis, or

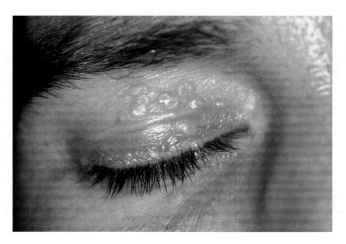

FIGURE 10.18 Multiple eyelid lesions of molluscum contagiosum in a 30-year-old man with AIDS. (Courtesy of Narsing Rao, MD.)

Antiretroviral Drugs	Mutations Detected	Resistance Predicted
NRTIs		
ZDV (zidovudine)	M41L, L210W, T215C, K291E	Yes
ABC (abacavir)	M41L, L74V, M184V, L210W, T215C, K219E	Yes
ddI (didanosine)	M41L, L74V, L210W, T215C, K219 E	Yes
3TC (lamivudine	M41L, V118I, M184V, L210W, K219E	Yes
FTC (emtricitabine)	M41L, V118I, M184V, L210W, K219E	Yes
d4T (stavudine)	M41L, L210W, K219E	Yes
TDF (tenofovir)	M41L, L210W, K219E	Yes
NNRTIs		
ETR (etravirine)	A98G, Y181C	Yes
EFV (efavarenz)	A98G, V108I, Y181C	Yes
NVP (nevirapine)	A98G, V108I, Y181C	Yes
RPV (rilpivirine)	Y181C	PROB
PIs		
FPV (fosamprenavir)	L10F, V32I, L33F, M46I, I47V, I54M, I62V, L63P, A71V, V82A, L90M	Yes
IDV (indinavir)	L10F, K20R, V32I, M36L, M46I, L63P, I64V, A71V, V82A, L90M	Yes
NFV (nelfinavir)	L10F, K20R, V32I, M36L, M46I, L63P, I64V, A71V, V82A, L90M	Yes
SQV (saquinavir)	L90M	Yes

FIGURE 10.22 Genotype panel of a highly resistant HIV demonstrating multiple mutations and limited treatment options. This scenario is best avoided by encouraging strict adherence and can be seen in very treatment experienced patients. NNRTIs, nonnucleoside reverse transcriptase inhibitors; NRTIs, nucleoside/nucleotide reverse transcriptase inhibitor; PIs, protease inhibitors. (Image credit Richard Serrao, MD.)

Drugs must always be used in combination. This principle became clear after the introduction of the NRTI zidovudine, also known as azidothymidine (AZT), as the first drug approved for the treatment of HIV in 1987. Still in use to this day, AZT was erroneously implicated by many to have contributed to AIDS deaths when in fact patients died because monotherapy always fails.

HIV is successfully treated via a "cocktail" approach, utilizing two—primarily three—drug combinations that disrupt viral replication through the various mechanisms. Hopes for a cure arose in the late 1990s with the introduction of the PI and NNRTI classes, finally pushing viral suppression to sustained undetectable levels. This created the semblance of viral eradication. Unfortunately, viremia will always rebound within weeks of medication withdrawal. Some patients can reexperience an acute HIV syndrome if viremic levels are extreme.

Until there is a cure, treating HIV amounts to a daily uninterrupted lifelong commitment. This is as simple as taking one pill once a day or as difficult as taking one pill once a day. This sentence appears erroneous, yet it emphasizes that one person's circumstances to adhere can vary greatly from another's. Complexities arise with haphazard adherence to ART, either from neuropsychiatric or psychosocial comorbidities or "chaos," or from problems of drug sustainability in resource-limited areas.

A patient's first regimen is their best regimen; regimens that need to be switched due to adverse reactions or resistance are done so typically at the expense of convenience and/or tolerability. Patients must be aware that treating HIV is unlike treating hypertension or diabetes; if insulin or antihypertensives are discontinued, they can be restarted with the expectation that their efficacy returns to their pre-cessation levels. ART, however, is interacting with a live virus, a virus that replicates *billions* of times per day, so that when less than 70% to 95% (depending on the drug combinations studied) of a regimen is consumed per month, virologic failure, namely detectable viral load with concomitant mutations leading to possible multidrug-resistant HIV, is likely to occur.[53] In many cases, ART is postponed until there is certainty that adherence is optimized for this very reason.

"Hit hard, hit early" reflected the practice in the late 1990s and early 2000s. Because HIV remained universally fatal and early retroviral cocktails demonstrated remarkable results, the goal was to get as many people on treatment. Unfortunately, viral load suppression during these years came at a cost. Peripheral neuropathy, pancreatitis, hepatitis, bone marrow suppression, and metabolic derangements like hyperlipidemia were common.

Many older NRTIs like didanosine and stavudine contribute to an increased risk for hepatic steatosis (fatty liver) associated with lactic acidosis, a potentially life-threatening disturbance of acid-base homeostasis associated with mitochondrial toxicity. Patients can present with nonspecific GI symptoms, malaise, and elevations in transaminase enzymes. Partly through this same mechanism, many of these older drugs contribute to lipodystrophy (abnormal fat) characterized by accumulation of visceral fat within the abdomen and loss of subcutaneous fat (lipoatrophy) on the extremities and face giving the appearance of a protuberant abdomen, pronounced veins in the limbs (due to relative fat wasting) and sunken cheeks, and fat accumulation behind the neck.

Many patients during the early 2000s expressed concern over the use of available regimens since they did not want to have an appearance that could give away their diagnosis to others. Injection of poly-L-lactic acid compounds into the subcutaneous tissues of the face to offset the atrophy has become less necessary nowadays. Many drugs like ritonavir, atazanavir, indinavir, and Bactrim are nephrotoxic or cause drug stones. Efavirenz, an early NNRTI, can exacerbate neuropsychiatric comorbidities and should therefore be avoided in patients with certain mental health comorbidities. Newer medications for HIV are not without their adverse reactions, but they certainly have improved with respect to side effect profile and barriers to resistance via novel mechanisms and pharmacokinetics.

Timing of ART and Potential Complications: IRIS

To offset the accumulating evidence that demonstrated harm, the hit hard, hit early approach receded in the early 2000s, and studies were performed to determine if patients can wait on ART and if allowing their CD4 count to drift downward is safe. Starting earlier potentially unnecessarily increased the time for toxicities to accumulate. For years, a CD4 cutoff of 350 to 500 was recommended to start, as starting earlier was not yet proven to offer a survival advantage. As drugs became safer, the hit hard, hit early approach returned, but finally within a different context. Hitting early, as early as HIV is diagnosed and even as early as the acute retroviral syndrome occurs, finally proved to offer survival benefit in 2015.[33]

Immune Reconstitution Inflammatory Syndrome

The cardinal signs and symptoms of inflammation orchestrated by a working immune response to a pathogen or injury are purulence, swelling, erythema, warmth, or pain. The inflammatory cascade also contributes to fever. In the nonimmunocompromised host, the location of these findings helps localize a source of an infection. For example, cough with productive sputum suggests pneumonia, a stiff neck and headache point toward meningitis, right lower quadrant abdominal pain and anorexia signal appendicitis, and so on.

In HIV/AIDS, these clues can be absent or subtle for some time before an OI sickens a patient. Within the context of commencing ART, the term IRIS reflects a paradoxical *worsening* of clinical stability during a time in which the obvious expectation for the patient is clinical improvement. This phenomenon typically occurs when ART causes a rapid CD4 count *rise* from a very low starting point, typically ≤100 where many OIs can incubate. As the immune system improves (and viral load rapidly drops), it can now recognize OIs and in so doing create symptoms that were brewing but silent so that a simmering tuberculosis or cryptococcal meningitis can become symptomatic.

Almost any pathogen can trigger IRIS; tuberculosis, MAC, PJP, and CMV are common. In resource-rich areas, IRIS is infrequent because patients are starting ART at much higher CD4 counts. It is recommended to start ART within 2 weeks of any HIV-positive patient not on ART even if they have an active OI after the treatment for the OI has been initiated except for those with active cryptococcal or tuberculous meningitis. Delaying ART in these conditions is preferred given the higher propensity for a severe IRIS phenomenon.

One manifestation of IRIS is an immune recovery uveitis. Like IRIS, immune-related uveitis is paradoxical clinical worsening of intraocular inflammatory reactions, attributable to improved immune functions after starting ART in HIV patients. It is also referred to as immune recovery vitritis and is most commonly seen in patients with CMV retinitis.

Since this condition can arise randomly in those at risk, clinicians must be on alert 1 week to several months after starting ART and hunt for and treat the OI causing the syndrome. It is preferable to continue ART; adjunctive glucocorticoids can be utilized to calm down the inflammation.

PEP and PREP

HIV medications can be used in the non–HIV-positive patient. The terms PEP and PREP refer to postexposure and preexposure prophylaxis. PEP was first introduced as an aim to reduce the risk to healthcare workers who are exposed (or potentially exposed) to HIV from percutaneous injury from sharps contaminated with blood. This was later expanded to nonoccupational exposures (NPEP) such as condomless sex. The risk is clearest when the source is known to be HIV+ and not on treatment.

The risk to the exposed is quantified based on the circumstances of the exposure. A healthcare worker, for example, whose exposure to blood from an HIV+ patient not on treatment is through a needle or sharp that had visible blood and penetrates through intact skin is at highest risk; a man who has insertive vaginal sex with a condom with a woman whose HIV status is unknown is at relatively low risk. Given the toxicities of older ART, this quantification of probable risk used to be crucial because early recommendations prioritized triple drug prophylaxis only for the highest of risk, but two drugs for a lower risk exposure, aiming to strike a favorable risk-benefit ratio. Since modern ART is very safe, a three-drug regimen is now recommended in all who are (or potentially) exposed for whom PEP is indicated since the risk-benefit ratio is now most favorable.

For PEP to be most effective, it should be started immediately. Animal studies demonstrate PEP has reduced efficacy if started >72 hours after exposure. PEP is continued for 1 month; testing for HIV at the time of exposure and at intervals post-PEP are done to establish negative serostatus (HIV testing is negative) at the time of exposure and subsequent to prophylaxis. All attempts at identifying the status of the source person should be made; if they are HIV negative, PEP/NPEP can be stopped.

What if HIV medications were taken prior to any exposure? Could it offer protection against HIV in those at risk for HIV infection but are not HIV positive? The question of whether PREP is effective at HIV prevention was answered in a series of studies.[54] For those at substantial risk based on sexual activity (eg, multiple partners with inconsistent use of barrier protection), daily or on demand PREP with tenofovir-emtricitabine has been shown to reduce the risk of HIV infection. The formulations of this drug and study populations vary, yet PREP's effectiveness is based on adherence, with those most adherent achieving a 90% risk reduction.[55]

Despite its efficacy, uptake of PREP has been low. Prescribers should provide ongoing counseling about safe sex practices to patients who seek or are recommended PREP. Those on PREP should have periodic blood work to ensure safety and be tested for HIV at regular intervals because ongoing use of tenofovir-emtricitabine, which comprises only two NRTIs, is inherently suboptimal treatment for HIV infection if HIV is acquired while taking PREP. Additionally, patients should receive ongoing screening for STIs because those on PREP are at inherently higher risk for other STIs.[56]

HIV Vaccines and Cure Strategies

The main function of our immune system is to fight off acute infections and develop a memory, or protective immunity, from future exposures to the same and sometimes similar pathogens. Vaccines work as a preemptive strike, priming the body with a humoral or cellular army. This is accomplished via intramuscular or subcutaneous injection, ingestion or mucosal application of *antigens*, and surface proteins from a killed organism or live, attenuated organisms. Some vaccines are more immunogenic, or more apt to induce an immune response, than others. Some require boosters to ensure lifelong protection, and some vaccines, like influenza, still require annual inoculations because antigenic components of this virus drift year to year.

Effective vaccines and a cure for HIV have been elusive for many decades. The most promising strategies come from unique approaches like immunotherapy now common in cancer treatments, novel gene editing technology, and insights garnered from patients who are innately immune and from those who have been cured. None of these approaches has been wholly successful or ready for prime time yet.

For chronic infections such as HIV, the immune system fails because HIV quickly bypasses cellular immunity and hides deep within cellular genetic structures further sequestering it from detection and elimination. Not only that, HIV's pathogenicity is uniquely geared to destroying the very immune cells necessary to fight it off. It wins every time. And like influenza, yet to an exponentially greater degree, HIV's immunogenic antigens are so varied that a universal vaccine homing in on critical targets is difficult to achieve.

Most eligible vaccine trials have utilized a "prime-boost" approach with one component of the vaccine priming the body and the other boosting the response to that. Common cold viruses (adenovirus) and more esoteric viruses like canarypox have been modified with HIV antigen targets to serve as a Trojan horse, so to speak.

The Army-led RV144 vaccine trial, in combination with the Thailand Ministry of Public Health, demonstrated a lowering of HIV infection by 31.2% compared to placebo.[57] Subsequent studies looked at the potential for booster injections or more focused targeting of specific surface proteins which could increase that response.[58] Three ongoing studies performed under the HVTN (HIV Vaccine Trials Network) umbrella continue to show promise. Unfortunately, one of these that began in 2016 that enrolled more than 5400 HIV-negative participants in South Africa has been terminated due to similar rates of new infections from the experimental vaccine versus placebo.[59]

As vaccine research makes sequential adjustments, two major approaches for a cure continue to be explored: sterilizing and functional cure. Despite peripheral viral load suppression achievable through ART, HIV evades eradication because it hides out in *reservoirs* in either a transcriptionally latent or active phase while taking advantage of the tissue microenvironments that sequester it that are challenging to sterilize or replace. These reservoirs include practically every tissue but are concentrated in lymphatic tissue within the GI tract, CD4 cells, macrophages, dendritic cells, and microglia within the brain, among other sites. A sterilizing cure is one in which all reservoirs are rendered sterile, free from virus; a functional cure is defined as a sustained ART-free virologic remission after ART is discontinued.

An inherently risky procedure and not feasible for curing HIV, bone marrow transplantation (BMT) traditionally aims to replace diseased hematopoietic cells with healthy ones. It is most commonly used to treat leukemias particularly when traditional chemotherapy fails. The procedure requires two major steps: myeloablative chemotherapy which removes as much of the leukemic patient's hematopoietic system (principally progenitor bone marrow cells), followed immediately by transplantation of matched healthy donor stem cells. The transplanted cells repopulate the diseased patient's native bone marrow, essentially replacing it. It is through myeloablation (myelo = bone marrow; ablation = removal) that scientists aim for sterilization ("shock and kill") of all the cells that harbor HIV, but ablation alone is ineffective. What matters most with this approach, however, is the *types* of cells doing the replacing.

In highly publicized cases of patients with HIV who were cured after a BMT, two patients underwent the procedure principally for concomitant leukemia and were engrafted with cells from matched donors who also had T-cells that lacked the CCR5 coreceptors, coreceptors necessary for their specific strains of HIV that were 100% CCR5 tropic to gain cell entry. With their bone marrow now replaced with cells no longer capable of granting entry to HIV, these patients had both their leukemia and HIV simultaneously cured.[60,61]

This approach is still impractical. However, a proof of concept study in 2014 demonstrated reductions in HIV viral load when patients received infusions of their own modified CD4 cells where the CCR5 gene was rendered permanently dysfunctional.[62] Because HIV infection is in many ways a genetic disease in that it is integrated into human DNA, another approach is to genetically splice out HIV genes from infected cells. The new CRISPR (clustered regularly interspaced short palindromic repeats) technology uses guided RNA to recognize and attach to specific areas of DNA which can then be cut and edited, leading to silencing of certain genes. In an experimental mouse model, ART modified in a crystalline structure that allows for better cell penetration called LASER ART (long-acting slow-effective release antiviral therapy) was used in combination with CRISPR, resulting in 30% of mice having no trace of HIV.[63] This approach, which shows tremendous promise, will be expanded to nonhuman primates prior to consideration of testing in humans.

CONCLUSIONS

Since the start of the HIV epidemic, 75 million people have become infected and 32 million people have died from AIDS-related illnesses. Yet, by 2019, 24.5 million people were accessing ART worldwide.[64] This access is promising, creating, if you will, a holding pattern for a plane that has been patiently waiting to land.

Many advancements in the prevention and treatment of many infectious diseases during the time HIV has existed on this planet have reinforced the notion that prevention is achievable, and a cure is always on the horizon. We should be reminded that it was not until recently that HPV vaccination gave us the potential to make many head and neck, cervical, and anal cancers recede, and turn an incurable disease like hepatitis C curable.

Until the same applies to how we ultimately manage HIV, we can revel in the accomplishments made thus far that have transformed a horrible disease into a manageable one for many, but not for all. Attention must continue to be paid to the existence, identification, prevention, and treatment of HIV on all—and from all—fronts until it too becomes a part of history.

REFERENCES

1. Faria NR, Rambaut A, Suchard MA, et al. HIV epidemiology. The early spread and epidemic ignition of HIV-1 in human populations. *Science*. 2014;346:56-61.

2. Centers for Disease Control. Pneumocystis pneumonia – Los Angeles. *MMWR Morb Mortal Wkly Rep*. 1981;30:250-252.

3. Serwadda D, Mugerwa RD, Sewankambo NK, et al. Slim disease: a new disease in Uganda and its association with HTLV-III infection. *Lancet*. 1985;2(8460):849-852.

4. https://www.cdc.gov/hai/pdfs/bbp/exp_to_blood.pdf.

5. Patel P, Borkowf CB, Brooks JT, et al. Estimating per-act HIV transmission risk: a systematic review. *AIDS*. 2014;28(10):1509-1519.

6. Gray RH, Wawer MJ, Brookmeyer R, et al. Probability of HIV-1 transmission per coital act in monogamous, heterosexual, HIV-1 disordant couples in Rakai, Uganda. *Lancet*. 2001;357:1149-1153.

7. *Global HIV & AIDS Statistics – 2019 Fact Sheet*. Accessed February 1, 2020. https://www.unaids.org/en/resources/fact-sheet.

8. Quinn TC, Wawer MJ, Sewankambo NK, et al. Viral load and heterosexual transmission of human immunodeficiency virus type 1. Rakai Project Study Group. *N Engl J Med*. 2000;342(13):921-929.

9. Fleming DT, Wasserstein JN. From epidemiological synergy to public health policy and practice: the contribution of other sexually transmitted diseases to sexual transmission of HIV infection. *Sex Transm Infect*. 1999;75(1):3-17.

10. Rodger AJ, Cambiano V, Bruun T, et al. Sexual activity without condoms and risk of HIV transmission in sero-different couples when the HIV-positive partner is using suppressive antiretroviral therapy. *J Am Med Assoc*. 2016;316(20):171-181.

11. *World Health Organization – Regional office for Africa*. Accessed February 1, 2020. https://www.afro.who.int/health-topics/hivaids.

12. Singh S, Song R, Johnson AS, et al. HIV incidence, HIV prevalence and undiagnosed HIV infections in men who have sex with men, United States. *Ann Intern Med*. 2018;168(10):685-694.

13. Centers for Disease Control. *Diagnoses of HIV Infection in the United States and Dependent Areas, 2018*. HIV Surveillance Report 2019; 30. Accessed February 9, 2020. https://www.cdc.gov/hiv/statistics/overview/ataglance.html

14. *HIV Among People Aged 50 and Older*. Accessed February 1, 2020. https://cdc.gov/hiv/group/age/olderamericans/index.html.

15. Liu R, Paxton WA, Choe S, et al. Homozygous defect in HIV-1 coreceptor accounts for resistance of some multiply-exposed individuals to HIV-1 infection. *Cell*. 1996;86(3):367-377.

16. Shoko C, Chikobvu D. A superiority of viral load over CD4 cell count when predicting mortality in HIV patients on therapy. *BMC Infect Dis*. 2019;19:169. doi:10.1186/s12879-019-3781-1.

17. Ananworanich J, Chomont N, Eller LA, et al. HIV DNA set point is rapidly established in acute HIV infection and dramatically reduced by early ART. *EBioMedicine*. 2016;11:68-72.

18. Selik RM, Mokotoff ED, Branson B, et al. Revised surveillance case definition for HIV infection – United States, 2014. *MMWR Recomm Rep*. 2014;63:1.

19. Focà E, Magro P, Motta D, et al. Screening for neurocognitive impairment in HIV-infected individuals at first contact after HIV diagnosis: the experience of a large clinical center in Northern Italy. *Int J Mol Sci*. 2016;17(4):434.

20. Sharma SK, Mohanan S, Sharma A. Relevance of latent TB infection in areas of high TB prevalence. *Chest*. 2012;142(3):761-773.

21. Menzies D, Gardiner G, Farhat M, Greenaway C, Pai M. Thinking in three dimensions: a web-based algorithm to aid the interpretation of tuberculin skin test results. *Int J Tuberc Lung Dis*. 2008;12:498-505.

22. *Global Tuberculosis Report 2019*. Accessed February 1, 2020. https://www.who.int/tb/publications/global_report/en/.

23. *TB Statistics South Africa – National, Incidence, Provincial*. Accessed March 2, 2020. https://tbfacts.org/tb-statistics-south-africa.

24. Wasserman A, Engel M, Griesel R, Mendelson M. Burden of pneumocystis pneumonia in HIV-infected adults in sub-Saharan Africa: a systemic review and meta-analysis. *BMC Infect Dis*. 2016;16(1):482.

25. Ganiem AR, Dian S, Indriati A, et al. Cerebral toxoplasmosis mimicking subacute meningitis in HIV-infected patients; a Cohort study from Indonesia. *Plos Negl Trop Dis*. 2013;7(1):e1994.

26. Smith JR, Cunningham ET Jr. Atypical presentations of ocular toxoplasmosis. *Curr Opin Ophthalmol*. 2002;13(6):387-392.

27. Palestine AG, Rodrigues MM, Macher AM, et al. Ophthalmic involvement in acquired immunodeficiency syndrome. *Ophthalmology*. 1984;91(9):1092-1099.

28. Tandon R, Kim KS, Serrao R. Disseminated *Mycobacterium avium-intracellulare* infection in a person with AIDS with cutaneous and CNS lesions. *AIDS Read*. 2007;17(11):555-560.

29. Currier JS, Williams PL, Koletar SL, et al. Discontinuation of Mycobacterium avium complex prophylaxis in patients with antiretroviral therapy-induced increases in CD4+ cell count: a randomized, double-blind, placebo-controlled trial. AIDS Clinical Trials Group 362 Study Team. *Ann Intern Med*. 2000;133(7):493-503.

30. Mui UN, Haley CT, Tyring SK. Viral oncology: molecular biology and pathogenesis. *J Clin Med*. 2017;6(12):111.

31. Farrall AL, Smith JR. Eye involvement in primary central nervous system lymphoma. *Surv Ophthalmol*. 2020;65:548-561.

32. Borges ÁH, Neuhaus J, Babiker AG, et al. Immediate antiretroviral therapy reduces risk of infection-related cancer during early HIV infection. *Clin Infect Dis*. 2016;63:1668-1676.

33. The INSIGHT START Study Group; Lundgren JD, Babiker AG, Gordin F, et al. Initiation of antiretroviral therapy in early asymptomatic HIV infection. *N Engl J Med*. 2015;373(9):795-807.

34. Gallant J, Hsue PY, Shreay S, Meyer N. Comorbidities among US patients with prevalent HIV infection – a trend analysis. *J Infect Dis*. 2017;216(12):1525-1533.

35. *World Health Organization HIV/AIDS HIV Self-Testing*. Accessed February 1, 2020. https://www.who.int/hiv/topics/self-testing/en/.

36. Razzak Chaudhary S, Workeneh B, Montez-Rath ME, Zolopa AR, Klotman PE, Winkelmayer WC. Trends in the outcomes of end-stage renal disease secondary to human immunodeficiency virus-associated nephropathy. *Nephrol Dial Transpl.* 2015;30:1734-1740.

37. Nadkarni G, Patel A, Yacoub R, et al. The burden of dialysis-requiring acute kidney injury among hospitalized adults with HIV infection: a nationwide inpatient sample analysis. *AIDS.* 2015;29:1061-1066.

38. Saylor D, Dickens AM, Sacktor N, et al. HIV-associated neurocognitive disorder – Pathogenesis and prospects for treatment. *Nat Rev Neurol.* 2016;12(4):234-248.

39. Hartzler B, Dombrowski JC, Crane HM, et al. Prevalence and predictors of substance use disorders among HIV care enrollees in the United States. *AIDS Behav.* 2016;21(4):1138-1148.

40. Siyahhan J, Auh S, Krakora R, et al. The association between post-traumatic stress disorder and markers of inflammation and immune activation in HIV-infected individuals with controlled viremia. *Psychosomatics.* 2016;57:423-430.

41. Shaikh S, Ta CN. Evaluation and management of herpes zoster ophthalmicus. *Am Fam Physician.* 2002;66(9):1723-1730.

42. *Clinical Advisory: Ocular Syphilis in the United States.* Accessed January 21, 2020. https://www.cdc.gov/std/syphilis/clinicaladvisoryos2015.htm.

43. Wickremasinghe S, Ling C, Stawell R, Yeoh J, Hall A, Zamir E. Syphilitic punctate inner retinitis in immunocompetent gay men. *Ophthalmology.* 2009;116(6):1195-1200.

44. Musher DM, Hamill RJ, Baughn RE, et al. Effect of human immunodeficiency virus (HIV) infection on the course of syphilis and on the response to treatment. *Ann Intern Med.* 1990;113(11):872-881.

45. Crabol Y, Catherinot E. Rifabutin: where do we stand in 2016? *J Antimicrob Chemother.* 2016;71(7):1759-1771.

46. McClung NM, Lewis RM, Gargano JW, Querec T, Unger ER, Markowitz LE. Declines in vaccine-type human papillomavirus prevalence in females across racial/ethnic groups: data from a national survey. *J Adolesc Health.* 2019;65(6):715-722.

47. National Institutes of Health. *Guidelines for the Prevention and Treatment of Opportunistic Infections in Adults and Adolescents with HIV.* Accessed February 1, 2020. https://aidsinfo.nih.gov/guidelines/html/4/adult-and-adolescent-opportunistic-infection/341/varicella-zoster-virus.

48. Harrison KM, Song R, Zhang X. Life expectancy after HIV diagnosis based on national HIV surveillance data from 25 states, United States. *J Acquir Immune Defic Syndr.* 2010;53(1):124-130.

49. Cohen MS, Chen YQ, McCauley M, et al. Prevention of HIV-1 infection with early antiretroviral therapy. *N Engl J Med.* 2011;365(6):493-505.

50. Eisinger RW, Dieffenbach CW, Fauci AS. HIV viral load and transmissibility of HIV infection: undetectable equals untransmittable. *J Am Med Assoc.* 2019;321(5):451-452.

51. Fauci AS, Redfield RR, Sigounas G, Weahkee MD, Giroir BP. Ending the HIV epidemic: a plan for the United States. *J Am Med Assoc.* 2019;321(9):844-845.

52. Margolis DA, Gonzalez-Garcia J, Stellbrink H-J, et al. Long-acting intramuscular cabotegravir and rilpivirine in adults with HIV-1 infection (LATTE-2): 96-week results of a randomised, open-label, phase 2b, non-inferiority trial. *Lancet.* 2017;390(10101):1499-1510.

53. Tarantino N, Whiteley L, Craker L, Brown LK. Predictors of viral suppression among youth living with HIV in the southern United States. *AIDS Care.* 2020;32:916-920.

54. Grant RM, Lama JR, Anderson PL, et al; iPrEx Study Team. Preexposure chemoprophylaxis for HIV prevention in men who have sex with men. *N Engl J Med.* 2010;363(27):2587-2599.

55. Molina J, Capitant C, Spire B, et al. On-demand preexposure prophylaxis in men at high risk for HIV-1 infection. *N Engl J Med.* 2015;373:2237-2246.

56. Traeger MW, Conelisse VJ, Asselin J, et al. Association of HIV preexposure prophylaxis with incidence of sexually transmitted infections among individuals at high risk of HIV infection. *J Am Med Assoc.* 2019;321(14):1380-1390.

57. Rerks-Ngarm S, Pitisuttithum P, Nitayaphan S, et al. Vaccination with ALVAC and AIDSVAX to prevent HIV-1 infection in Thailand. *N Engl J Med.* 2009;361:2209-2220.

58. Robb ML, Rerks-Narmada S, Nitayaphan S, et al. Risk behaviour and time as covariates for efficacy of the HIV vaccine regimen ALVAC-HIV (vCP1521) and AIDSVAX B/E: a post-hoc analysis of the Thai phase 3 efficacy trial RV 144. *Lancet Infect Dis.* 2012;12(7):531-537.

59. National Institute of Allergy and Infectious Diseases. *Experimental HIV Vaccine Regimen Ineffective in Preventing HIV.* Accessed February 3, 2020. https://www.niaid.nih.gov/news-events/experimental-hiv-vaccine-regimen-ineffective-preventing-hiv.

60. Hütter G, Nowak D, Mossner M, et al. Long-term control of HIV by CCR5 Delta32/Delta32 stem-cell transplantation. *N Engl J Med.* 2009;360(7):692-698.

61. Allers K, Hütter G, Hofmann J, et al. Evidence for the cure of HIV infection by CCR5Δ32/Δ32 stem cell transplantation. *Blood*. 2011;117(10):2791-2799.

62. Tebas P, Stein D, Tang WW, et al. Gene editing of CCR5 in autologous CD4 T cells of persons infected with HIV. *N Engl J Med*. 2014;370:901-910.

63. Dash PK, Kaminski R, Bella R, et al. Sequential LASER ART and CRISPR treatments eliminate HIV-1 in a subset of infected humanized mice. *Nat Commun*. 2019;10(1):2753.

64. https://www.unaids.org/en/resources/fact-sheet.

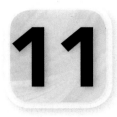

Rheumatology

Courtney Stull, Emily Purcell, Shiv Sehra, and
Rachel C. Druckenbrod

LEARNING OBJECTIVES

Rheumatologic conditions represent a range of disorders that reflect abnormal function of
the immune system, most with joint involvement. In addition, the majority of systemic rheumatologic diseases are associated with ocular manifestations. This chapter will cover the most
common rheumatologic diseases encountered in clinical practice, with an emphasis on the
ocular manifestations.

KEY CONCEPTS

- Assessment of rheumatologic disease and
  the common rheumatologic blood tests
- Individual diseases and their ocular
  manifestations:
  - Giant cell arteritis (GCA)
  - Polymyalgia rheumatica (PMR)

- Rheumatoid arthritis (RA)
- Systemic lupus erythematosus (SLE)
- Sjogren syndrome (SS)
- Sarcoidosis
- Spondyloarthropathies (SpA)
- Osteoarthritis (OA)
- Systemic sclerosis (SSc)

ASSESSMENT OF RHEUMATOLOGIC DISEASE AND COMMON RHEUMATOLOGIC TESTS

Rheumatologic conditions are primarily suspected based on history and examination. Blood tests
and imaging have varying degrees of sensitivity and specificity; thus they act only as adjuncts for
diagnosis. Because rheumatologic tests are not specific, the testing should be ordered only if the clinical suspicion for disease is high, with an aim to help confirm an already-suspected diagnosis, and
should not be used for "screening" purposes.

The assessment of a rheumatologic disease begins with a comprehensive history and examination.
The clinician should ask for the onset, duration, progression, and details of each patient symptom as
well as for each associated symptom. Patients may sometimes not volunteer information on otherwise
common or minor complaints, which may often hold a clue to the diagnosis. For example, patients
with Sjogren syndrome tend to have eye dryness and mouth dryness for an average for 3 years before
a diagnosis is made. Thus a complete review of systems should be obtained in every patient being
evaluated for a rheumatologic disease. Similarly, a full physical examination should be performed at

every initial consult for a systemic rheumatologic disease and at subsequent visits for every systemic rheumatologic process, since these diseases have the potential to involve all organ systems.

Testing for rheumatologic diseases is a relatively newer area of medicine. The first such test, called the rheumatoid factor (RF), was discovered in the 1940s. Since then, the number of immunologic tests for rheumatologic diseases has slowly expanded. The most commonly used immunological and nonimmunological tests that help clinical evaluation of rheumatologic diseases now include

- Rheumatoid factor
- Anti-citrullinated protein antibody (ACPA or anti-CCP)
- Antinuclear antibodies (ANAs)
- Anti–double stranded DNA antibodies (anti-dsDNA) and extractable nuclear antigens (ENAs)
- Anti-neutrophil cytoplasmic antibodies (ANCAs), anti–myeloperoxidase antibody (anti-MPO), and anti–proteinase 3 antibody (anti-PR3)
- Complete blood count (CBC), erythrocyte sedimentation rate (ESR), and C-reactive protein (CRP)

Testing for the antibodies is either achieved by indirect immunofluorescence (IIF) or by enzyme-linked immunosorbent assay (ELISA).

Rheumatoid factor (RF) was first discovered as an "activating factor" that could augment the agglutination of sheep red blood cells. Currently, the terminology is used to describe antibodies to the Fc (gamma) portion of the human antibody. The antibody might be of the IgA, IgG, IgM, or the IgE type, but usually the IgM type is commercially tested. Though termed "rheumatoid" factor, the RF is not specific for rheumatoid arthritis. As above, any antibody to the Fc (gamma) portion of a human antibody can give a positive test for the RF. **TABLE 11.1** below summarizes the rates of RF positivity in common rheumatologic ailments. In addition, RF positivity has been noted in chronic infections such as tuberculosis and syphilis, and high rates of positivity are also seen in hematologic malignancies, without having a diagnostic role. Thus RF should only be checked in patients where a positive test would be clinically relevant.

Anti-citrullinated protein antibodies (ACPAs or anti-CCPs) are antibodies to citrullinated peptides, which are some of the major antigens to which antibodies are directed in patients with rheumatoid arthritis (RA). These antibodies are as sensitive as or more sensitive than the RF, with studies reporting up to 94% prevalence in patients with RA. Presence of high-titer antibody in patients without features of RA has been associated with a higher incidence of RA later in life. Presence of high-titer ACPA antibody in patients with RA is associated with more severe disease, thus helping in prognosis in addition to diagnosis. Initially, ACPAs were felt to be very specific for RA; however,

TABLE 11.1 Likelihood of a Positive Rheumatoid Factor (RF) Test	
Condition	**Positive RF**
Normal human population	1%-10% (depending on race, age, ethnicity)
Rheumatoid arthritis	70%
Primary Sjogren syndrome	40%-70%
Mixed cryoglobulinemia (eg, from Hepatitis C)	Up to 100%
Mixed connective tissue disease	70%
Systemic lupus erythematosus	20%

TABLE 11.2   Conditions in Which ANA Can Be Positive With a Higher Incidence in the General Population

Category	Diseases with positive ANA at a higher incidence in the general population
Rheumatologic autoimmune diseases	Systemic lupus, drug-induced lupus, scleroderma, Sjogren syndrome, myositis, rheumatoid arthritis, mixed connective tissue disease
Nonrheumatologic autoimmune diseases	Hashimoto thyroiditis, Graves disease, inflammatory bowel disease
Malignancies	Almost any solid organ or hematologic malignancy
Infections	Chronic infections such as tuberculosis and syphilis

more study has shown that these antibodies can be seen in multiple other conditions such as Sjogren syndrome, psoriatic arthritis, and even leukemia.

ANAs include any antibody directed toward a normally occurring antigen in the cell nucleus. The gold standard of testing for ANAs is through IIF. When performed by IIF, ANAs are highly sensitive for ANA-associated rheumatologic diseases such as systemic lupus erythematosus (SLE), scleroderma, and myositis, among others. ANAs are very nonspecific antibodies. Historically they have been associated with a diagnosis of SLE; however, positive ANAs can be seen in a host of diseases, some of which are outlined in **TABLE 11.2**. When ANAs are detected with an IIF, both a titer and a pattern are reported. Antibody titer represents the greatest sample dilution for which antibody is still detectable and is reported as a ratio of sample:dilutant. As the titer rises, the ANA test result becomes more specific, with low titers being very common in otherwise normal humans (eg, ANA of 1:40 can be seen in up to 30% of normal humans, while ANA of 1:640 is seen in <1% of normal humans). The positive ANA cutoff is decided by the performing laboratory, and the usual cutoff is 1:160. If the ANA is positive at 1:160 and above with clinical features suggestive of an ANA-associated rheumatologic disease, the rheumatologist will usually order ELISAs for the antibodies more specific for the suspected disease.

Anti–double stranded DNA antibodies (anti-dsDNA) and extractable nuclear antigens (ENAs) may be ordered in patients who have a positive ANA (usually a titer of > or = 1:160) and clinical features suggestive of an autoimmune rheumatologic disease. Anti-dsDNA antibody is 98% specific for SLE. The antigens for the ENAs are present within the cell nucleus and are extracted from the nucleus for testing, thus the term "extractable nuclear antigens." The commonly tested ENAs include

- Anti-SSA/SSB antibodies: Usually seen in Sjogren syndrome and SLE
- Anti-Smith antibodies: >95% specific for SLE
- Anti-ribonucleoprotein (RNP) antibodies: Usually seen in mixed connective tissue disease (MCTD) and SLE
- Anti-Scl70 antibodies: Usually seen in scleroderma
- Anti-Jo1 antibodies: Usually seen in inflammatory myositis

Similar to the ANA, anti-neutrophil cytoplasmic antibody (ANCA) is tested in the lab using IIF, and this is the initial screening test for the ANCA-associated rheumatologic diseases. Instead of antibodies directed to antigens in the nucleus, ANCAs are directed toward antigens in the cytoplasm of neutrophils. Again, like with other rheumatologic antibodies, ANCAs are nonspecific and can be seen with a host of autoimmune, infectious, and malignant processes. The clinical utility of ANCA is only when testing for ANCA-associated vasculitides, namely granulomatosis with polyangiitis (GPA, formerly called Wegener granulomatosis), microscopic polyangiitis, eosinophilic granulomatosis with polyangiitis (formerly called Churg-Strauss syndrome), and renal-limited ANCA vasculitis. If any of these diseases is suspected and an ANCA is positive, the rheumatologist would then order an anti-myeloperoxidase antibody (anti-MPO) and/or an anti–proteinase 3 antibody (anti-PR3) by ELISA as a confirmatory test. If both of these are negative, then a positive ANCA is considered to be nonspecific and without clinical relevance. Another increasingly recognized cause of positive ANCA/MPO/PR3 is the use of cocaine. Cocaine is often "cut" with the antihelminthic drug levamisole (banned in the United States and Canada due to adverse effects), which can cause a vasculitis like presentation and give a positive ANCA/MPO/PR3 result. Given the growing nature of this problem, the clinician should be aware of this association.

Complete blood count (CBC), erythrocyte sedimentation rate (ESR), and C-reactive protein (CRP) are the commonly used laboratory tests that are helpful in the diagnosis of all types of inflammatory processes, including autoimmune disease, infections, and malignancies. In inflammation, the white blood count tends to rise with a neutrophil predominance, along with an elevated platelet count, and a normocytic, normochromic anemia. Caution should be exercised when interpreting an elevated white cell count, since this is also commonly present in infections. The ESR and CRP are two other tests that tend to rise with increased inflammatory disease activity. An upward trending ESR and CRP suggest increasing inflammation and tend to signify worsening disease. CRP is more sensitive and specific than ESR, has a shorter half-life (thus mirrors disease activity more closely), and is less influenced by age; it is therefore arguably a superior test to ESR. In addition to inflammation, ESR can be elevated due to a number of other factors. Conditions that cause a decrease in the albumin-to-globulin ratio in the blood can increase ESR, such as multiple myeloma and other monoclonal gammopathies. ESR is also dependent on the number of red blood cells present and tends to rise in patients with anemia. In addition, patients with chronic kidney disease almost universally have an elevated ESR. In contrast, CRP is more specific for inflammation.[1]

The normal range for ESR should be set to maximize the sensitivity and specificity. As the ESR value increases, it is more likely to indicate underlying pathology, although the differential diagnosis is broad, including rheumatologic inflammation such as GCA, serious infections such as endocarditis (Chapter 4), or malignancy. Women tend to have a higher ESR, and increasing age is also associated with an increasing ESR in the absence of clinical disease; thus normal may be defined in terms of age and gender. The following useful formulas estimate the maximum normal ESR value for 98% of the population aged 20 to 89 years[2]:

Male normal ESR (mm/hr): Age $\div$ 2
Female normal ESR (mm/hr): (Age + 10) $\div$ 2

For patients over the age of 65, the formulas may slightly underestimate the normal maximum normal value.[3]

An ESR result over 100 has a 99% specificity for identifying a *sickness index* (including malignancy, infection, and noninfectious inflammatory conditions) but a low sensitivity for each condition category (36% for infection; 25% for malignancy; 21% for noninfectious inflammatory diseases).[4]

CRP values also correlate with cardiovascular disease risk, with higher levels correlating with higher risk, even with in the range of normal.[5] The high-sensitivity CRP (hsCRP) test allows for accurate measurements of CRP < 1.0 mg/dL. The hsCRP reference ranges are therefore defined according to cardiovascular disease risk (Chapter 3).[6]

Elevated cardiovascular disease risk/low-grade inflammation: CRP 0.3 to 1.0 mg/dL
Clinically significant inflammation: CRP >1.0 mg/dL

It is important to recognize there is no uniformity in reported units for CRP across laboratories, and some use mg/dL while others use mg/L.

RHEUMATOLOGIC DISEASES AND THEIR OCULAR MANIFESTATIONS

GIANT CELL ARTERITIS

Giant cell arteritis (GCA), also known as temporal arteritis, is an inflammatory disorder of unknown etiology that affects medium- and large-sized arteries of the head and neck, most commonly the extracranial branches of the carotid artery. It is the most common form of systemic vasculitis in adults and usually occurs in persons aged 50 years or older (mean age at onset 79 years).[7] The most feared complication of GCA is sudden painless loss of vision. The incidence of GCA varies widely between populations. In 2008, it was estimated that 228,000 United States residents had GCA, and incidence is estimated at 18 per 100,000. The incidence of GCA is highest in persons of northern European or Scandinavian descent. The greatest risk factor for GCA is age, as well as gender (more than twice as common in women compared with men) and tobacco use.[7] There is a strong relationship between GCA and polymyalgia rheumatica (PMR), which is a common inflammatory disease characterized by morning stiffness and pain in the shoulders and hip girdles and affects a similar demographic as GCA. PMR occurs in 50% of patients with GCA, whereas approximately 15% of patients with PMR will develop GCA.[8]

Signs and Symptoms of Giant Cell Arteritis

The onset of GCA is usually insidious, with progression of symptoms over weeks to months, but in some cases the disease begins abruptly. The classically described presentation of GCA includes

- Constitutional symptoms
- New headaches (unilateral or bilateral)
- Scalp tenderness
- Jaw claudication
- Vision abnormalities (vision loss or diplopia)

The constitutional symptoms are nonspecific and similar to those seen in PMR, such as fatigue, fever, weight loss, and anorexia. The character of the headache is variable, and pain may localize to any part of the skull. The most consistent characteristic is that the headache is new or different from prior headaches. On examination, half of patients may have abnormalities of the temporal artery (enlargement, beaded/nodular swelling, tenderness, or decreased pulse), and others may report tenderness of the scalp.[7] The inflammation within the vascular wall restricts the luminal diameter. As a result, claudication (or pain caused by ischemia) may occur in the muscles of mastication (jaw claudication), extremities, and occasionally the muscles of the tongue or those involved in swallowing. In the jaw muscles, discomfort is noted especially when chewing meat, which requires relatively prolonged chewing.[7] It is important to distinguish jaw claudication (characterized as a pain due to muscle fatigue with poor blood flow) from other, more common causes of jaw pain; for example, jaw pain due to temporomandibular joint disorder may occur with immediate onset of chewing and may be accompanied by other features such as jaw "popping" or clicking, jaw clenching, or teeth grinding. Other rare symptoms and ischemic cranial complications in GCA include tinnitus/hearing loss, facial pain or swelling, tongue pain or necrosis, throat pain, and scalp necrosis.[9–11] Large vessel aneurysms and/or stenoses are potential short and/or long-term complications of GCA and can be associated with chest pain, limb claudication, and stroke. Atypical disease manifestations include fever of unknown origin (a fever in absence of a known diagnosis), respiratory symptoms (dry cough), and neurologic manifestations (TIAs, strokes). While both anterior and posterior circulation strokes rarely occur in GCA, vertebrobasilar involvement is the most common.[12] Death from GCA is also not common and is usually due to rupture of an aortic aneurysm or aortic dissection. Most aortic complications from GCA are diagnosed 5 years or more after original disease diagnosis. At this time, guidelines are unclear about the role for aortitis/aortic aneurysm screening among patients with GCA.[13]

Ocular Giant Cell Arteritis

Vision loss is the most-feared complication of GCA though is rarely the initial symptom, usually following other symptoms by several weeks or months. Overall, visual symptoms occur in 20% to 25% of GCA with some studies reporting rates as high as 50% or more.[14] Permanent vision loss occurs in about 5% of patients in the era of corticosteroids.[15] Because permanent vision loss is usually preceded by visual symptoms for an average of 8.5 days[16] and vision loss may be prevented in 90% or more of cases with prompt recognition and treatment,[17] visual symptoms due to GCA are considered an ocular emergency.

Visual symptoms in GCA include (in decreasing frequency)

- sudden painless vision loss
- amaurosis fugax/transient monocular vision loss
- diplopia
- eye pain

All of varying severity and two or more may occur contemporaneously. Amaurosis fugax is an ominous sign of impending visual loss in GCA.[14] Diplopia occurs in up to 10% of patients and is due to extraocular muscle or cranial nerve ischemia. Arteritic diplopia usually begins as a transient symptom that progresses to constant and is accompanied by other typical GCA symptoms or clinical signs in nearly all cases.[18] Vision loss due to GCA may be unilateral or bilateral (less common), transient or permanent, and partial or complete. Risk for involvement of the second eye in unilateral cases is very high if not promptly treated.

The ocular signs in GCA are ischemic in nature due to thrombosis of one or more of the arteries supplying the globe and/or the orbit by granulomatous inflammation. The most common manifestation (by far) is arteritic anterior ischemic optic neuropathy (AAION) due to involvement of the posterior ciliary artery (**FIGURE 11.1**), occurring in over 80% of cases, though the entire ophthalmic artery or any of its branches can be affected.

On funduscopy, AAION appears as a pallid optic nerve head edema that must be differentiated from nonarteritic anterior ischemic optic neuropathy (NAAION), an unrelated, similarly appearing, and much more common disease entity. The pathophysiology of NAAION is entirely distinct and involves temporary hemodynamic insufficiency (hypoperfusion) of the posterior ciliary artery. Vision loss is often noted upon first awakening from sleep. NAAION generally affects older patients with systemic vascular risk factors (including hypertension, diabetes, and sleep apnea) and local ocular risk factors (including small cup-to-disc ratio and the presence of optic disc drusen) and shares many clinical features with AAION.[19] Though not absolute, features which are suggestive of NAAION rather than AAION include[20]

- absence of typical systemic GCA symptoms
- absence of significantly elevated inflammatory biomarkers
- absence of diffuse choroidal nonfilling on fluorescein angiogram
- lack of visual symptoms preceding vision loss (ie, lack of amaurosis fugax)
- less severe vision loss at initial onset
- appearance of hyperemic rather than pallid optic disc swelling (**FIGURE 11.2**)
- absence of signs indicating central retinal artery involvement (eg, cotton wool spots, central retinal, or cilioretinal artery occlusion)

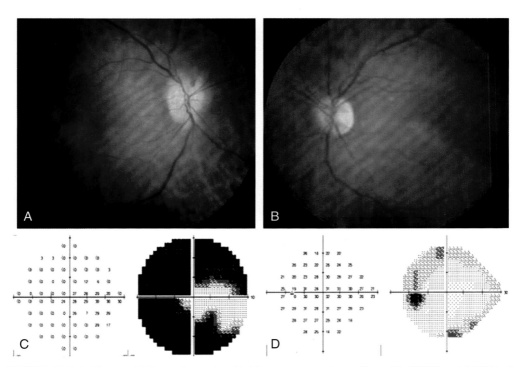

FIGURE 11.1 A 69-year-old Caucasian male with biopsy-proven giant cell arteritis (GCA) and AAION of the right eye (A), with permanent visual field loss (HVF 10-2) (C). The left eye remained unaffected (B) with full visual field (HVF 24-2) (D) after prompt initiation of intravenous steroids. Note the chalky white disc edema of the right optic nerve in (A), typical for GCA. (Image credit: Rachel Druckenbrod, OD [VA Boston Healthcare System].)

Other possible ocular ischemic manifestations in GCA include (in order of decreasing frequency) cilioretinal artery occlusion, central retinal artery occlusion, ophthalmoplegia, posterior ischemic optic neuropathy, and (rarely) anterior segment ischemic signs such as neovascular glaucoma, anterior uveitis, ocular hypotony, marginal corneal ulceration, scleritis, episcleritis, and orbital pseudotumor.[14] This pattern of involvement is best appreciated through understanding the pathogenesis of the disease. Based upon histological grounds, the disease appears to be an autoimmune response to a component of the elastic laminae of involved arterial vessels. Vessels without an elastic lamina, such as arterioles, are unaffected. The posterior ciliary arteries and the short posterior ciliary arteries serving the optic nerve head are arteries. The central retinal artery, despite its name, is an arteriole, except near its point of origin.

Choroidal ischemic lesions can also develop with occlusion of the posterior ciliary arteries, that later appear as chorioretinal degenerative lesions on the ocular fundus examination (**FIGURE 11.3**).[14] If the ocular fundus examination does not demonstrate frank ischemic injury (eg, in patients experiencing transient visual loss), fundus fluorescein angiography is useful to identify delayed or incomplete filling of the posterior ciliary arteries, which is present in nearly all patients with symptoms of vision loss due to GCA[14] (**FIGURE 11.4**).

Giant Cell Arteritis Diagnosis

GCA diagnosis is made by a thorough history, physical examination, laboratory evaluation, and histopathological evaluation of an arterial biopsy specimen. The history may reveal the typical symptoms

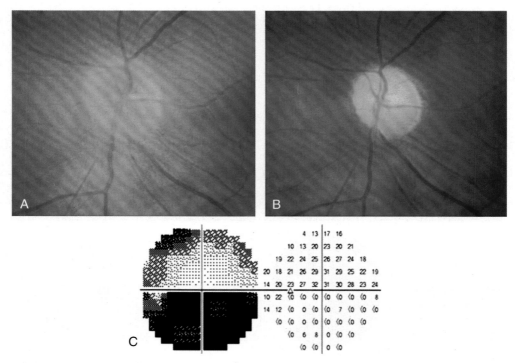

FIGURE 11.2 Nonarteritic anterior ischemic optic neuropathy (NAAION) with hyperemic disc edema and peripapillary hemorrhages at acute presentation (A) and optic atrophy upon resolution (B). The patient suffered a permanent inferior altitudinal visual field defect (C). (Image credit: Rachel Druckenbrod, OD [VA Boston Healthcare System].)

associated with GCA as discussed above. Physical examination may show scalp tenderness, temporal artery abnormalities (beading, tenderness, enlargement, loss of pulse), tenderness of the shoulder and hip girdle muscles when PMR is also present, and/or eye findings. The most common laboratory abnormality is elevated inflammatory markers (ESR and CRP). ESR and CRP are elevated in more than 95% of GCA cases, but normal ESR and CRP do not exclude a diagnosis of GCA. Thrombocytosis is common and, when present, is slightly predictive for AAION versus NAAION.[21] Patients can also present with a normochromic, normocytic anemia. The "gold standard" diagnostic test for GCA is histopathological analysis of a temporal artery biopsy (TAB) with specimen length of at least 1 cm (ideally 2 cm), revealing histopathologic features of temporal arteritis which include intimal hyperplasia, disruption of the internal elastic lamina (as evidenced by use of an elastic stain), granulomatous infiltration of the media and adventitia with or without multinucleated giant cells, and tissue necrosis (**FIGURE 11.5**).

Several important considerations for clinical management exist surrounding the TAB. First, treatment initiation should not be delayed while awaiting biopsy, and thus TAB should be obtained promptly with risk for false-negative results if delayed. Several robust studies agree that the incidence of positive TAB in GCA obtained within 2 to 4 weeks is not altered by pretreatment.[22] Second, in GCA, inflammation is found most often in medium-sized muscular arteries that originate from the arch of the aorta and tends to affect the arteries in a segmental fashion, which may result in so-called "skip lesions."[7] The biopsy specimen of the temporal artery shows vasculitis in about 80% of patients with GCA as long as an adequate length of vessel is sampled.[23] About 20% of patients with GCA may have a biopsy specimen of the artery that is negative; this may occur due to

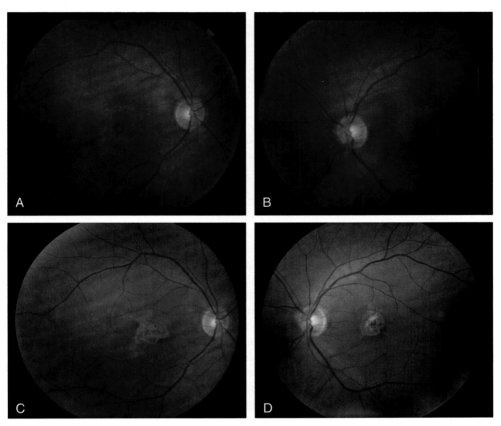

FIGURE 11.3 A 64-year-old Caucasian male with bilateral macular infarction due to choroidal thrombosis in biopsy-proven giant cell arteritis. Fundus appearance OD (A) and OS (B) 2 weeks after symptomatic central vision loss. Fundus appearance 1 year later, with macular scarring OD (C) and OS (D). (Image credit: Rachel Druckenbrod, OD (VA Boston Healthcare System).)

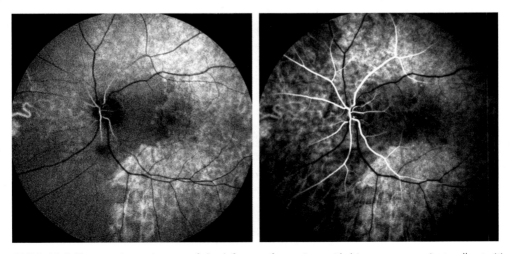

FIGURE 11.4 Fluorescein angiogram of the left eye of a patient with biopsy-proven giant cell arteritis demonstrates significantly delayed arteriolar filling. Left: Choroidal filling is patchy and highly delayed at 52 seconds, indicating posterior ciliary artery ischemia with risk for arteritic anterior ischemic optic neuropathy. Note that the retinal arteriolar phase has just begun, indicating there is also significant ischemia of the retinal circulation with risk for arteritic central retinal artery occlusion. Right: By 60 seconds, there is still incomplete filling of the choroid and the retinal arteriovenous phase has yet to begin. (Image credit: Rachel Druckenbrod, OD, VA Boston Healthcare System.)

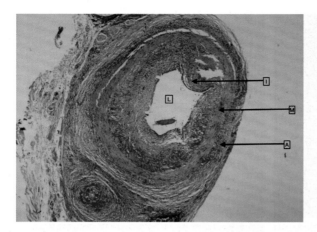

FIGURE 11.5 Intima (I) hyperplasia compromises the lumen (L) of this temporal artery biopsy specimen; further luminal narrowing can trigger ischemia. Also shown are vascular media (M) and adventitia (A). (Photo credit: John Perry, MD. Department of Pathology, Mount Auburn Hospital, Cambridge, MA.)

the disease sparing this vessel or due to a patchy distribution of disease activity, so that the biopsy did not reveal the disease.[23] Therefore, a negative TAB does not rule out disease in a patient with a concerning clinical presentation. When GCA is strongly suspected but biopsy is negative, a second biopsy (eg, of the other side of the head) or an imaging test should be considered. Standard MRI or CT can show aortic involvement, and high-resolution 3T MRI can show intracranial and superficial cranial arteritis. Among patients with ocular GCA, MRI may show optic nerve parenchymal enhancement, perineural sheath enhancement, and/or nonspecific orbital enhancement.[24] Color doppler ultrasound has been considered as a potential noninvasive and inexpensive alternative to TAB and MRI, with reported 80% sensitivity and 90% specificity for GCA.[25] However, reported sensitivity rates are highly variable, accurate diagnosis is dependent on the expertise of the ultrasonographer, and abnormalities typically disappear after only 3 days of glucocorticoid treatment; thus the use of temporal artery ultrasound has not replaced the TAB in clinical practice.[8] The management of patients with high clinical suspicion, but two negative biopsies and normal vascular imaging should be considered in conjunction with a rheumatologist. GCA can at times be diagnosed solely based upon the clinical presentation.

Classification criteria for GCA exist (BOX 11.1) to help confirm the diagnosis of GCA.[26] However, it should be noted that validity of these criteria has been called into question with potential for both missed diagnosis and overdiagnosis; the diagnosis of GCA should thus be approached with full consideration of all historical, clinical, laboratory, and biopsy or imaging data.[27] Differential diagnosis of GCA is broad and includes occult infections, malignancy, systemic amyloidosis, and other forms of systemic vasculitis.

BOX 11.1 The 1990 ACR Classification Criteria for GCA Include:

Three out of the five criteria below usually required for diagnosis, however it is possible to make a diagnosis without meeting three criteria.

- Age at onset greater than 50 years old
- A new headache
- Temporal artery abnormality (tenderness to palpation or decreased pulsation)
- Elevated ESR (≥50 by Westergren method)
- Abnormal TAB (showing vasculitis characterized by a predominance of mononuclear cell infiltration or granulomatous inflammation usually with multinucleated giant cells)

Giant Cell Arteritis Treatment

Glucocorticoids such as prednisone are the therapy of choice for GCA and should be started as soon as the diagnosis of GCA is strongly suspected. An oral dose of steroids at 40 to 60 mg/day is often sufficient, though higher dose steroid at 80 mg/day orally or intravenous dosing at 1 mg/kg/day for 3 days (followed by oral taper) is often advocated in the presence of visual symptoms or vision loss.[17] As previously mentioned, therapy should be started even before the biopsy is performed since the diagnostic yield of the TAB is not altered by corticosteroid therapy for at least 2 weeks, maybe longer.[7] Patients will require months of treatment with glucocorticoid therapy and should be monitored for side effects which include osteoporosis, pathological bone fractures, gastroesophageal reflux disease, peptic ulcer disease, opportunistic infections, hypertension, diabetes, cataracts, weight gain, and mood disorders which can be complicated by steroid-induced psychosis.[8] Patients at risk for gastrointestinal bleeding from high-dose steroids may benefit from prophylactic treatment with a proton pump inhibitor or histamine H2 receptor antagonist (Chapter 7) while treated with steroids. Patients with diabetes mellitus or prediabetes should be educated that blood glucose levels may rise with the initiation of high-dose steroids, and this should be integrated into the overall management of comorbidities. Steroids are usually continued at the initial effective dose until all reversible symptoms, signs, and laboratory abnormalities (elevated ESR, CRP) have reverted to normal, which usually takes 2 to 4 weeks, and a slow taper can be initiated after this. Inflammatory markers are monitored throughout the treatment course, and if they rise again as steroid is withdrawn, the patient is returned to the higher dose. Most patients have a chronic disease that requires prednisone treatment for at least 1 year and often for several years.[7] Relapse rates range from 34% to 74% and usually occur during the first year of treatment and in patients who are on prednisone doses less than 20 mg daily.[8] Steroid-sparing agents should be considered, especially in patients with contraindications to prolonged high-dose corticosteroid therapy. These agents include methotrexate, an antifolate antimetabolite, or tocilizumab, a humanized monoclonal antibody against the IL-6 receptor. Other agents that may be promising include azathioprine, ustekinumab, cyclophosphamide, dapsone, and leflunomide.[8] GCA is a lifelong disease and requires frequent monitoring by both a rheumatologist and an eye care provider. The return of lost vision caused by AAION is extremely uncommon, even after treatment.[8] Patients should be counseled that vision loss that is present at diagnosis may continue to progress despite treatment, which occurs in 10% of patients.[8,17]

In summary, GCA poses a significant diagnostic challenge due to its variable, nonspecific symptom profile and the occasional challenge when standard confirmatory diagnostic test results are at odds with the clinical impression. Due to the potential vision-threatening consequences of GCA, its early diagnosis and treatment are critical and a low threshold for evaluation by all healthcare providers is imperative. Fortunately, with early diagnosis and treatment, the overall prognosis for survival and vision can be favorable. Patients require frequent and chronic monitoring in rheumatology and/ or primary care along with eye care specialists for signs of disease activity and adverse effects from treatment.

POLYMYALGIA RHEUMATICA

PMR is an inflammatory condition involving the proximal joints of the upper and lower extremities. It is considered the most frequent inflammatory articular condition in patients above age 50, with a lifetime prevalence in the range of 2.4% for women and 1.7% for men.[28] While "-myalgia" is a component of the disease name and suggests muscle pathology, the actual pathology involves the joint, including bursitis, synovitis, and tenosynovitis. These can be detected on soft tissue imaging such as MRI or ultrasound. An assessment for myositis with a serum CK level should be normal in cases of PMR. In patients presenting with symptoms suggesting PMR, in addition to the diagnosis and treatment of PMR, clinicians should be alert to the concurrent risk for GCA, which is reported to occur in 20% or more of patients with PMR and carries risk for permanent vision loss (unlike PMR itself). However, only about half of patients with PMR have GCA.[29] All patients with suspected PMR should thus be assessed for cranial and ocular symptoms of GCA, as the intensity of treatment for the two conditions varies; treating PMR alone (which requires low-dose steroids) can allow GCA to progress with irreversible vision loss as noted above.

PMR (and GCA) typically occur in patients older than 50 years old, with the peak incidence between ages 60 and 70. The disease occurs more frequently in females, with about a threefold increase in risk versus males.[30] There are genetic factors, including population and HLA associations; Scandinavia has the highest rate of disease with a lower incidence in southern European countries, as well as non-European populations.

Signs and Symptoms of Polymyalgia Rheumatica

Typical PMR symptoms include soreness and stiffness in the shoulder girdle, neck, and proximal lower extremities (hip girdle). Patients may have difficulty with tasks that involve raising the arms above the shoulders, such as putting on a shirt or coat; with more severe symptoms, arising from bed is difficult due to hip pain. As with other inflammatory rheumatologic conditions, morning stiffness is typical, with decreasing symptoms during daily activities. Prolonged rest can allow symptoms of stiffness to flare. Subjective symptoms of weakness may be present due to the periarticular inflammation and pain that can limit motion; however, true muscle weakness is not present. In addition, as noted above, findings of myositis with serum CK elevation would indicate an alternate diagnosis. Constitutional symptoms including fatigue and malaise are also common. When symptoms of GCA (as reviewed above) including headache, jaw claudication, visual symptoms (especially amaurosis fugax or unilateral vision loss), or high fevers are present, prompt evaluation should be initiated along with empiric glucocorticoid therapy for GCA to prevent vision loss (preserving the fellow eye if unilateral vision loss has already occurred).

Polymyalgia Rheumatica Diagnosis

In addition to a thorough history and comprehensive examination, lab evaluation should center on an assessment for inflammation. While the sed rate (ESR) has been the traditional test of choice, with a level above 40 mm/hr suggesting PMR (with or without GCA), testing for CRP has been found to have a higher sensitivity and specificity at diagnosis. Thus, CRP is currently considered the test of choice by many rheumatologists[31]; the ESR adds little additional diagnostic discriminatory power and many physicians no longer order it. Additional testing including CBC, renal and electrolytes, and thyroid assessment with TSH are commonly ordered. Other rheumatological tests such as RF and CCP are indicated to aid in the differential diagnosis; in PMR they are typically normal or negative. Based upon clinical findings and lab results of elevated inflammatory markers without indications of another disease process offering a more likely explanation for the history and examination findings, the diagnosis of PMR can be made. Imaging and biopsy are not indicated when suspecting PMR. However, when GCA is suspected, TAB should be performed.

Polymyalgia Rheumatica Treatment

Treatment of PMR entails glucocorticoid therapy as doses of 15 to 20 mg of prednisone daily. This is substantially lower than typical doses commonly used to treat GCA (in the range of 40-60 mg daily), thus underscoring the importance of ascertaining with a high degree of clinical certainty that GCA is not present before treating PMR alone. Markers of inflammation (CRP, ESR) should return to normal after initiation of treatment. Over time, glucocorticoid dose should be slowly tapered with monitoring of inflammatory markers and clinical symptoms. A flare in symptoms or increase in inflammatory markers during the steroid taper usually indicates an excessively rapid taper, necessitating an increase in dose with a slower taper. Patients often remain on a slow glucocorticoid taper for 1 to 2 years.

Older literature has linked the diagnosis of PMR to higher rates of cancer diagnosed in the following months. While newer data have not consistently reinforced this finding, there remains some uncertainty in this area.[32] While current guidelines do not advocate aggressive imaging for which there are no data to support improved outcomes (such as full body CT scanning), status of routine age and gender-appropriate cancer screening should be reviewed, with recommendations to maintain regular screening as appropriate.

Rheumatoid Arthritis

Rheumatoid arthritis (RA) is a chronic systemic inflammatory disorder of unknown cause characterized by symmetric polyarticular pain, swelling, and morning stiffness. The disease involves acute and chronic inflammation in the synovium of joints (synovitis) which can lead to significant and irreversible joint damage without appropriate treatment. RA is understood to be the most common inflammatory arthritis, affecting from 0.5% to 1% of the population worldwide, with a female to male ratio between 2:1 and 3:1. In the United States, the disease prevalence is around 1% and the median observed incidence is approximately 40 cases per 100,000.[33] Overall, the disease appears to be less common in Asia and Africa than in the United States and Europe. RA can affect individuals of any age, including infants and the elderly, but most commonly occurs in the 40 to 60 age range. The precise cause of RA is unknown, but many studies have demonstrated a link between disease and genetic and environmental factors. There is a 15% concordance in monozygotic twins, which is four times greater than the rate in dizygotic twins, suggesting a genetic component.[34] The genes with the greatest impact are in the class II major histocompatibility complex (MHC) locus, with a strong association of RA with a specific sequence of select human leukocyte antigen (HLA)-DR haplotypes. The strongest known environmental risk factor for RA is cigarette smoking, with the risk of RA increasing with the quantity and duration of cigarette use. There is also some evidence linking obesity to increased risk of RA.

Signs and Symptoms of Rheumatoid Arthritis

RA most commonly presents insidiously, with gradually progressive pain, swelling, and stiffness in several joints over weeks to months. Occasionally, it can present acutely with severe symptoms and accompanying systemic symptoms. The hallmark symptoms of RA are pain, morning stiffness, and swelling of joints. Classically, it involves small joints of the hands and feet in a symmetric distribution. Specifically, it tends to affect the metacarpophalangeal and proximal interphalangeal joints of the fingers, the wrists, and the metatarsophalangeal joints of the toes (**FIGURE 11.6**). It can also commonly affect other synovial joints of the upper and lower extremities, including elbow, shoulder, hip, knee, and ankle joints. Axial joint involvement is less common, but can occur in 20% to 50% of patients.[35] Aside from joints, rheumatoid arthritis can involve other components of the musculoskeletal system (muscles, bones) as well as many other organ systems. Extraarticular manifestations of RA occur in around 40% of patients with RA over the course of the disease. Age, positive serum RF or ANA, and smoking are risk factors for extraarticular involvement.[36]

Ocular Rheumatoid Arthritis

There are several eye-related conditions that can occur in patients with RA. The most common is dry eyes, or keratoconjunctivitis sicca (KCS), which occurs in 10% to 25% of patients. If dry eye is confirmed in the setting of RA and no alternative explanation identified, patients are considered to have secondary Sjogren syndrome. Artificial tears and/or ointments are first-line treatment for dry eye

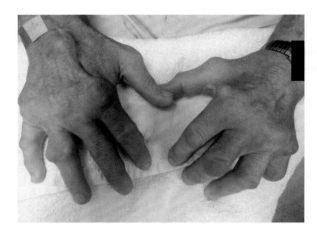

FIGURE 11.6 Severe rheumatoid arthritis. Note involvement of the proximal small joints of the hand, including the proximal interphalangeal and metacarpophalangeal joints with swelling and deformity. There is muscle wasting adjacent to the thumbs. The distal interphalangeal joints are spared. (Image credit Shiv Sehra, MD.)

syndrome, though severe forms may require advanced therapies including topical steroids, topical cyclosporine, oral secretagogues (presently used off-label), topical autologous serum, punctal occlusion, and/or therapeutic contact lenses.[37] Management of dry eye disease is also discussed within the section on Sjogren syndrome.

Episcleritis and scleritis are important but uncommon ocular manifestations of RA, occurring in up to 3% and up to 6% of patients, respectively.[38] Because episcleritis often features a benign course and may go unrecognized, its prevalence may be underestimated. It is important to recognize that while these complications are uncommon in RA, RA is among the most common identifiable causes for both episcleritis and scleritis, and patients presenting with these ocular findings should be questioned about existing RA diagnosis or symptoms of RA in cases of undiagnosed disease. Since the most severe inflammatory ocular complications of RA can be sight-threatening and usually require oral steroids and/or oral immunosuppressive therapies, management should involve an experienced eye care specialist as well as a rheumatologist.

Episcleritis is relatively more sudden in onset versus scleritis, with symptoms of discomfort and "salmon pink" sectoral conjunctival hyperemia. It is bilateral in 40% of cases and visual acuity is usually unaffected. RA-associated episcleritis is indistinct in its clinical features from other causes of episcleritis and both simple and (less commonly) nodular forms may occur. Instillation of a topical vasoconstrictor (eg, phenylephrine or an alpha-1 agonist such as apraclonidine) may be used diagnostically to demonstrate complete or near-complete blanching of the superficial episcleral vessels (FIGURE 11.7), which will not occur in scleritis. Episcleritis is often treated with palliative surface lubrication or topical steroids in the case of moderate/severe disease and uncommonly requires oral nonsteroidal antiinflammatory drugs (NSAIDs) or steroids.[38]

Scleritis presents more insidiously and is accompanied by more intense redness, pain, and photophobia.[39] Scleritis involves inflammation and congestion of the deep episcleral vascular plexus, creating scleral edema and a bluish-red coloration which is most apparent under natural sunlight. Tissue thinning in more severe forms may also create a blue/gray coloration due to visibility of the underlying uvea (FIGURE 11.8). RA-associated scleritis tends to occur in a bilateral distribution and in older patients compared with scleritis due to nonrheumatic disease, and any form of scleritis may occur (eg, diffuse, nodular, or necrotizing anterior forms, or posterior scleritis).[40,41] Scleromalacia perforans, an often asymptomatic and severe form of noninflammatory necrotizing scleritis that can lead to scleral perforation due to extreme tissue thinning, is also highly associated with (longstanding) RA. Among all systemic disease causes of scleritis, rheumatic disease is most common, and RA is the most prevalent of the rheumatic associations (eg, 40% of cases in one series, followed

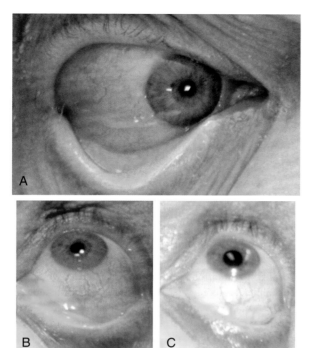

FIGURE 11.7 A, Episcleritis of the right eye, demonstrating "salmon pink" hyperemia. B, Inferior sectoral episcleritis of the left eye at baseline, and after instillation of topical phenylephrine 2% (C), demonstrating blanching of superficial episcleral vessels. (Image credit: Rachel Druckenbrod, OD (VA Boston Healthcare System).)

by systemic vasculitis in 25% and SLE in 11%).[42] Scleritis is more commonly seen in RA patients with long-standing disease and seropositivity (RF and/or ACPAs), and it is quite unusual for scleritis to be an initial manifestation of RA[23]; indeed, a majority of patients diagnosed with RA-associated scleritis already have a known RA diagnosis.[42] Scleritis in RA is associated with poorer disease prognosis and increased mortality.[43] Treatment of RA-associated scleritis usually requires oral steroids at an initial dose of 1 mg/kg/day, though some minor cases may respond to oral NSAIDs. A "loading dose" with intravenous steroid may precede oral steroid therapy in severe cases. Scleritis in RA often benefits from a second immunosuppressive agent in addition to steroid (either for disease control or

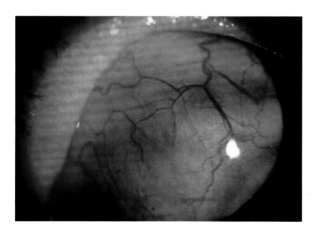

FIGURE 11.8 Necrotizing scleritis. An 82-year-old patient with long-standing rheumatoid arthritis presenting with necrotizing scleritis. (Reprinted from Garg SJ. *Uveitis.* 2nd ed. Philadelphia, PA: Wolters Kluwer; 2018.)

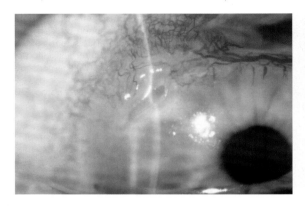

FIGURE 11.9 Peripheral ulcerative keratitis in rheumatoid arthritis. (Reprinted with permission from Rapuano CJ. *Wills Eye Institute – Cornea.* 2nd ed. Philadelphia, PA: Wolters Kluwer; 2011.)

steroid-sparing), such as cyclophosphamide, methotrexate, azathioprine, mycophenolate mofetil, or ciclosporin. Limited case series and reports show benefit in using the biologic agents infliximab and rituximab.[38]

Peripheral ulcerative keratitis (PUK) is a severe inflammation of the juxtalimbal cornea which can occur along with or independent of scleritis (usually necrotizing scleritis), with risk for corneal ulceration, thinning, and perforation (**FIGURE 11.9**). A pathognomonic, crescent-shaped corneal ulceration occurs with epithelial break and underlying stromal thinning. Patients report ocular redness and pain, and progressive astigmatism or corneal opacification may contribute to reduced vision. Up to 40% of PUK occurs in association with RA, while up to 3% of RA cases may develop PUK.[38] Like scleritis, the presence of PUK in RA is a harbinger of poor disease prognosis. Treatment of PUK is similar to scleritis.

Finally, RA is an uncommon cause of acquired Brown syndrome, which occurs secondary to inflammation of the bursa between the orbital trochlea and the superior oblique tendon (a tenosynovitis).[39] Patients complain of a painful, intermittent diplopia worst on upward-medial gaze and sometimes a "clicking" sensation in the region of the trochlea. Ocular motility examination shows apparent inferior oblique palsy. Inflammatory Brown syndrome is responsive to oral steroids.[44]

Rheumatoid Arthritis Diagnosis

There is no single pathognomonic physical finding or laboratory test result that defines the disease. The current standard for RA disease classification is the 2010 American College of Rheumatology (ACR) and European League Against Rheumatism (EULAR) classification criteria.

The diagnosis of RA is based on a clinical syndrome of inflammatory arthritis defined by at least one joint with definite synovial swelling (synovitis) that is not better defined by a different disease, blood tests including the serologies of RF and ACPA as well as inflammatory markers ESR and CRP, and duration of symptoms >6 weeks.[33] Notably, positive autoantibodies (RF and ACPAs) are neither universally present nor required to make the diagnosis of RA; RF and/or ACPAs are present in approximately 80% of patients with RA. Additionally, they can be found in the sera several years before clinical symptoms in patients who will go on to develop RA and can also be found in normal, healthy patients.

Rheumatoid Arthritis Treatment

Treatment of RA is aimed toward controlling joint inflammation and preventing joint damage that can occur over time with uncontrolled inflammation. The principles of treatment of RA include early recognition and diagnosis, care by an expert in the treatment of rheumatic disease, early use of disease modifying antirheumatic drugs (DMARDs), importance of tight control with a treat-to-target strategy aiming for remission or low disease activity, and use of anti-inflammatory medications such as NSAIDs and glucocorticoids only as adjuncts to therapy. There has been a significant improvement in the outcomes of RA with the application of these principles of treatment. DMARDs include conventional synthetic agents such as hydroxychloroquine (HCQ), sulfasalazine, and methotrexate; biologic agents including, but not limited to, TNF-alpha inhibitors, interleukin-1 receptor antagonists, and interleukin receptor antagonists; and targeted synthetic DMARDs including JAK inhibitors. Standard practice is to initiate therapy with one of the conventional DMARDs, most commonly methotrexate if there is not a contraindication to its use, while treating active inflammation with an anti-inflammatory agent such as glucocorticoids or NSAIDs. If there is an inadequate response to initial DMARD therapy, combination therapy with multiple DMARDs is warranted. During treatment, patients need to be regularly evaluated for clinical response, disease activity, and laboratory monitoring for drug toxicities.

SYSTEMIC LUPUS ERYTHEMATOSUS

SLE is a widely studied rheumatologic condition, often viewed as the prototype systemic autoimmune disease. SLE results from chronic and recurrent activation of the immune system that yields production of antibodies and other protein products that contribute to inflammation and tissue damage. Specifically, SLE is characterized by a systemic loss of self-tolerance, with production of pathogenic autoantibodies against nucleic acids and their binding proteins. Like many rheumatologic conditions, this aberrant immune system activation occurs in the milieu of genetic susceptibility and environmental triggers.[45]

It occurs predominantly in young women in their childbearing years. The skewed gender in lupus is dramatic, with a 9:1 female predominance, which suggests a role for both hormones and as-yet uncharacterized sex-related factors in disease pathogenesis. Lupus also has a predilection for nonwhite groups, with higher rates in blacks, Asians, and Hispanics compared with whites.[45]

Signs and Symptoms of Systemic Lupus Erythematosus

The aberrantly activated immune system in SLE can cause damage to virtually any organ system or tissue. The presentation is variable, ranging from mild joint and skin involvement to life-threatening renal, hematologic, or central nervous system involvement. Furthermore, the clinical course of SLE is variable and may be characterized by unpredictable disease flares and remissions. Given the heterogeneous nature of the disease, it is helpful to consider clinical features of SLE by organ system.

- Constitutional symptoms including fatigue, malaise, myalgia, and weight loss are extremely common and occur in most patients at some point during the course of disease.
- The musculoskeletal system is involved in 90% of patients, with arthralgias (joint pains) and arthritis (joint swelling) being most common and often some of the earlier manifestations of disease.
- Most patients with SLE have skin and mucous membrane lesions at some point in the course of disease; there is a great degree of variability in type of skin involvement but the most classic feature characteristic of SLE is a malar rash (also known as "butterfly rash") that presents as erythema over the cheeks and nose (sparing nasolabial folds) after sun exposure (FIGURE 11.10). Patient should be asked about photosensitivity, oral and nasal ulcers, hair loss, and any rashes or skin changes, which all can be seen in SLE.
- The cardiovascular system can be involved in SLE; the most common cardiac manifestation is pericarditis, but the myocardium, valves, conduction system, and coronary arteries can also be

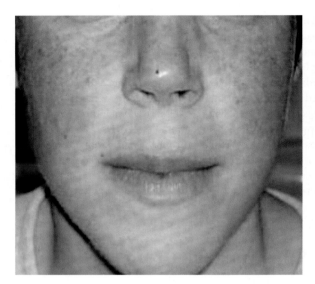

FIGURE 11.10 The malar or butterfly rash (erythema over the cheeks in the shape of a butterfly) is typical in systemic lupus erythematosus. This is distinguished from the heliotrope rash of dermatomyositis in which the rash includes the upper and lower lids and spares the bridge of the nose. (From Ricci SS. *Maternity and Pediatric Nursing.* 2nd ed. Philadelphia, PA: Wolters Kluwer; 2012.)

involved. Raynaud phenomenon is a vasculopathic process characterized by reversible skin color changes induced by cold. Vasculitis can occur in SLE patients, with a broad spectrum of manifestations depending on the size of the vessels that become inflamed. Thromboembolic disease, both arterial and venous, can be present in SLE, particularly when antiphospholipid antibodies are present.

- Renal involvement, including several forms of glomerulonephritis, is commonly seen in SLE and associated with significant morbidity and mortality.
- Gastrointestinal involvement in SLE can include esophagitis, protein losing enteropathy, lupus hepatitis, and mesenteric vasculitis.
- Pulmonary involvement manifests as pleuritis with or without pleural effusions, interstitial lung disease, pneumonitis, pulmonary hypertension, shrinking lung syndrome, and alveolar hemorrhage.
- The central nervous system can be involved in lupus with a broad array of manifestations including cognitive dysfunction, "brain fog," psychosis, seizures, headache, neuropathies, and occasionally myelitis and aseptic meningitis.
- Hematologic abnormalities are frequently encountered in SLE and can be seen in any of the three blood cell lines.[46]

Ocular Systemic Lupus Erythematosus

Although not necessarily a primary target of immune-mediated damage in SLE, the eye can be affected in a variety of ways. In a recent series of 161 SLE patients enrolled at a tertiary referral center, 31.1% had at least one ocular manifestation.[47] SLE can involve any ocular structure including the eyelid, ocular adnexa, sclera, cornea, uvea, retina, and optic nerve. Ocular manifestations of SLE often correlate to systemic disease activity and tend to improve with treatment of the underlying SLE.

KCS is the most common ocular manifestation of SLE, occurring in approximately 25% to 35% of patients, often as part of a secondary Sjogren syndrome.[23,39] After KCS, retinal involvement in the form of lupus retinopathy is the second most common ocular manifestation of SLE, with a reported incidence between 3.3% and 28%.[48] Fortunately, the incidence of posterior segment disease may be declining with improved systemic disease control in the era of modern treatment options.[47] The classic finding of SLE retinopathy is the cotton wool spot, an ischemic infarct in the retinal nerve fiber

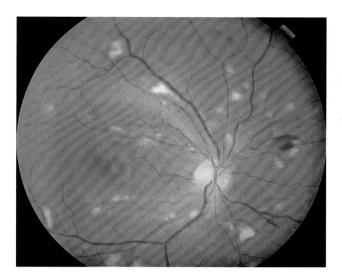

FIGURE 11.11 Right fundus of a 25-year-old woman with an acute exacerbation of systemic lupus erythematosus shows cotton wool spots and retinal hemorrhages. (Credit: From Gold DH, Weingeist TA. *Color Atlas of the Eye in Systemic Disease.* Baltimore, MA: Lippincott Williams & Wilkins; 2001.)

layer, which may result from immune complex deposition or other mechanism(s) contributing to microangiopathy. There are often multiple in number and accumulated in the posterior pole, sometimes in a "Purtscher-like" distribution around the optic nerve head, with or without associated intraretinal or retinal nerve fiber layer hemorrhages (FIGURE 11.11).

Although, as noted, retinal hemorrhages may be present, cotton wool spots in the absence of other retinal findings should always bring SLE to mind, even though this finding is not pathognomonic for lupus. Severe cases (associated with more severe systemic disease activity) may also feature macular edema and optic disc edema with risk for optic atrophy.[49] A second form of SLE retinopathy involves retinal vascular disease, either vascular occlusions (arteriolar and/or venular) or (less commonly) a primary vasculitis. The pathophysiology of retinal vascular disease in SLE is unclear and considered complex, with several contributing mechanisms hypothesized, including immune-complex deposition, the presence of antiphospholipid antibodies, accelerated atherosclerosis in SLE patients, and contributions from systemic SLE drug therapy.[50] Retinal vascular disease occurs most commonly in the setting of systemic disease activity with central nervous involvement. Lupus choroidopathy, manifested by areas of serous or exudative retinal detachment, detachment of the retinal pigment epithelium, or retinal pigment epitheliopathy can occur independently of or with lupus retinopathy.

The periocular skin can be involved in lupus, especially in discoid lupus erythematosus, presenting with symmetrical erythema and edema of the outer third of the lower eyelids and lesions that tend to heal with scarring, atrophy, and loss of eyelashes. SLE is a rare cause of anterior uveitis and can also be associated with posterior uveitis.[51]

In addition to ocular complications from SLE itself, a common reason for patients with SLE to seek ocular evaluation is for monitoring of potential ocular side effects of drugs used to treat SLE, namely steroids and antimalarials. Patients managed on HCQ are at risk for maculopathy, which can result in permanent, bilateral, paracentral vision loss if not detected early (FIGURE 11.12). At recommended (low-risk) doses of HCQ, maculopathy risk is <1% at 5 years and <2% at 10 years but rises to 20% or more after 20 years of drug use. A number of risk factors substantially increase the likelihood of maculopathy, including daily HCQ doses >5 mg/kg, cumulative doses >1000 g, longer duration of drug use, renal disease, pre-existing macular disease, and concomitant use of tamoxifen.[52] HCQ retinal toxicity presents as a pathognomonic "Bull's eye" maculopathy with concentric degeneration of the perifoveal photoreceptors, best-visualized in its early stages using spectral-domain optical coherence tomography. Fundus examination alone is insufficient for early detection. It is important to recognize that Asian patients may show areas of extrafoveal rather than perifoveal degeneration. In 2016,

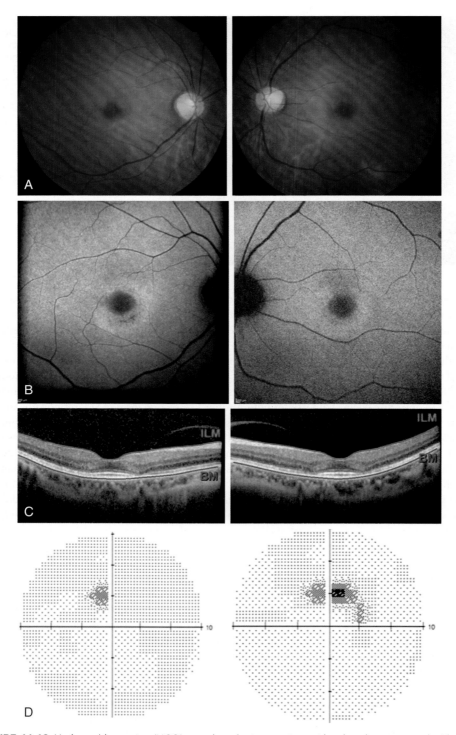

FIGURE 11.12 Hydroxychloroquine (HCQ) maculopathy in a patient with scleroderma treated with high-dose HCQ (11 mg/kg/day). A, Fundus photos demonstrate perifoveal arcuate retinal depigmentation most prominent at the inferior foveas. B, Autofluorescence imaging shows circinate hyperautofluorescence of damaged perifoveal retinae. C, Optical coherence tomography imaging shows perifoveal thinning with loss of the outer retinal layers. D, Visual field testing (HVF 10-2) shows superior paracentral scotomas consistent with retinal damage. (Image credit: Dr. Tak-Yin Chau, OD (VA Boston Healthcare System).)

TABLE 11.3	Screening for the Detection of Chloroquine and Hydroxychloroquine Retinopathy: 2016 American Academy of Ophthalmology Recommendations
Frequency	• Baseline examination within 1 yr of drug initiation • Annual screening beginning after 5 yr of drug use, in the absence of maculopathy and major risk factors • More frequent screening in the presence of major risk factors
Recommended testing	**Primary tests** • Automated visual fields: 10-2 or 24-2 (for Asian race) • Spectral domain optical coherence tomography **Adjunctive testing when available** • Multifocal electroretinography • Fundus autofluorescence **Insufficient screening tests** • Fundus examination • Time-domain optical coherence tomography • Fluorescein angiography • Full-field electroretinography • Electrooculogram • Amsler grid • Color vision testing

Marmor MF, Kellner U, Lai TY, Melles RB, Mieler WF. Recommendations on screening for chloroquine and hydroxychloroquine retinopathy (2016 revision). *Ophthalmology*. 2016;123(6):1386-1394.

the American Academy of Ophthalmology (AAO) released updated screening recommendations for HCQ maculopathy (**TABLE 11.3**).[52] If HCQ maculopathy is detected, the drug should be stopped to prevent progressive damage, though some patients will continue to progress and remain at risk for vision loss for several years, due to slow clearance of the drug from the body.[53] Serial eye examination should continue every 3 months until stability is reached.

Systemic Lupus Erythematosus Diagnosis

Given the wide array of symptoms, signs, and laboratory findings with which SLE can present, the diagnosis can be challenging. In addition to a detailed clinical history, physical examination, and review of systems, laboratory tests help in diagnosis of SLE. Basic laboratory tests should be obtained including complete blood count (CBC) to evaluate for cytopenias; complete metabolic panel (CMP) to assess renal and hepatic function; and urinalysis (UA) to evaluate for proteinuria, cellular casts, and hematuria. In addition to routine blood work, other laboratory tests that can support the diagnosis of SLE include ANA and, if positive, other specific autoantibodies such as anti-dsDNA, anti-Smith, antiphospholipid antibodies, and anti-RNP. Additionally, spot urine protein-to-creatinine ratio should be obtained to quantify proteinuria and assess severity of glomerular disease, and complement levels C3 and C4 checked to evaluate for hypocomplementemia, which can all be seen in SLE. Additional tests such as imaging or biopsy of a potentially involved organ may also be necessary to help distinguish SLE from another process. There is no pathognomonic feature, test, or diagnostic criteria for SLE, and therefore clinicians often use SLE classification criteria, designed for inclusion in research studies, to guide diagnosis. The 2019 European League Against Rheumatism (EULAR)/American College of Rheumatology (ACR) classification criteria for SLE requires the presence of a positive ANA as an entry criterion; additive criteria consist of seven clinical (ie, constitutional, hematologic, neuropsychiatric, mucocutaneous, serosal, musculoskeletal, renal) and three immunologic (ie, antiphospholipid antibodies, complement proteins, SLE-specific antibodies) categories, each of which are weighed from 2 to 10. A classification of SLE is given with a score of 10 or more points. SLE can mimic other autoimmune, infectious, and malignant conditions, and the diagnosis requires consideration and exclusion of alternative diagnoses.[46]

Systemic Lupus Erythematosus Treatment

The goals of treatment in SLE are to achieve the lowest possible disease activity, prevent organ damage, minimize drug toxicity, improve quality of life, and avoid long-term complications. Essentially any new symptom or sign should be considered as potentially related to underlying SLE and worked up with additional studies accordingly (imaging, biopsy, etc.). An important component of management is monitoring for disease activity with routine labs including CBC, CMP, UA, spot urine protein:creatinine, dsDNA titers (which can often fluctuate with disease activity), and complement levels C3 and C4 which, when low, can indicate active lupus. Generally speaking, there is no utility in repeating or trending ANAs or other specific antibodies, aside from the anti-dsDNA antibodies. Treatment of SLE is tailored to the individual, based on disease activity, disease severity, patient preference, and comorbidities. The comprehensive management of SLE includes nonpharmacologic measures such as sun protection in the form of daily sunscreen and avoidance of direct sun and UV light; exercise; smoking cessation; appropriate immunizations; and monitoring for and treatment of comorbid conditions such as increased atherosclerosis risk, pulmonary hypertension, antiphospholipid antibody syndrome, osteopenia, and depression. Given the epidemiology of SLE, affecting predominantly young women, birth control and pregnancy planning is another important component of SLE management. Women should be counseled to avoid pregnancy during active disease due to the high risk of miscarriage and exacerbation of SLE. Furthermore, many of the pharmacologic therapies used in SLE are not safe in pregnancy, and medication changes should be made to avoid high-risk medication use during pregnancy whenever possible. With regard to pharmacologic therapy, generally speaking, all patients with SLE and any degree of disease activity should be treated with an antimalarial such as HCQ, which can help relieve constitutional symptoms, musculoskeletal manifestations, and skin and mucosal disease. Additional pharmacologic therapy depends on the severity of disease and combination of manifestations. Patients with moderate SLE involvement with significant but nonorgan threatening disease, such as constitutional, cutaneous, musculoskeletal, and hematologic involvement, can be managed with HCQ and low-dose prednisone and potentially a steroid-sparing immunosuppressive agent such as azathioprine or methotrexate. With more severe or organ-threatening manifestations such as renal or central nervous system involvement, the approach to treatment often starts with induction therapy with more intense immunosuppression such as high-dose IV glucocorticoids ("pulse" methylprednisolone) to rapidly reduce inflammation, and initiation of another steroid-sparing immunosuppressive agent such as mycophenolate, azathioprine, cyclophosphamide, or rituximab (a biologic).[54]

SJOGREN SYNDROME

Sjogren syndrome (SS) is a chronic autoimmune inflammatory disorder that affects the exocrine glands of mucus membranes and other organs. It is characterized by lacrimal and salivary gland dysfunction that results from lymphocytic infiltration and results in the sicca complex. KCS refers to dryness of the cornea and conjunctiva (dry eyes) and xerostomia refers to subjective symptoms of dry mouth, both of which comprise the sicca complex. It can exist as a primary syndrome or secondary to another autoimmune disease, such as SLE, rheumatoid arthritis, scleroderma, or polymyositis.[55] SS is considered the second most common autoimmune disease after rheumatoid arthritis, with a prevalence estimated at 1%, and incidence of 7 per 100,000 in the United States.[51] It is more common in women with a female to male ratio of 9:1, and a peak incidence in the fifth and sixth decades of life.[51,55]

Signs and Symptoms of Sjogren Syndrome

The most common clinical presentation (80% of patients) includes the sicca syndrome (dry mouth and dry eyes).[56] Often, optometrists and ophthalmologists are the initial providers to see these patients and are in a unique position to make an early diagnosis. The usual clinical presentation is dry eyes followed by dry mouth. Patients may report a gritty, sand-like feeling in the eyes, and may notice daily or nocturnal oral dryness, finding themselves constantly drinking water, or waking up at night to do so. Complications of dry eye are discussed below. Oral complications include oral sores, difficulty chewing/swallowing dry foods, dental caries, chronic oral candida infection, salivary gland swelling, and recurrent sialadenitis (bacterial infection of the salivary glands).

SS can affect virtually any organ, some of the more common extraglandular features of SS include inflammatory joint and muscle pain, chronic fatigue, swollen salivary glands, gastrointestinal tract involvement (reflux, difficulty swallowing, chronic constipation), pulmonary complications (chronic cough, interstitial lung disease), neuropathies, or lab abnormalities (anemia, leukopenia, lymphopenia). Patients with SS are at a higher risk of developing lymphomas and should undergo regular screening.

Ocular Sjogren Syndrome

KCS, or dry eye, is the most common manifestation of SS, but SS can also lead to other vision-threatening complications including corneal melts, uveitis, scleritis, optic neuritis, and vision loss.[51] Dry eye disease is usually symptomatic, although more than 40% of patients with objective eye disease can be asymptomatic.[37] Common symptoms of dry eye include a burning sensation, gritty sensation, itching, redness, mucus exudate, tearing, itching, and photophobia.[51] Patients may experience transient episodes of blurred vision that improve with resting or blinking the eyes. As the disease progresses, patients may report a significantly reduced quality of life.

SS causes dry eye due to autoimmune destruction of the lacrimal glands, leading to aqueous-deficient dry eye, which is exacerbated by concurrent meibomian gland dysfunction. The tear film functions to maintain ocular surface health by maintaining clear vision and serving as a protective barrier and consists of three layers: the aqueous, lipid, and mucin layers. Abnormalities in any layer can lead to unstable tear film and dry eye disease (**FIGURE 11.13**).[51] Dry eye disease can be separated into two major categories: aqueous-deficient (characterized by reduced tear production, primarily related to lacrimal gland dysfunction and secondarily to meibomian gland dysfunction) and evaporative dry eye disease (related to meibomian gland dysfunction/blepharitis and changes in the lipid component of tears, which result in faster aqueous tear evaporation).[57] Untreated dry eye disease can lead to distortion of patient's vision, decreased quality of life from bothersome symptoms, and increased risk for serious ocular disease such as bacterial and fungal ocular infections, corneal ulcers, corneal melting/ulceration, and endophthalmitis.[51] Another disabling complication is filamentary keratitis, which involves strands of mucous and debris from epithelial cells adhering to the corneal surface. Blinking leads to disruption of these filaments which causes pain, foreign body sensation, photophobia, and decreased vision.[51] Routine contact lenses should be used with caution in patients with SS, as they are at higher risk for worsening symptoms due to the irregular ocular surface.[51] Management of dry eye syndrome in SS is discussed below.

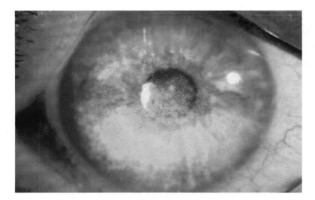

FIGURE 11.13 Severe superficial punctate epitheliopathy is present centrally and inferiorly in this patient with severe dry eye syndrome. Inferiorly the keratopathy is confluent. (From Rapuano CJ. *Wills Eye Institute – Cornea.* 2nd ed. Philadelphia, PA: Wolters Kluwer; 2011.)

Sjogren Syndrome Diagnosis

The diagnosis of SS can be challenging given that extraglandular features of SS often overlap with other autoimmune conditions, and it may be difficult to distinguish primary from secondary SS. The goal in the diagnostic evaluation is to document objective evidence of dry eyes and dry mouth/salivary gland involvement and to prove autoimmunity. The serologic tests that are commonly associated with SS include positive anti-SSA (anti-Ro), anti-SSA/SSB (anti-La), or positive rheumatoid factor (RF) plus positive ANA.

Symptomatic dry eye can be assessed by a positive response to one of the following three questions:

1. Have you had daily, persistent, troublesome dry eyes for >3 months?
2. Do you have a recurrent sensation of sand or gravel in the eyes?
3. Do you use tear substitutes >3 times per day?[57]

Schirmer test is an objective measurement of tear production (**FIGURE 11.14**). It is performed by placing a paper test strip into the lower portion of a patient's eyelid, then measuring the length of moistened paper after 5 minutes have elapsed. A result less than or equal to 10 mm/5 min is abnormal, and a result less than or equal to 5 mm/5 min in each eye is highly suggestive of KCS. Alternative screening for dry eyes includes vital dye staining of the ocular surface with either fluorescein-sodium, lissamine green, or rose Bengal stains.[56] Sialometry is an objective measurement of saliva production. After a 60-minute fast, the patient is asked to expectorate into a container for 15 minutes. This amount is calculated as a salivary flow rate, with a normal rate 0.3 to 0.5 mL/min and a flow rate less than 0.1 mL/min providing objective evidence of dry mouth. A nuclear medicine salivary scan can

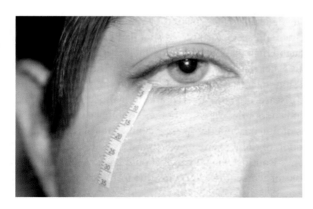

FIGURE 11.14 Schirmer strip testing objectively assesses for dry eye syndrome. (From Bennett ES. *Clinical Manual of Contact Lenses.* 5th ed. Philadelphia, PA: Wolters Kluwer; 2019.)

also be used to document objective evidence of abnormal salivary gland function. It is important to perform these tests only after the patient has stopped all anticholinergic medications. Labial minor salivary gland biopsy is most useful in seronegative patients or those who may have more than one explanation for xerostomia (ie, medications). A report of focal lymphocytic sialadenitis with a focus score of at least 1/4 mm^2 is diagnostic of Sjogren syndrome. It is important to consider other causes of sicca symptoms, most importantly medication-related dryness, as well as anxiety/depression, viral infections, mouth breathing, sarcoidosis, systemic lupus, and rheumatoid arthritis.

Sjogren Syndrome Treatment

There is no cure for SS. The goal of therapy includes amelioration of sicca symptoms, prevention of complications, and treatment of extraglandular manifestations. A comprehensive dry eye examination should be performed by a cornea specialist or optometrist specializing in dry eye mangement, which involves assessment of tear production, tear film stability, tear osmolarity, lid margin disease, and ocular surface staining for damage.[56] Therapy is based on the severity of the dry eye disease and the patient response to therapy. Patients with mild symptoms can be managed with modification of their environment and activities, by avoiding systemic medications that cause reduced tear secretion. The first-line therapy for dry eye involves use of "artificial tears," which add volume to the tear lake and increase the residence time of the tear supplement on the ocular surface.[37] There are several commercially available products that differ in their composition. These products include the addition of electrolytes (to help prevent ocular surface damage), hypotonic solutions (given hyperosmotic tear film is pro-inflammatory), viscous agents (to increase residence time of tear supplement), and lipid-like substances (to mimic lipid component of tears). Some of these additives may cause blurred vision, depending on the viscosity of the lubricant. Ocular ointments are another option, typically used before bedtime. Among the wide variety of supplements, none is clearly superior. It is recommended that, when supplements are used more than 4 to 6 times daily, patients should use preservative-free formulations due to the toxicity associated with frequent use of preservatives.[37] Other treatment considerations include topical corticosteroids, topical cyclosporine, omega-3 essential fatty acids, punctal occlusion of the tear duct, topical autologous serum, and therapeutic contact lenses.[37] Off-label use of the oral secretagogues for dry eye disease has shown benefit in some reported cases.[37]

Dental health is also important given the abnormal saliva production, and patients should have regular dental care to prevent caries. Dry mouth symptoms can be treated with artificial saliva or agents that stimulate salivary flow (sugar-free lozenges or oral secretagogues such as pilocarpine or cevimeline).

Treatment of systemic manifestations (musculoskeletal symptoms, fatigue, other extraglandular symptoms) may involve the use of HCQ as first-line therapy followed by methotrexate, and in some cases, short courses of low-dose corticosteroids.[56] Treatment strategies for other organ-specific disease manifestations are considered in the context of the severity of involvement and the individual patient's preferences. As discussed in the section on management of SLE, patients with rheumatic disease managed on HCQ should undergo regular screening with an eye care specialist to monitor for HCQ maculopathy.

SARCOIDOSIS

Sarcoidosis is a systemic and clinically heterogeneous disorder that is characterized by the development and accumulation of noncaseating granulomas in any organ system. The etiology is unclear, but environmental, genetic, and infectious causes have been suggested. While any organ system can be involved, the lungs are involved in 90% of cases.[58] Lymph node involvement is common as well, especially in the hilar regions of the lungs. Due to the clinical heterogeneity and variation in diagnostic criteria internationally, the worldwide prevalence and incidence of sarcoidosis have been difficult to estimate. The highest annual incidence has been observed in northern European countries (5-40 cases per 100,000), with lower incidence in Japan. The incidence may vary between races, with a higher annual incidence (more than three times) in black than in white Americans.[58,59] The disease is more acute and severe in black patients, while asymptomatic and chronic disease is more frequent in white patients.[60] Sarcoidosis affects slightly more women than men and women are more likely to have ocular and neurologic manifestations. Sarcoidosis affects people of any age, with median age of onset around 40 years.[60]

Signs and Symptoms of Sarcoidosis

Patients may be asymptomatic or present with a wide range of nonspecific symptoms, as sarcoidosis can affect every organ system. Sarcoidosis often first comes to attention when abnormalities are detected on a chest radiograph that may be performed for another indication. The most common manifestations are pulmonary (eg, cough, shortness of breath, or incidentally found hilar lymphadenopathy on chest imaging), and while isolated pulmonary sarcoidosis can occur, pulmonary disease is often accompanied by extrapulmonary involvement. Common extrapulmonary manifestations include joints (arthritis), eyes (uveitis, retinal vasculitis, and orbital disease), liver (abnormal liver function tests), lymph nodes (lymphadenopathy, especially in the hilar region), cardiac (conduction abnormalities, arrhythmias, heart failure), and skin (sarcoid granulomas, erythema nodosum, and scar sarcoidosis [tattoos]). Additional symptoms include fatigue, night sweats, weight loss, small fiber neuropathy, and cognitive dysfunction. Lofgren syndrome, an acute presentation consisting of arthritis, erythema nodosum, and bilateral hilar lymphadenopathy, occurs in 9%–34% of patients. Heerfordt syndrome (also called uveoparotid fever) represents 5% of acute presentations and includes uveitis, fever, and swelling of the parotid glands that can lead to compression of CN VII within the parotid bed and a facial nerve palsy.

Ocular Sarcoidosis

Ocular disease may be the initial manifestation of sarcoidosis in as many as 30% of cases[61] and may progress to severe vision impairment or blindness. The most common ocular symptom is dry eye. Other ocular complications in sarcoid most commonly include granulomatous anterior uveitis (30%-70%), followed by conjunctival nodule formation (40%), followed by posterior, intermediate, or panuveitis, though any part of the eye, orbit, and adnexa can be involved.[60,62,63]

Granulomatous conjunctival nodules are common in sarcoidosis but may be asymptomatic and most typically involve the palpebral conjunctiva, but the bulbar conjunctiva can also be involved (FIGURE 11.15).[61]

Scleritis due to sarcoidosis is possible, but uncommon. Though also relatively uncommon, sarcoidosis should be included in the differential diagnosis for inflammatory orbital lesions, especially with lacrimal gland involvement (dacryoadenitis) (FIGURE 11.16). CT imaging in sarcoidosis dacryoadenitis shows diffuse enlargement of the gland with homogenous enhancement. Orbital fat, extraocular muscles, and the optic nerve sheath can also be involved. Extensive orbital disease may lead to eyelid/periorbital edema, ptosis, proptosis, globe displacement, ophthalmoplegia, optic nerve dysfunction, and symptoms of diplopia, reduced vision, or severe dry eye.[60,61] Sarcoid induced inflammatory myositis may resemble Graves ophthalmopathy. These types of manifestations respond well to topical therapy.

Sarcoidosis-associated uveitis is the most frequently encountered ocular manifestation and is usually anterior, bilateral, chronic, and granulomatous. It not only presents with pain, photophobia, lacrimation, blurred vision, or redness but can also be asymptomatic, and patients may develop permanent ocular damage before sarcoidosis is diagnosed.[60] While anterior uveitis associated with

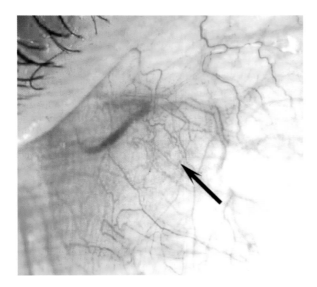

FIGURE 11.15 One of many bilateral yellow pearly granulomas (black arrow) of the bulbar conjunctiva presenting in a 55-year-old, asymptomatic Caucasian woman, later proven to have sarcoidosis. (Courtesy Dr. Thomas Freddo.)

sarcoidosis is always due to a granulomatous disease process, it is important to note that the presentation may actually be more consistent with so-called "nongranulomatous" anterior uveitis in some cases (eg, early on in the disease course, with less severe disease, or with successful treatment), lacking typical granulomatous signs; in fact, anterior chamber cells and flare may be the only signs.[61] As with any chronic anterior uveitis, anterior and posterior synechia may result in a distorted iris and pupil, with risk for intraocular pressure elevation. Granulomatous uveitis occurs in 80% of cases, with typical granulomatous signs including large, "mutton-fat" keratic precipitates, iris or trabecular meshwork nodules, or choroidal granuloma on posterior examination[61] (**FIGURE 11.17**). Granulomatous and severe cases of chronic uveitis carry risk for secondary cataract, glaucoma, macular edema, and keratopathy.[60] With intermediate, posterior, or panuveitis, ocular fundus examination can show

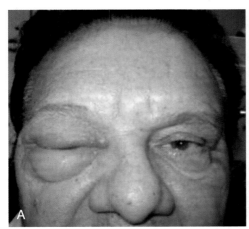
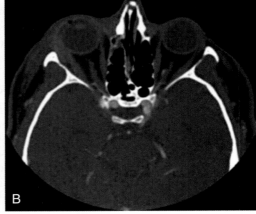

FIGURE 11.16 Sarcoidosis dacryoadenitis of the right orbit in a 69-year-old man with inactive pulmonary sarcoidosis and remote history of recurrent bilateral anterior uveitis related to sarcoidosis. A, Periorbital soft tissue edema related to sarcoid dacryoadenitis. B, Noncontrast orbital CT showing homogenous enlargement of the right lacrimal gland with slight enhancement. (Image credit: Rachel Druckenbrod, OD (VA Boston Healthcare System), with permission from the patient.)

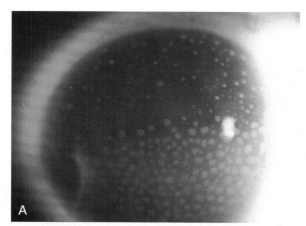

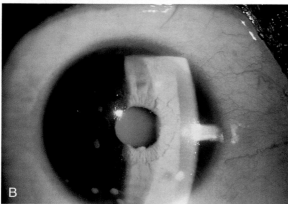

FIGURE 11.17 A, There are large, granulomatous-appearing (mutton-fat) keratic preciptates in this patient with sarcoidosis. B, Busacca nodules in the iris stroma and Koeppe nodules along the iris border are typically associated with diseases causing granulomatous uveitis, such as sarcoidosis. There are Koeppe nodules along the iris border at the 1, 4, and 8 o'clock positions in this patient. (Credit: From Tasman W, Jaeger E. *The Wills Eye Hospital Atlas of Clinical Ophthalmology.* 2nd ed. Philadelphia, PA: Lippincott Williams & Wilkins; 2001.)

various degrees of vitritis, retinal periphlebitis (usually midperipheral), multifocal chorioretinitis, and unifocal or multifocal choroidal granuloma formation.[61,62] Vasculitis in sarcoidosis is generally not associated with significant vascular occlusion. Retinal vasculitis can be diagnosed based on perivascular sheathing along a vessel seen on fundoscopic examination, with intraretinal hemorrhages and fluorescein angiography indicating increased vascular permeability.[23] In addition to vitritis and chorioretinitis, macular edema is a common cause for vision loss in sarcoidosis. Depending on the extent and severity of inflammation, sarcoidosis uveitis may be treated with one or a combination of therapies including topical steroids and cycloplegics, ocular and periocular corticosteroid injections or implants, and systemic agents including steroids, immunosuppressants (eg, methotrexate and azathioprine), or biologics (specifically the tumor necrosis factor alpha [TNF-α] inhibitors).

Posterior segment involvement in sarcoidosis is considered a risk factor for neuro-ophthalmological sarcoidosis. Cranial neuropathy from granulomatous infiltration involving the optic nerve or the facial nerve is the most common manifestation of neurosarcoidosis.[61] Sarcoidosis optic neuropathy may result from direct optic nerve infiltration with visible optic nerve head granuloma, optic sheath granuloma, optic neuritis/edema, or optic atrophy. Optic neuropathy may also result secondarily from raised intracranial pressure or severe posterior uveitis.[23] Involvement of the optic nerve is an indication for systemic therapy. Pupillary abnormalities, visual field loss, nystagmus, or other disorders of eye movements are also possible with central nervous system sarcoidosis.

Interestingly, the classic systemic vasculitides are rarely associated with retinal vasculitis.

TABLE 11.4	Key Findings on Clinical Evaluation and Diagnostic Testing in Inflammatory Joint Disease	
Disease	**Usual Differentiating Clinical Features**	**Key Lab/Imaging Findings**
Ankylosing spondylitis	Family history, symmetric disease	HLA-B27-positive
Psoriatic arthritis	Personal history of psoriasis or family history of psoriatic arthritis	Asymmetric changes in the sacroiliac joints
Reactive arthritis	History of recent infection, need to rule out active infection	Unilateral sacroiliac joint disease
IBD-associated arthritis	History of IBD	Asymmetric changes in the sacroiliac joints
Undifferentiated spondyloarthropathy	None specific other than low back pain and stiffness, does not fit any other category	Variable

with long-standing axial SpA is the development of syndesmophytes, which occur with ossification of intervertebral ligaments and, in the most severe form, convert the entire vertebral column into a rigid "bamboo spine," so termed because of the radiographic appearance resembling a stalk of bamboo. Other imaging findings that suggest SpA but are not specific include erosive joint disease and enthesitis. The radiographic changes that can develop in PsA are relatively a more specific pattern, characterized by concurrent erosive changes and new bone formation in the same joint and a propensity for involvement in the distal interphalangeal (DIP) joints.[70]

Spondyloarthritis Treatment

The goal of treatment for axial and peripheral SpA are to relieve symptoms, maintain functional capacity, and prevent complications of musculoskeletal and extraarticular manifestations of disease. Patients should be followed regularly for monitoring of disease activity as well as medication safety. An important component of treatment is nonpharmacological, including patient education, physical therapy and exercise, and smoking cessation. The pharmacologic treatment of axial and peripheral SpA includes NSAIDs, conventional (nonbiologic) disease-modifying antirheumatic drugs (DMARDs), and biologic DMARDs. The initial pharmacologic therapy for most patients with symptomatic SpA is NSAID therapy. Many patients will have symptom control with maximum dose NSAID monotherapy. Each NSAID (eg, naproxen, celecoxib, ibuprofen, etc.) should be assessed for efficacy for 2 to 4 weeks before switching to a different NSAID. If effective, a given NSAID should be used as needed per symptoms. In patients with an inadequate response to trial of at least two NSAIDs at maximum dose for several weeks, the next steps depend on whether the disease is predominantly axial or peripheral. For axial SpA, the next step after failure of NSAIDs is a TNF-α inhibitor, such as adalimumab, infliximab, etanercept, certolizumab, or golimumab, or an IL-17 inhibitor such as secukinumab. If the initial TNF-α inhibitor yields adequate response, the next step is a switch to a second TNF-α inhibitor or to IL-17 inhibitor. Of note, patients with underlying IBD/enteropathic arthritis should be managed preferentially with TNF-α inhibitor given lack of efficacy of IL-17 inhibitors in IBD.[70] In patients with peripheral SpA who do not respond to an adequate NSAID trial, the next step is a nonbiologic DMARD such as sulfasalazine, methotrexate, or leflunomide. If peripheral SpA is resistant to nonbiologic DMARD, a biologic DMARD such as TNF-α inhibitor should be used.[70]

OSTEOARTHRITIS

Osteoarthritis (OA) is the most common form of arthritis in the United States and worldwide.[71,72] Traditionally, it was believed to be a noninflammatory form of arthritis; however, more recent studies have demonstrated subclinical inflammation in osteoarthritic joints. The disease usually affects individuals over the age of 40 with an increasing incidence in older ages. However, it can affect adults in almost all age groups. Obesity is a risk factor in OA of weight-bearing joints (such as knees and hips). Along with the weight-bearing joints, DIP joints of the fingers and the spine are commonly affected (FIGURE 11.22). Distal digital joint involvement is often noted due to the presence of osteophytes (bony nodules) on examination; osteophytes are also seen with x-ray imaging. Previous trauma to joints also predisposes to the development of OA, which may be more severe or develop earlier than atraumatic joint disease. OA, especially involvement of the hand joints, can be familial.

Signs and Symptoms of Osteoarthritis

As a (primarily) noninflammatory arthritis, there are no associated ocular or other organ system manifestations of OA. Patients present with pain and occasionally bony changes of the joints. Joint effusions can develop with more severe joint involvement, often in the knees. Progressive joint degeneration leads to functional impairment due to loss of range of motion and pain. Classically, the pain is worse with activity and better with rest. OA is usually least symptomatic in the morning upon awakening and worse as the day progresses. The exact mechanism of pain in OA is not well understood, and the joint structures that trigger pain symptoms (bone, bursa, tendon, etc.) likely vary among patients. Imaging and clinical examination findings do not always correlate with the degree of pain that patients report.[71]

Osteoarthritis Diagnosis

The diagnosis is made with a thorough history and joint examination; when inflammatory findings or constitutional symptoms are present, another etiology for joint symptoms should be considered (such as rheumatoid arthritis or other immune or infectious conditions). X-ray imaging can

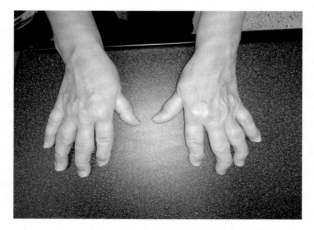

FIGURE 11.22 Osteoarthritis commonly involves the distal, small joints of the hands, seen here with nodules in the distal interphalangeal (DIP) joints of both hands (Heberden nodes), which are due to bony overgrowth. (Image credit Shiv Sehra, MD.)

be helpful in differentiating OA from other causes of joint pain and diminished range of motion. Affected joints reveal degenerative changes, sclerosis of articular surfaces, and osteophyte formation, findings which help confirm the diagnosis. In contrast to the bone growth of osteoarthritic osteophytes, joint imaging in rheumatoid arthritis reveals periarticular erosions and osteoporosis. In the distal upper extremities, OA usually involves finger DIP joints while RA is seen more commonly in the MCP joints, along with the presence of inflammation and deformity in more advanced disease. There is no ocular involvement in OA.

Osteoarthritis Treatment

Treatment is geared toward maintaining function, flexibility, and muscle strength. Advice to stay active and perform home exercises is simple, but sound guidance; if needed, referral for physical therapy can be helpful for patients to get started and to assist with disease exacerbations or recovery after injury or a period of immobility. Weight loss (for overweight and obese individuals) may slow down the progression of the disease in the large weight-bearing joints (hips, knees) and can improve symptoms and function. Pain relief with acetaminophen and NSAIDs is the mainstay of treatment, though these therapies are often not ideal. Some patients experience limited benefit from acetaminophen and the total daily dose must be monitored to avoid toxicity (with hepatic failure in overdose). In older patients who are most often affected by OA pain, NSAIDs carry a higher risk of gastrointestinal toxicity. The topical NSAID diclofenac is available, and for some patients it offers benefit; skin reactions are the most common adverse effect.[73] However, topical use is not practical for hips or across multiple joints. Local therapies that are more invasive include intra-articular injections of corticosteroids and hyaluronic acid derivatives, though there is debate on the benefit of these treatments. Joint replacement, for hips and knees most often, is the last resort in treatment of the disease. When successful, patients experience improvement in pain and function, though range of motion may not return to the pre-arthritis baseline.

SYSTEMIC SCLEROSIS

Systemic sclerosis (SSc) is a multiorgan disorder of unclear etiology which is characterized by progressive fibrosis of the skin and other organ systems, along with vascular dysfunction. Scleroderma, the term applied when disease is limited to the skin, is derived from the Greek words sclerosis (hardening) and derma (skin). When the disease involves additional organ systems, it is referred to as SSc. There are two forms of systemic sclerosis: limited SSc and diffuse SSc. The signs and symptoms for each are discussed separately below.

Limited Systemic Sclerosis: Signs and Symptoms

In limited systemic sclerosis, the dermatological findings include skin fibrosis limited to the regions distal to the elbows and the knees, though it may sometimes involve the face. Skin fibrosis in the digits may restrict flexion, causing sclerodactyly. The occurrence of Raynaud phenomenon is extremely common (99%) in limited SSc, the criteria for which includes color change in the digits from blue to white in the cold (due to vasoconstriction), followed by return of red coloration upon rewarming. While typically fully reversible with warming, severe complications in Raynaud phenomenon such as skin ulcers and digital ischemia can result. Skin telangiectasias (small visible dilated capillaries in the skin) are common. Dystrophic calcification may also occur, with deposition of subcutaneous calcium crystals that grow into nodules (known as calcinosis) (**FIGURE 11.23**).[74]

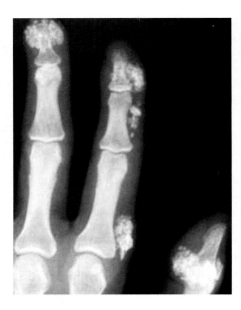

FIGURE 11.23 Close-up hand roentgenogram of a 46-year-old woman with limited cutaneous systemic sclerosis. Note extensive subcutaneous calcinosis. (Reprinted from Koopman WJ. *Arthritis and Allied Conditions*. 15th ed. Philadelphia, PA: Wolters Kluwer; 2004.)

Involvement of other organs is also typical in limited SSc. Gastroesophageal reflux and esophageal dysmotility are present in 67% of patients, with dysphagia impacting eating and digestion. Pulmonary fibrosis is seen in 37% of affected patients.[74] Pulmonary hypertension is a complication of advanced disease, with high levels of morbidity and mortality; 31% of patients are affected. The ANA titer is usually highly positive (>90%) and anticentromere antibodies are usually positive in a high titer as well. The older acronym CREST syndrome bears mention, as it remains in clinical use in many settings as a mnemonic for the usual manifestations of calcinosis, Raynaud phenomenon, esophageal dysmotility, sclerodactyly, and telangiectasias.

Ocular involvement in SSc is rare (for both limited and diffuse forms), and if the eyes are involved, it is usually in the form of inflammatory eye disease such as scleritis and uveitis.

Diffuse Systemic Sclerosis: Signs and Symptoms

In diffuse systemic sclerosis, the dermal thickening extends proximal to the elbows and knees and may involve the chest, back, and the trunk. Raynaud phenomenon is also very common (97%); joint involvement is more common (98%) as compared to limited disease (78%), while rates of esophageal dysmotility are similar (67%).[74] Sclerosis of other organ systems is also common. Renal involvement, rare in the limited form of SSc, occurs more often in diffuse disease, with scleroderma renal crisis occurring in 17% of patients.[74] Severe hypertension and progressive renal failure develop, requiring prompt management to avoid serious complications. Testing for ANA is usually positive (>90%) in a nucleolar pattern. Patients may have positive anti-Scl70 antibodies (associated with higher incidence of interstitial lung disease) or positive anti-RNA Pol III antibodies (associated with higher incidence of scleroderma renal crisis).

Skin findings are an almost universal feature, though the diagnosis can occasionally be made without sclerosis of the skin. The skin thickening begins distally—starting from the finger tips and the toes and progressing proximally (**FIGURE 11.24**). If the skin is thickened proximally, but not distally, then another diagnosis should be sought. As noted above, while Raynaud phenomenon is an almost universal feature, this phenomenon alone is not diagnostic as it can be seen in other autoimmune conditions, as well as in isolation as Raynaud syndrome.

12 Neurology

Vanessa S. Cooper, Jeffrey J. Dewey, and
Rachel C. Druckenbrod

LEARNING OBJECTIVES

The visual system is closely linked to the central nervous system. Indeed, the optic disc is the only directly visible extension of the central nervous system. Numerous neurologic conditions may present with visual symptoms, and referrals to neurologic care from optometry clinics are quite common. Moreover, visual symptoms can be the sole manifestations of neurologic pathology or harbingers of more widespread dysfunction which may progress acutely with devastating consequences. Thus, a firm grasp on the aspects of neurologic disease relevant to the visual system is a necessity for the practicing optometrist.

KEY CONCEPTS

Cerebrovascular disease
Ocular vascular disease
    Retinal artery occlusion
    Ischemic optic neuropathy
Bell palsy
Myasthenia gravis
Horner syndrome

Neoplasms
Headache syndromes
    Primary headache
    Secondary headache
Optic neuritis
    Multiple sclerosis

CEREBROVASCULAR DISEASE

Introduction

Cerebrovascular diseases affect the integrity of the vascular structures of the brain and/or cerebral blood flow. Clinically, most cerebrovascular diseases manifest as stroke or cerebrovascular accident (CVA). In the United States, both men and women have a lifetime risk of CVA of about 25%. The highest risk of stroke is generally at younger ages for men and older ages for women.[1,2] Nonmodifiable risk factors for stroke include older age, African American race, and genetic determinants. Major modifiable risk factors include[3,4]:

- Hypertension
- Diabetes mellitus

- Smoking
- Dyslipidemia
- Physical inactivity
- Heavy alcohol use
- Hypercoagulable states
- Chronic inflammation
- Prothrombotic medications (ischemic CVA)
- Anticoagulant and antiplatelet medications (hemorrhagic CVA)

Approaches to minimize the impact of these risk factors include medications and lifestyle modifications, which are an integral part of stroke prevention and management. For medications that increase stroke risk, a comprehensive assessment of the risks and benefits is important. The pathophysiology and management of hypertension, diabetes, dyslipidemia, and coagulopathies are reviewed in detail elsewhere in the text (Chapters 2, 3, 5, and 8).

A majority of strokes are classified as ischemic (80%)[5] (**FIGURE 12.1**). Mechanisms of ischemic CVA include thrombosis (localized arterial clot), embolism from a nonlocal source (most often atherosclerotic plaque or cardioembolic), hypoperfusion or watershed infarction (so-called due to involvement of the *watershed* regions between the large vessel territories), small lacunar infarcts (associated with chronic hypertension), or various less common insults such as vasculitis, prothrombotic states, and vasospasm. The most common presentations of ischemic stroke are due to atheromatous embolism from an internal carotid artery plaque causing occlusion of the middle cerebral artery. Indeed, carotid stenosis and the presence of carotid plaque are significant risk factors for stroke (Chapter 3). Cardiac arrhythmias (most often atrial fibrillation) and in some situations the presence of a patent foramen ovale also pose significant stroke risk due to formation of platelet-fibrin emboli in the setting of disrupted cardiac blood flow. Similarly, turbulent flow from a carotid artery dissection can result in a stroke due to thromboembolism. As listed below, symptoms and clinical findings in acute CVA will differentiate the anterior cerebral circulation (carotid arteries and

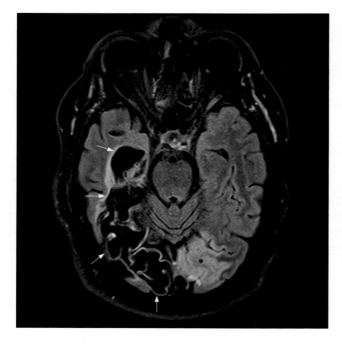

FIGURE 12.1 Noncontrast T2-weighted MRI showing extensive ischemic cerebrovascular accident (CVA) in a 64-year-old man with cardiomyopathy, hypertension, and hyperlipidemia. There is right-sided encephalomalacia (tissue shrinkage) from an old ischemic CVA in the occipital, parietal, and frontal lobes (white arrows). There is left-sided hyperintensity of the occipital lobe indicating more recent ischemic CVA in the division of the left posterior cerebral artery (black asterisk). (Image credit: Dr Rachel Druckenbrod, OD, VA Boston Healthcare System.)

branches) from the posterior cerebral circulation (vertebral arteries and branches, which also supply the brainstem) (**FIGURE 12.1**).[6]

- Anterior circulation CVA signs/symptoms
  - Aphasia (inability to comprehend and/or produce language)
  - Unilateral central facial palsy ("facial droop")
  - Unilateral motor weakness
  - Unilateral sensory deficits
- Posterior circulation CVA signs/symptoms
  - Dizziness/vertigo
  - Nausea/vomiting
  - Ataxia (uncoordinated movement)
  - Gait instability
  - Dysarthria (slurred speech)
  - Crossed motor and sensory deficits
  - Visual field loss
  - Diplopia/eye movement abnormalities

It is important to distinguish between transient ischemic attack (TIA) and fulminant cerebral infarction (CVA). TIA is an acute episode of neurological dysfunction that is a significant risk factor for CVA; it signifies the presence of tissue ischemia without infarction. Criteria require imaging (typically MRI) without acute ischemia and symptom resolution within 24 hours (though most resolve within 4 hours).[5] Initially, the presenting symptoms of acute TIA and CVA are indistinguishable. Amaurosis fugax is considered a form of visual TIA (just as a retinal infarction in retinal artery occlusion [RAO] is considered a *stroke of the eye*). TIA is clinically relevant because it is a strong predictor of CVA in the next 90 days (8%-10%), most occurring within 7 days.[4]

Hemorrhagic CVA represents 20% of all strokes and is broadly caused by impaired vascular integrity (**FIGURE 12.2**). Unlike ischemic CVA, initial symptoms of hemorrhagic CVA may involve more generalized symptoms such as headache, loss of concentration, and vomiting due to mass effect of the blood collection; focal neurologic deficits may also be present. Hypoperfusion of brain tissue may lead to a secondary ischemic CVA (and focal deficit) in some cases, and neurological deficits may also result from brain tissue toxicity from prolonged exposure to blood products. Increased intracranial pressure from an intracranial hemorrhage may produce transient neurological deficits (including transient homonymous visual field loss) which improve or resolve once blood is resorbed or surgically evacuated. Hemorrhagic CVA is typically subdivided into intraparenchymal hemorrhage (IPH) and subarachnoid hemorrhage (SAH).[5] Primary IPH results from spontaneous rupture of susceptible small blood vessels (most often due to vascular impacts of chronic hypertension), while secondary IPH is due to etiologies such as vascular malformations, aneurysms, or coagulopathies. The most common cause of SAH is head trauma. Blood is generally restricted to cortical areas in these cases and may cause neurologic symptoms if sufficient area of cortex is involved (**FIGURE 12.2**). Spontaneous SAH most commonly results from rupture of an intracranial aneurysm and can be neurologically devastating; other etiologies include hypertension, brain tumors, vascular malformations, or drug abuse (eg, amphetamines). SAH may contribute to Terson syndrome (TS), which involves intraocular hemorrhaging concomitant with intracranial hemorrhage. SAH and TS are covered in more detail below (see headache disorders).

When patients present with symptoms concerning for acute stroke, clinical assessment determines hemodynamic stability and establishes a differential diagnosis. When a clinical diagnosis of acute stroke is confirmed, the next step is to differentiate between ischemic and hemorrhagic etiologies. CT (computed tomography) scan of the brain is the preferred modality to evaluate for acute hemorrhage, and it has an advantage of rapid scanning time (Chapter 15). When CT reveals no

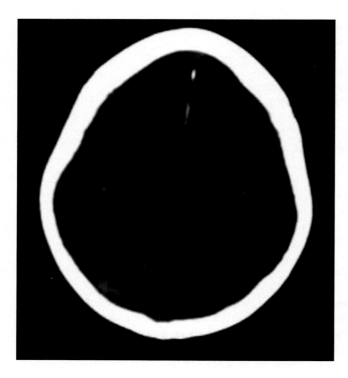

FIGURE 12.2 Noncontrast head CT demonstrating subarachnoid hemorrhage (SAH) overlying the right parietal and occipital lobes in an 81-year-old man. His presenting symptoms were headache, nausea/vomiting, left-sided arm weakness, and dysarthria. An extensive workup did not reveal a specific etiology for the SAH. (Image credit: Dr Rachel Druckenbrod, OD, VA Boston Healthcare System.)

bleeding or intracranial mass, patients with stroke may be offered thrombolysis, often with tissue plasminogen activator (tPA). As opposed to anticoagulants which prevent propagation of established clot, thrombolytic agents lyse established clots, thereby restoring perfusion and reversing cerebral ischemia to viable brain tissue which minimizes ischemic tissue damage and improves long-term clinical outcomes. However, thrombolytic use carries substantial risk for hemorrhagic complications, and the risks and benefits must be carefully weighed together with each patient. Since there is a narrow window of time after which thrombolysis has been shown to lose benefit, it is imperative for patients to seek emergency care immediately with stroke symptom onset, and the emergency evaluation must be efficient. Many hospitals have acute stroke teams to expedite the medical evaluation and deliver thrombolysis to eligible patients as rapidly as possible.

Acute stroke requires hospital admission for further management, which involves close monitoring along with a workup to determine the stroke etiology and mitigate risks to decrease risk of recurrent events. Patients with significant physical limitations may require physical rehabilitation once medically stable. Many patients suffer persistent poststroke disabilities which require long-term outpatient management.

Approach to Vision Loss From Cerebrovascular Disease

Sudden-onset vision loss, either transient (amaurosis fugax) or permanent, raises concern for a vascular event. Vascular pathology affecting the eyes and visual pathways can be localized by the phenomenology of visual symptoms. This depends on an accurate history, specifically addressing the onset and duration of symptoms, binocularity (vs monocularity), as well as distribution of changes in the visual fields. Corroboration with examination is a must, as often the subjective experience can be difficult for patients to describe (especially when transient), and many patients will not instinctively use maneuvers to clarify the pattern of their visual loss. Reliable localization can significantly narrow the differential diagnosis and expedite proper workup.

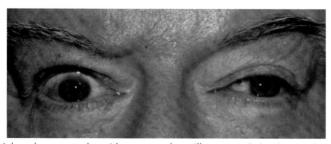

FIGURE 12.6 Partial oculomotor palsy with preserved pupillary constriction in a patient with diabetic third nerve palsy. The affected left eye deviated outward and slightly downward at neutral gaze and left-sided ptosis is present.[7] (From Liu GT, Volpe NJ, Galetta SL. *Liu, Volpe, and Galetta's Neuro-Ophthalmology*. 3rd ed. New York, NY: Elsevier Inc; 2019:39-52. doi:10.1016/B978-0-323-34044-1.00003-1.)

neurological signs and symptoms.[16] For instance, Weber syndrome involves infarct of the third cranial nerve nucleus and adjacent descending corticospinal tracts, resulting in ipsilateral third nerve palsy and contralateral hemiparesis. Injury to the sixth nerve nucleus causes ipsilateral lateral rectus palsy but can also involve muscles of facial expression controlled by the adjacent seventh nerve nucleus, which when accompanied by contralateral body hemiparesis is known as Raymond-Foville syndrome. One-and-a-half syndrome is a disorder of conjugate gaze that occurs due to infarct of the pontine medial longitudinal fasciculus and nearby paramedian pontine reticular formation, causing ipsilateral conjugate gaze paresis and slowed adduction of the ipsilateral eye with abducting nystagmus of the fellow eye on contralateral gaze. Similarly, nystagmus can be seen in infarcts of the pons, medulla, or cerebellum, but is often associated with vertigo, facial palsy, and/or ataxia depending on the exact localization. A detailed review of brainstem and cerebellar syndromes involving eye movements is outside the scope of this text, but the key lesson for the practicing optometrist is to be wary of oculomotor abnormalities when associated with other neurologic signs or symptoms, or when deficits of conjugate gaze are present.

Though not a true stroke, cavernous sinus thrombosis should be considered in the differential of cerebrovascular oculomotor palsies. Cranial nerves III, IV, and VI travel through the cavernous sinus, in addition to some sensory branches of cranial nerve V (V1 and V2), the sympathetic pupillary fibers, and the internal carotid artery (**FIGURE 12.7**). At its worst, a cavernous sinus thrombosis causes ipsilateral total monocular paresis, associated with numbness on the ipsilateral upper and middle thirds of the face due to trigeminal involvement. Blurred vision, optic disc edema, proptosis, and ocular pain can also occur. Thrombosis is generally secondary to infection, but can be spontaneous or related to a disorder of coagulation[17] (Chapter 8). Suspicion for cavernous sinus thrombosis mandates urgent evaluation with cerebral venous imaging. Many other pathologies of the cavernous sinus may contribute to ophthalmoplegia (including pituitary tumor invasion and various inflammatory causes), and the presentation of simultaneous, ipsilateral deficits of cranial nerves III, IV, and/or VI, or a Horner syndrome along with ophthalmoplegia, should immediately raise concern for cavernous sinus pathology with indication for prompt neuroimaging (Chapter 15).

Oculomotor defects do not necessarily implicate the cranial nerves or their nuclei and can be due to lesions rostral to (above) the brainstem. Defects due to pathology above the cranial nerve nuclei are referred to as "supranuclear" eye movement disorders. The most common cortical oculomotor deficit is the unilateral horizontal gaze restriction resulting from infarcts in the MCA territory. The right frontal eye field, which lies in the visual premotor cortex, initiates gaze to the left of midline, and vice versa. Patients with infarcts affecting a frontal eye field will have a so-called gaze preference toward the side of the lesion, as they cannot initiate contralateral gaze, despite having intact extraocular muscle function. In cases of a dense preference, this cannot be voluntarily overcome, but the oculocephalic reflex (or vestibulo-ocular reflex) is preserved. This reflex may be demonstrated by the examiner moving the patient's head to the opposite side of the direction of deficient gaze while the

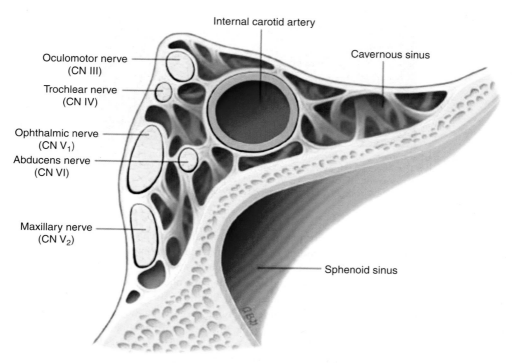

FIGURE 12.7 Cross-sectional anatomy of the cavernous sinus (UpToDate: https://www.uptodate.com/contents/images/ID/65634/Cavernous_sinus_anatomy.jpg.)

patient is asked to fixate on the examiner's face (the so-called doll's head maneuver). With intact oculocephalic reflex, the eyes move reflexively into the direction of deficient voluntary gaze, indicating nuclear control of extraocular muscles is intact.

CLINICAL PEARLS
- Restrictive ophthalmoplegia is an important differential for vascular causes of ophthalmoplegia
- In restrictive ophthalmoplegia, there is a mechanical limitation to full extraocular muscle movements, often due to orbital pathology such as thyroid eye disease, orbital masses, and orbital inflammation
- Clinical exam findings suggestive of a restrictive cause for ophthalmoplegia include:
  - Positive forced duction test (examiner is unable to push or pull the globe into the direction of inaction)
  - Proptosis
  - Vertical or horizontal displacement of the globe
  - Resistance to retropulsion of the globe
  - Concomitant signs of optic nerve compression (eg, relative afferent pupillary defect, dyschromatopsia, optic disc edema or pallor)
  - Concomitant signs of orbital vascular congestion (eg, conjunctival hyperemia and chemosis, engorged or "corkscrew" episcleral vessels, raised intraocular pressure, orbital bruit)

Transient Monocular Vision Loss

Transient monocular vision loss (TMVL) can be due to retinal ischemia from carotid or cardiac embolization to the retinal circulation.[18] This is perhaps the most common use of the term *amaurosis fugax*, though this term can apply to either monocular or binocular events. Onset is generally painless and lasts a few minutes, the latter distinguishing it from transient vision loss due to disc edema and disc drusen, which last no more than a few seconds (this short-duration transient vision loss may be referred to as *transient visual obscuration* [TVO]). TMVL is sometimes subjectively experienced as an altitudinal (respecting the horizontal) deficit, lowering down from the top of the field or rising up from the bottom, the former described as a "curtain coming down."[19] Visual resolution occurs gradually, in an altitudinal direction opposite to its emergence. Symptoms of this description are suggestive of regional optic nerve or retinal ischemia and are concerning for carotid stenosis or cardiac embolic event (most often atrial fibrillation, Chapter 4) and should be approached as a form of TIA.

Diffuse or concentric TMVL is less associated with embolic disease and instead suggests a generalized hemodynamic insufficiency of the retinal and choroidal circulation, often from severe ipsilateral carotid artery stenosis, or other mechanisms such as thrombotic posterior ciliary artery occlusion in the setting of giant cell arteritis (GCA; see below and Chapter 11).[20] Symptoms may be precipitated by mechanisms that reduce ocular perfusion pressure, for example, eating a large meal (ie, shunting blood away from the eye to the gut), bending over or sitting up quickly, or placing external pressure on the eye. Patients with nocturnal hypotension may notice vision loss upon waking that subsequently improves after getting out of bed.[21] Diffuse TMVL that is precipitated by exposure to bright light, especially with symptoms of dull eye pain, often heralds severe ipsilateral carotid stenosis.[20]

It is important to recognize significantly elevated intraocular pressure (especially with concomitant low systemic blood pressure) as a noncardiovascular source of TMVL.[20] These patients may notice postural vision loss, or, in the case of closed-angle ocular hypertension, vision loss in situations that cause pupillary mydriasis, such as dim lighting, sexual intercourse, or exercise. Thorough optometric exam will detect this subset of patients, and extensive systemic workup may not be necessary.

Retinal Artery Occlusion

The central retinal artery is a continuation of the ophthalmic artery, which is in turn the first intracranial branch of the internal carotid artery (**FIGURE 12.8**). The central retinal artery ultimately divides into four branches that each serve a quadrant of the retina. As above, emboli from proximal sources can lodge in the central retinal artery or its terminal branches, leading to TMVL when the embolus is transient and retinal infarction when occlusion is prolonged. This is analogous to the pathology of cerebral ischemic strokes and is influenced by the same cardiovascular risk factors.[22]

The precise incidence of stroke after retinal embolization or TMVL is controversial (range 2%-25%) and is generally considered much lower than the risk after hemispheric TIA.[23,24] RAO is classified as central retinal artery occlusion (CRAO) or branch retinal artery occlusion (BRAO), each of which is further subdivided. All forms should be considered ophthalmologic emergencies when they present acutely and symptomatically and require prompt evaluation for stroke risk.

CRAO describes an occlusion of the retinal artery prior to any of the retinal branch points. Four unique clinical subtypes have been described[25]:

- nonarteritic CRAO (NACRAO)
- transient NACRAO
- NACRAO with cilioretinal sparing
- arteritic CRAO due to GCA

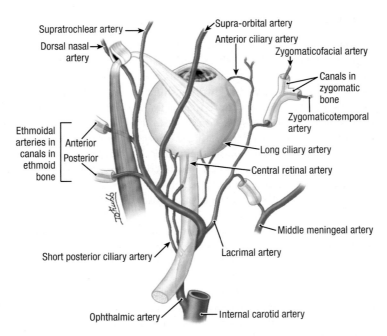

Supratrochlear artery

Dorsal nasal artery

Supra-orbital artery

Anterior ciliary artery

Zygomaticofacial artery

Canals in zygomatic bone

Zygomaticotemporal artery

Ethmoidal arteries in canals in ethmoid bone — Anterior / Posterior

Long ciliary artery

Central retinal artery

Middle meningeal artery

Short posterior ciliary artery

Lacrimal artery

Ophthalmic artery

Internal carotid artery

FIGURE 12.8 Anatomy of the ophthalmic artery and its branches. (From Agur AMR. *Grant's Atlas of Anatomy.* 15th ed. Philadelphia, PA: Wolters Kluwer; 2020.)

NACRAO is the most common subtype, generally secondary to thrombotic or embolic events related to underlying cardiovascular conditions as noted earlier. Hypertension; diabetes mellitus; tobacco smoking; and history of coronary artery disease, TIAs, or cerebral strokes all portend higher risk. Ipsilateral carotid artery atherosclerosis is particularly common and is considered the most common source of emboli, though the aorta and cardiac arrhythmias are also important sources of fibrin-platelet and calcific emboli. Less commonly, hypoperfusion secondary to severe carotid stenosis also results in NACRAO. Ocular risk factors include optic nerve drusen and elevated intraocular pressure, presumably due to increased resistance in retinal vessels and secondarily decreased perfusion pressure. In younger patients, coagulopathies, vasculitis, and myeloproliferative or sickle cell disease may contribute (Chapter 8).[22,25] NACRAO and transient NACRAO are likely manifestations of the same pathologic process, though in the latter case the symptoms fully resolve, by definition. A passing embolus or a drop in ocular perfusion pressure that then recovers may result in transient NACRAO. BRAO is also divided into permanent and chronic subtypes and is usually due to embolization. Occlusion of the cilioretinal artery is recognized as a form of BRAO, though it is important to note that the cilioretinal artery branches from the choroidal circulation (and thus the posterior ciliary artery), not the central retinal artery. NACRAO with cilioretinal sparing simply represents NACRAO in a patient with a patent cilioretinal artery, which can preserve some degree of visual acuity.[26]

RAO presents with sudden, painless monocular vision loss, either sectoral (BRAO) or more diffuse (CRAO). Markedly decreased visual acuity occurs in the majority of CRAO; the presence of collateral flow from a cilioretinal artery, a normal anatomic variant, accounts for most cases of preserved acuity. Visual field deficits in BRAO correspond to a retinal vascular territory, and acuity is more commonly spared.[27] The most common acute finding in CRAO is a cherry red spot at the fovea, with or without associated retinal whitening, though optic disc edema and retinal pallor can be seen (**FIGURE 12.9**). Cherry red spot occurs due to the normal anatomical absence of inner retinal layers at the fovea, and thus lack of inner retinal swelling (whitening) at the fovea, with visibility of the reddish underlying choroid. Fundoscopic examination in BRAO shows signs of retinal ischemia correlating to a branch perfusion territory (**FIGURE 12.9**). It is important to examine the fundus carefully for retinal emboli in order to distinguish embolic RAO from nonembolic causes of RAO; emboli frequently migrate and

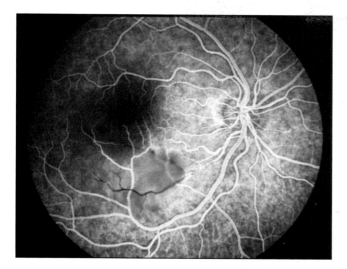

FIGURE 12.9 Fluorescein angiogram reveals retinal arteriolar and capillary nonperfusion in the distribution and inferior-temporal branch retinal artery occlusion. (From Fineman MS. *Retina*. 3rd ed. Philadelphia, PA: Wolters Kluwer; 2018.)

may be seen more distally in a retinal branch (**FIGURE 12.9**).[25] While the absence of a visible embolus does not fully exclude embolic RAO (due to the possibility of embolus migration), the presence allows nonembolic causes of RAO to be excluded. Identifying an embolus in the case of CRAO is especially important as it eliminates suspicion for nonembolic CRAO due to GCA. Emboli in CRAO are often lodged within the vasculature on the surface of the optic disc and can be technically difficult to observe. Though the retina typically appears normal in the period after CRAO, optic atrophy is commonly seen. Neovascularization can result from all types of RAO though is much more typical of CRAO.[25,28,29] Diagnosis of RAO is sometimes aided with fluorescein angiography, which can reveal central or branch occlusion (**FIGURE 12.10**); this may be especially helpful in cases of partial or incomplete RAO.

Outcomes in RAO directly correlate with retinal reperfusion time. When the central retinal artery is experimentally clamped to create a complete CRAO in the Rhesus monkey, no retinal damage occurs if CRAO lasts 97 minutes or less, while massive, irreversible retinal damage results after 240 minutes.[30] In clinical practice, it is impossible to know exactly how long or to what extent the retinal blood flow has been compromised in RAO, so attempts may be made to reperfuse the eye, especially in the case of CRAO. Previous common treatment attempts have included hyperbaric oxygen, ocular massage, vasodilatory medication, and anterior chamber paracentesis.[22,31] No high-quality evidence exists to support any intervention, though a recent prospective case series suggested potential benefit from thrombolysis with intravenous tPA given up to 4.5 hours after symptom onset.[32] These findings are similar to other recent small-scale studies of thrombolysis within varying time windows.[31] The risk of severe bleeding as a complication of thrombolysis should be weighed against the possibility of visual recovery. Unfortunately, significant residual visual impairment is common despite treatment attempts, partly because diagnosis and intervention are usually delayed and the window of opportunity for visual restoration is short. Workup and management of the risk factors described above is critical for secondary prevention. Transient CRAO is a TIA of the eye and should be approached like a cerebral TIA, that is, as a possible harbinger of future ocular/cerebrovascular events. Anterior segment neovascularization is a common long-term sequela that can lead to glaucoma, necessitating long-term monitoring after CRAO.[22]

Anterior Ischemic Optic Neuropathy

Anterior ischemic optic neuropathy (AION) describes a collection of vascular syndromes affecting the optic nerve head. It can further be subdivided into nonarteritic (NAAION) and arteritic (AAION) types.

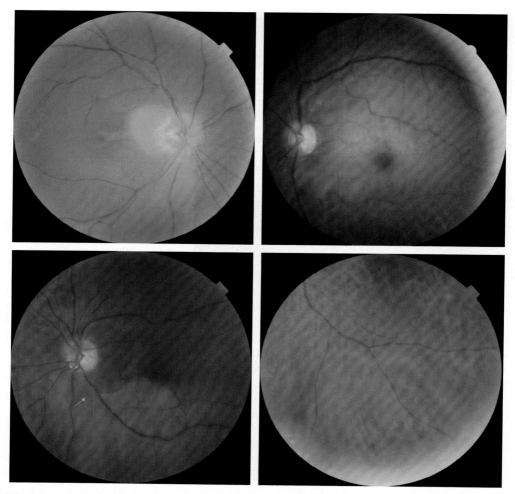

FIGURE 12.10 Central retinal artery occlusion (CRAO) (top panels) and branch retinal artery occlusion (BRAO) (bottom panels). Top-left: Complete CRAO with cherry-red spot; note the attenuation of retinal arterioles; there is no visible embolus at the disc. Top-right: Partial CRAO with "watershed" whitening (ischemia) of the macula; there is no embolus visible at the disc. Bottom-left: Inferior BRAO with associated retinal whitening; note the embolus within the proximal inferior-temporal arteriole as it branches at the disc (asterisk) and severe attenuation of the same arteriole distal to the embolus (arrow). Bottom-right: Nonoccluding retinal arteriolar plaque lodged within a distal branch of the inferior-temporal arteriolar tree. (Image credit: Rachel Druckenbrod, OD, VA Boston Healthcare System.)

NAAION is far more common than AAION, comprising approximately 85% of cases. Despite this relative frequency, the exact pathophysiology remains unknown. NAAION probably results from a hemodynamic disturbance that leads to transient hypoperfusion of the optic nerve, which results in tissue infarction. It is clear that a small optic cup-to-disc ratio, implying anatomic crowding of the prelaminar and/or retrolaminar retinal ganglion cell axons as they form the optic nerve, is a risk factor for NAAION.[33] Hypertension, hyperlipidemia, diabetes mellitus, obstructive sleep apnea, and cigarette smoking are also known risk factors.[34] NAAION classically presents as sudden onset, painless, altitudinal monocular visual field loss, often noticed first upon awakening, which can be immediately at maximal severity or progress over days in a gradual or stepwise fashion. The disc will appear swollen and hyperemic (**FIGURE 12.9**). Rarely, patients present asymptomatically with incipient NAAION, an incomplete form of NAAION which progresses to fulminant NAAION in 25% of cases.[35]

High-quality evidence for effective treatment of NAAION is lacking, though evidence exists that high-dose systemic steroids may be beneficial.[36] Adverse effects of high-dose steroids should be weighed against the likelihood of visual recovery. Even without treatment, patients do often experience modest improvement in vision, but can be left with permanent field cuts or decreased acuity.[33] As the risk factors for NAAION are systemic, the opposite eye is at elevated risk, though recurrence in the same eye is rare likely due to atrophy of infarcted axons.[37,38] Secondary prevention depends on risk factor modification.

AAION is due to GCA, also known as temporal arteritis. It is critically important to identify this etiology early on, as widespread consequences can ensue, including extensive monocular or binocular retinal damage and systemic complications of vasculitis including large-territory cerebral infarcts. Though the presentation can sometimes be identical to NAAION, there are features which are suggestive of AAION rather than NAAION[39]:

- systemic GCA symptoms, including headache, jaw claudication, scalp tenderness, and malaise
- elevated inflammatory biomarkers
- diffuse choroidal nonfilling on fluorescein angiogram
- visual symptoms preceding vision loss (ie, amaurosis fugax)
- severe vision loss at initial onset
- pallid optic disc swelling (**FIGURE 12.9**)
- absence of signs indicating central retinal artery involvement (eg, cotton wool spots, central retinal or cilioretinal artery occlusion)

As in NAAION, visual field loss in AAION is frequently altitudinal and can progress gradually, though is often severe at initial onset. Fundoscopic examination reveals a swollen disc that is pale, in contrast to the hyperemic appearance in NAAION (**FIGURE 12.11**).[33] The gold standard for diagnosis is temporal artery biopsy. Expeditious treatment with corticosteroids can prevent further ischemia and should be initiated immediately upon suspicion of AAION, prior to biopsy. Patients often require long-term corticosteroid therapy. GCA and AAION are discussed in more detail in Rheumatology (Chapter 11).

Posterior Ischemic Optic Neuropathy

Posterior ischemic optic neuropathy (PION) is far less common than AION; in a large series of 1400 patients diagnosed with ION between 1973 and 2008, 96% of all ION was AION while only 4% represented PION.[40] There are arteritic and nonarteritic forms (analogous to AION), and it is also seen in the perioperative setting. Spinal surgery (especially when performed in the prone position) is often cited, though other procedures including ophthalmic, cardiothoracic, abdominal, and orthopedic surgeries have also been implicated.[41] Postsurgical cases are often bilateral with significant visual loss. Pattern of field deficit is more variable than with AION and central field loss may be most common.[42] The optic nerve appears normal on fundus exam in acute PION and may be differentiated from optic neuritis due to the absence of pain and the older age of patients typically affected. MRI is often employed to differentiate PION from optic neuritis or bilateral cerebral causes such as posterior reversible encephalopathy syndrome (PRES). No therapy is supported by quality evidence in the absence of GCA; similar to NAAION, for nonarteritic, nonsurgical PION, high-dose steroids are controversially of benefit and their use should be considered with caution.[42]

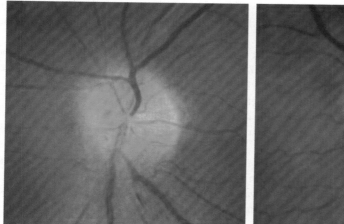
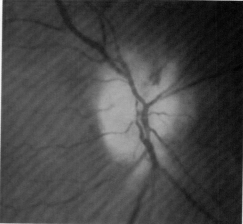

FIGURE 12.11 Fundoscopic image following nonarteritic anterior ischemic optic neuropathy (NAAION) (left) versus arteritic anterior ischemic optic neuropathy (AAION) (right). In NAAION, the disc is hyperemic, as opposed to the pallid disc seen in AAION. (Image credit: Dr Rachel Druckenbrod, OD, VA Boston Healthcare System.)

BELL PALSY

Bell palsy refers to the acute onset of unilateral facial nerve paresis without identifiable cause and constitutes a majority of facial palsy cases encountered in clinical practice. Identifiable causes of facial nerve paralysis should not be referred to as Bell palsy, although in common parlance the term is often (inaccurately) ascribed to facial palsy in general.

The facial nerve, or cranial nerve VII, innervates the muscles of facial expression and stapedius muscle of the inner ear (which regulates volume of sound transmission) and carries fibers innervating the lacrimal and salivary glands, as well as afferent taste fibers from the anterior two-thirds of the ipsilateral tongue. Bell palsy occurs when a segment of the facial nerve becomes inflamed and function is impaired. Patients experience weakness of almost all facial muscles, notably including the forehead, as well as altered taste, abnormally loud sound in the ipsilateral ear, and irritation of the ipsilateral eye (**FIGURE 12.12**). Weakness of the orbicularis oculi is noteworthy for the optometrist, as impaired eye closure (lagophthalmos) can lead to significant dry eye and also leaves the patient vulnerable to corneal abrasion.[43]

While most cases of facial paralysis represent idiopathic peripheral or Bell palsy, this is a diagnosis of exclusion, and other causes must first be considered, including inflammatory (Chapter 11), infectious (most often Lyme disease and herpes simplex virus—Chapter 9), and neoplastic (Chapter 8) causes. Any dysfunction of other cranial nerves should immediately raise concern for an alternate diagnosis. Careful history, review of systems, and physical examination will often provide clues to an alternative cause, which is then confirmed with further testing. Stroke should also be considered as a cause of unilateral facial weakness, even in the absence of other symptoms. Most cases of facial paralysis from stroke are due to cerebrovascular accident of the motor cortex and create what is known as a *central* seventh nerve palsy (or upper motor neuron palsy), as opposed to the *peripheral* (or lower motor neuron) palsy that occurs in Bell palsy (and other peripheral causes). A key differentiating feature of central facial palsy is sparing of the forehead muscles, as these are dually innervated by upper motor neurons from both hemispheres (**FIGURE 12.13**). Prompt neurologic evaluation is key to expediting evaluation for potentially sinister etiologies of a central palsy.

Speculation as to a viral cause for Bell palsy exists, and the treatment often involves a combination of oral antiviral (such as valacyclovir) as well as a course of oral steroid. Even without

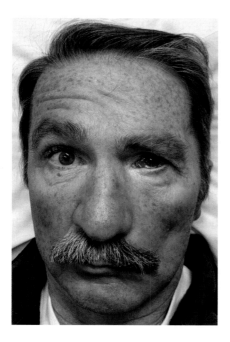

FIGURE 12.12 Patient with a chronic left seventh nerve palsy. The weakness of the left frontalis muscle, seen as asymmetric wrinkling of the forehead when asked to raise his eyebrows, indicates this is a lower motor neuron disorder. Note also the severe left eye irritation from inability to fully close the eye (despite weighting of the eyelid). (Image credit Dr Jeffrey J Dewey, MD, Yale School of Medicine.)

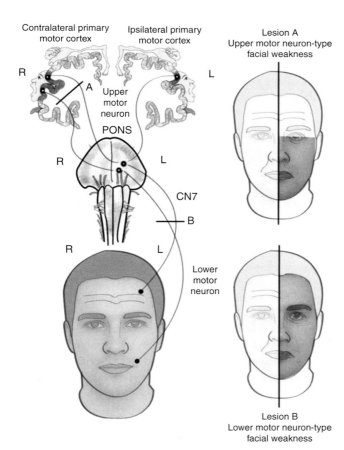

FIGURE 12.13 Central and peripheral CN VII palsy schematic representing the clinical differences of central (upper motor neuron, lesion A) and peripheral (lower motor neuron, lesion B) lesions. The muscles of the forehead receive bilateral cortical innervation that is carried through the ipsilateral lower motor neuron, while the rest of the muscles of facial expression are innervated by the contralateral cerebral cortex. Thus, central brain lesions causing facial nerve palsy will cause facial palsy with sparing of the frontal region due to bilateral cortical innervation of the frontal muscles. Conversely, a peripheral or lower motor neuron lesion to CN VII, such as Bell palsy, will cause complete ipsilateral facial hemiparesis, including the frontal muscles. (From Hasso AN. *Diagnostic Imaging of the Head and Neck.* Philadelphia, PA: Wolters Kluwer; 2011.)

treatment, the natural history of Bell palsy involves a high percentage of complete or partial spontaneous recovery within 1 year (60% to more than 90%, depending on baseline severity), but early treatment with oral steroid increases the chance of full recovery and speeds the rate of recovery versus no treatment.[44,45] Data from robust clinical trials argues that the addition of antiviral is of no benefit, though data also exist from smaller studies showing a benefit for patients with increasing severity of facial nerve paralysis.[46] Since antivirals are generally well-tolerated (with the exception of patients with renal disease), it is common to give both antiviral and steroid in clinical practice when treating Bell palsy.

Aggressive lubrication with topical ophthalmic lubricating drops and/or ointments during the daytime and overnight are important until orbicularis oculi function sufficiently recovers. A protective eye shield or moisture goggles provide corneal protection from injury, especially important overnight or when engaging in activities that pose risk for eye injury. Patients with a robust Bell phenomenon (aka palpebral oculogyric reflex) are naturally at decreased risk for corneal compromise in the setting of reduced orbicular oculi function, but lubrication and protective measures should still be implemented. In patients who do not recover eyelid function, surgical placement of a gold weight in the upper eyelid or permanent partial or complete surgical eyelid closure with tarsorrhaphy may be indicated. Even with full recovery of Bell palsy, there are two notable sequelae which may result: chronic upper eyelid retraction and aberrant regeneration of facial nerve fibers. Upper eyelid retraction creates continued lagophthalmos even after recovery of the orbiulcaris oculi and may be caused by chronic stiffening of the levator palpebral superiorus muscle from unopposed action while the orbicularis oculi was weak.[47] Aberrant regeneration occurs when healing fibers of the facial nerve incorrectly innervate peripheral muscle groups such that aberrant branches simultaneously innervate what are normally distinct subdivisions of the facial nerve; this can result in a phenomenon known as synkinesis, or muscular co-contraction of previously independent muscles, whereby intentional contraction of one muscle results in unintentional contraction of another. Examples include involuntary mouth movement during eyelid closure (or vice versa) and tearing with salivation (the so-called crocodile tears phenomenon). Synkinesis, which is decreasing quality of life, may be managed with options such as surgery or botulinum toxin injections.[48]

MYASTHENIA GRAVIS

Myasthenia gravis (MG) is an autoimmune disease affecting electrochemical transmission in the neuromuscular junction of skeletal muscle via attack on neurotransmitter receptor complexes in the postsynaptic muscle membrane. Clinically, this manifests as fatigable weakness in the affected muscles. Symptoms in MG tend to be better upon awakening and worse at the end of the day but may improve after periods of rest. Ocular MG is defined as disease restricted to muscles of eye movement and/or eyelid muscles (creating symptoms of diplopia and/or ptosis), while generalized MG involves bulbar, limb, and/or respiratory muscles (creating symptoms such as dysphagia, dysarthria, dyspnea, and/or weakness of muscles in the face, neck, arms, hands, or legs). Diplopia in ocular MG can present due to involvement of a single ocular muscle; signs of ocular misalignment on examination are often variable and in a pattern that cannot be localized to a single cranial nerve. The combination of new eyelid ptosis and diplopia should prompt consideration for MG. It is important to recognize that pupillary muscles are always spared, as they are under autonomic control, so MG should not be considered in neurologic eye disease which involves pupillary dysfunction. More than 50% of patients present with ocular symptoms initially, and more than 50% of these patients will develop generalized MG within a 2-year time period. MG generally affects women younger than 40 years and men older than 50 years.[49] Respiratory failure is a feared cause of mortality among MG patients, and thus inquiry about symptoms of dyspnea is important at every patient encounter. Neck flexion or extension weakness, as well as dysarthria or dysphagia, can be indicators of impending respiratory weakness.

Several in-office clinical evaluations may be useful for identifying ocular MG. Cogan lid twitch is a sensitive and specific sign elicited by asking the patient to look downward, then upward, then straight ahead; a positive test results when a small upward twitch (overshoot) of the eyelid is observed just after the patient returns to primary gaze.[50] The "rest test" can be performed in any optometry office on patients with ptosis and suspected MG. It involves documenting a patient's ptosis, ideally photographically, before and after a 2- to 5-minute period of resting with the eyes closed. The test is considered positive when ptosis improves by 2 mm or more immediately after rest.[51] It is important to recognize that the duration of improvement may be very brief, often lasting only seconds. Though the sensitivity of this test is controversial, specificity is greater than 90%, and as such a positive result should raise suspicion for MG.[51,52] The rest test can be augmented by placing an ice pack over the affected eye, known as the "ice pack test," which may lead to more dramatic improvement (**FIGURE 12.14**).[53,54] Alternatively, a "sustained upgaze test" can be employed to demonstrate fatigability of the eyelid; the patient is asked to sustain upgaze for a duration of 60 to 120 seconds, and magnitude of eyelid ptosis is measured pre- and posttesting. Ptosis that worsens by 1.5 mm or more may be considered suspicious for MG.[55] Orbicularis oculi fatigability can similarly be demonstrated by asking the patient to forcibly close the eyelids for a duration of time (or alternatively, to repeatedly open and forcibly close the eyelids). Patients with a clinical picture suspicious for MG should undergo

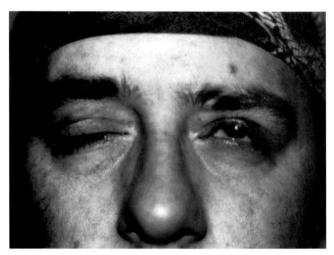

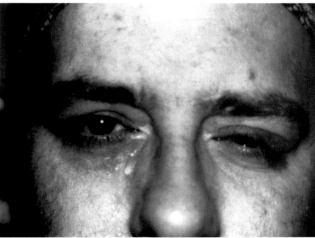

FIGURE 12.14 Diagnostic response to an ice pack test. Patient had significant right ptosis prior to application of ice pack for 2 to 3 minutes (top) that dramatically improved immediately after removal of ice. These findings will be short-lived as temperature of the neuromuscular junction rapidly returns to normal.[53] (From Golnik KC, Pena R, Lee AG, Eggenberger ER. An ice test for the diagnosis of myasthenia gravis. *Ophthalmology.* 1999;106(7):1282-1286. doi:10.1016/S0161-6420(99)00709-5.)

confirmatory testing as below and be referred to a neurologist or neuro-ophthalmologist for management. If breathing or swallowing are affected, urgent evaluation in the emergency setting may be required.

MG is confirmed with serologic antibody screening and electrophysiologic testing. Acetylcholine receptor antibody (AChR-Ab) testing is now widely available and is highly specific for MG, though it is important to recognize that not all cases of MG will be seropositive; this is especially true for ocular MG, where AChR-Ab positivity occurs in only about 50% of patients. Three separate AChR-Ab tests are currently available, with varying sensitivities for generalized MG[56-58]:

- Binding AChR-Ab: 80% to 90+% sensitive
- Modulating AChR-Ab: 86% sensitive
- Blocking AChR-Ab: 52% sensitive

Addition of modulating AChR-Ab to the binding antibody test increases sensitivity of testing by <5%, and in most cases ordering the binding AChR-Ab alone is sufficient. A fourth antibody screening test is available, known as anti–muscarinic tyrosine kinase (MuSK) antibody, which is positive in about 40% of MG cases that are seronegative for the AChR-Abs.[58] Though not common, anti-MuSK may also be positive in some cases of ocular MG which are otherwise seronegative.[59]

Electrophysiology is still considered the gold standard for MG diagnosis and can confirm the diagnosis in the absence of antibody seropositivity. Repetitive nerve stimulation (RNS) involves the use of a recording electrode to record a muscle's compound action potential amplitude over a period of repeated stimulation; in MG, a decrement in amplitude occurs over 4 to 5 stimulations, depending on frequency of testing. Responses are often recorded from intrinsic hand muscles innervated by the median or ulnar nerve, as well as orbicularis oculi or nasalis innervated by the facial nerve. Sensitivity of RNS for MG diagnosis can be as high as 80%; generally, RNS is less sensitive for more distal muscles and for ocular MG.[60,61] Single-fiber electromyography (SFEMG) is more technically challenging than RNS but has emerged as the most sensitive electrophysiological test for MG, detecting more than 90% of generalized MG and more than 80% of ocular MG. A single-fiber needle electrode is inserted into the muscle and variability in transmission time across the neuromuscular junction is analyzed. It is common to test the frontalis, orbicularis oris, and extensor digitorum communis (of the forearm) in generalized disease and the orbicularis oculus in ocular MG.[60]

Cholinesterase inhibitors such as pyridostigmine can be both diagnostic and therapeutic. These medications inhibit breakdown of acetylcholine at the postsynaptic terminal, prolonging the activity of this neurotransmitter and increasing muscle activation. A positive response to one of these medications is supportive of the diagnosis of MG in the proper clinical circumstances, and oral formulations can be continued indefinitely for symptomatic treatment. More severe cases are also managed with long-term immunosuppression, and in many cases an asymptomatic or pauci-symptomatic state can be achieved. For patients with persistent diplopia, prismatic optical correction is challenging due to the fluctuating nature of symptoms in MG. However, in undertreated chronic MG, fixed eye movement deficits can lead to stable diplopia. These patients are often good candidates for prism lens correction. Similarly, a ptosis crutch can be helpful for patients with ptosis that does not respond to medical management.[62] Corrective surgery for strabismus or ptosis can also be performed.[63] It is important to recognize that many drugs are relatively or absolutely contraindicated in MG due to risk for disease exacerbation; collaboration with the patient's neurologist is advisable prior to initiating any new medication. Some of the more commonly prescribed systemic medications which may adversely affect MG include beta-blockers, fluoroquinolone antibiotics, aminoglycoside antibiotics, corticosteroids, and anticholinergic agents. Adverse effect from topical administration of anticholinergics is uncommon, but has been reported.[64]

Especially for patients diagnosed with seropositive MG, it is important to pursue investigations for thymoma with computed tomography (CT) of the chest. Up to 75% of seropositive MG will demonstrate either thymic hyperplasia (most common) or thymic tumor (thymoma), the latter of which can be malignant.[65] Evidence suggests a therapeutic benefit from thymectomy in patients with MG younger than 65 years, regardless of the presence of a thymoma.[66] A thymoma should be resected regardless of patient age. Since other forms of autoimmune disease occur with higher frequency in MG patients versus the general population (such as thyroid dysfunction, rheumatoid arthritis, and systemic lupus erythematosus), directed physical and other diagnostic testing for these entities is also recommended. Detailed discussion of these entities is included in Endocrinology and Rheumatology (Chapters 6 and 11).

HORNER SYNDROME

Horner syndrome, or oculosympathetic paresis, describes the triad of unilateral miosis and ptosis combined with ipsilateral facial anhidrosis (decreased sweating). These signs rarely affect vision and are often observed by others before the patient is symptomatic. Horner syndrome results from sympathetic denervation of the eye and face on the affected side. The sympathetic pathway begins in the hypothalamus and synapses with second-order neurons in the lower cervical and upper thoracic spinal cord (C2-T8). These travel through the upper thoracic cavity, traversing the region of the brachial plexus and upper apex of the lung, and ascend to synapse with third-order neurons within the superior cervical ganglion, located near the carotid artery bifurcation (at the level of the angle of the jaw). These final axons in the pathway form a plexus traveling rostrally on the surface of the internal carotid artery and ultimately join other orbital nerves to reach the pupil and Muller muscles of the upper and lower eyelids (**FIGURE 12.15**).[67] Lesions at any point along this pathway can cause Horner syndrome, and etiologies are classified as localizing to first-order (central), second-order (preganglionic), or third-order (postganglionic) regions. Up to 40% of cases have no identifiable cause despite extensive imaging; among identifiable causes, a majority of cases involve a pre- or postganglionic lesion (44% and 43%, respectively) while a minority of Horner syndrome is central (13%). Wallenberg syndrome (lateral medullary syndrome) from infarction of the brainstem is the most common first-order lesion, and these patients present with a multitude of additional neurological symptoms. Second-order Horner syndrome tends to result from trauma (often iatrogenic, eg, from brachial plexus injury due to the use of forceps during childbirth) or tumors of the lung or mediastinum; Pancoast syndrome describes Horner syndrome combined with shoulder/arm pain due to an apical lung mass (Chapter 8). There are many causes of third-order Horner syndrome; pertinent examples include carotid artery dissection (a medical emergency, often accompanied by neck pain) and cavernous sinus pathology (which may also present with ophthalmoplegia). Some headache syndromes can contribute to third-order Horner syndrome (discussed later in the chapter). The decision to pursue emergent versus timely workup of Horner syndrome is guided by clinical history/context and examination findings which provide etiological clues.[68]

On examination, anisocoria is present, usually not more than 1.5 mm. The magnitude of anisocoria is more pronounced when measured in dim lighting versus bright lighting, implicating the miotic pupil as pathologic. This magnitude of difference in pupil size in dim versus bright light between the Horner pupil and fellow pupil is often small (eg, 0.5 mm).[69] Slow, partial dilation of the Horner pupil, known as dilation lag, can be seen when lighting is dimmed due to passive relaxation of the parasympathetically innervated pupillary sphincter. This may best be observed with serial infrared photography or videography, and when present it is the most pathognomonic clinical sign of Horner syndrome (**FIGURE 12.16**). The Horner pupil may require as long as 10 to 12 seconds to achieve 90% of its dilation potential (25 seconds for full dilation), while a normal pupil requires only 5 seconds (maximum 10-12 seconds).[70]

Subtle upper eyelid ptosis is present on the side of miosis, usually not more than 2 mm since it is Muller muscle and not the levator palpebrae superioris which is affected (**FIGURE 12.17**). Subtle "reverse ptosis" of the lower eyelid may be observed as inferior eyelid retraction (and thus increased

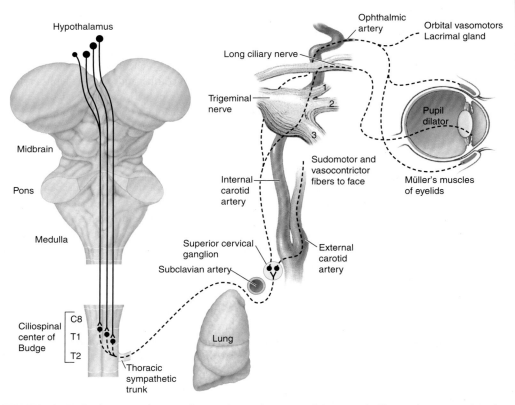

FIGURE 12.15 Ocular sympathetic pathways. Sympathetic stimuli begin with "first-order neurons" in the hypothalamus, descending through the brainstem to reach the intermediolateral column of the spinal cord at levels C8-T2. This region is termed the ciliospinal center of Budge. The second-order neuron follows the sympathetic chain to the superior cervical ganglion where these "preganglionic" sympathetic fibers synapse. Third-order neurons (postganglionic fibers) leave the ganglion as a plexus surrounding the internal carotid artery and are distributed to the orbit via the ophthalmic artery and ophthalmic division of the trigeminal nerve. (From Freddo TF. *Anatomy of the Eye and Orbit*. Philadelphia, PA: Wolters Kluwer; 2017.)

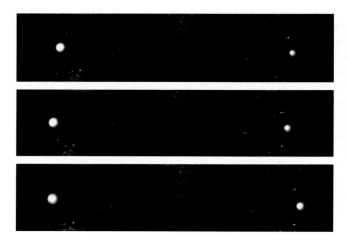

FIGURE 12.16 Dilation lag of a left-sided Horner pupil as documented by serial infrared photography. Pupil dilation was imaged at 5 seconds (top panel), 10 seconds (middle panel), and 25 seconds (bottom panel) after room lights were turned off. The normal right pupil reaches maximal dilation within 10 seconds, while the left Horner pupil requires 25 seconds to reach maximal dilation. (Photo credit: Dr Druckenbrod.)

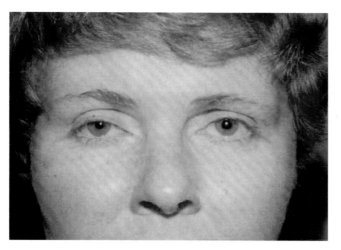

FIGURE 12.17 Manifestations of Horner syndrome. Patient has ptosis and miosis on the right. The miosis may appear more exaggerated in dim light. Abnormal sweating on the right half of the face may be seen but is often difficult to observe in practice. (Reprinted from Campbell WW. *DeJong's The Neurologic Examination.* 8th ed. Philadelphia, PA: Wolters Kluwer; 2019, with permission.)

visibility of the inferior sclera) due to loss of tone of the inferior Muller muscle (**FIGURE 12.17**). Iris heterochromia is often present in congenital cases of Horner syndrome since sympathetic signaling is required for normal iris pigmentation; dark-eyed patients have a lighter-colored iris on the affected side while blue-eyed patients may have a darker-colored iris on the affected side. Anhidrosis is the least common finding, due not only to its difficult detection without special testing but also since nerves responsible for facial sweating branch off at the carotid bifurcation (and thus will not be affected by third-order lesions).

In-office pharmacologic testing can be used to both confirm and localize a suspected Horner syndrome (**TABLE 12.1**), though in clinical practice the testing is usually limited to diagnostic confirmation; in the era of magnetic resonance imaging, pharmacologic localization has fallen out of practical use. It is also impractical to attempt to both confirm and localize a Horner syndrome with same-day pharmacological testing as drug interference creates testing bias. Academically, a first- or second-order Horner syndrome may be differentiated from a third-order Horner syndrome with topical 0.5% hydroxyamphetamine, which releases norepinephrine into the postsynaptic cleft of the third-order neuron when sympathetic signaling is intact; thus, a first- or second-order Horner pupil will dilate in response to hydroxyamphetamine, while a third-order Horner pupil will not. Sympathetic denervation is confirmed by instilling topical apraclonidine (0.5% or 1%), a weak alpha-1 agonist, into both eyes and reevaluating the pupils after 1 hour. In Horner syndrome that has been present for 2 weeks or more, the pupillary dilator in the affected eye becomes exquisitely sensitive to (weak)

TABLE 12.1	Pharmacologic Testing in Horner Syndrome: Topical Agents, Mechanisms of Action, and Mydriatic Effects on the Affected Pupil	
Pharmacologic Agent	**Mechanism of Action**	**Clinical Effect on Horner Pupil**
Cocaine 10%	Norepinephrine reuptake inhibitor	No dilation
Apraclonidine 0.5%-1%	Weak direct alpha-1 stimulation	Dilation
Hydroxyamphetamine 0.5%	Release of norepinephrine from postsynaptic terminal	First- and second-order Horner: no dilation Third-order Horner: dilation

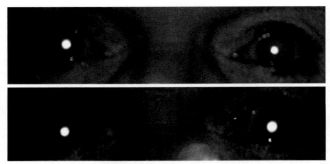

FIGURE 12.18 Pharmacological diagnosis of Horner syndrome with topical apraclonidine 0.5% drops, documented by infrared photography. Top panel: Pre-apraclonidine, the left Horner pupil is miotic compared to the normal right pupil. Bottom panel: The left pupil dilated in response to apraclonidine while the right pupil did not, creating "reversal of anisocoria" which is indicative of Horner syndrome. Note also the resolution of the right upper lid ptosis post-apraclonidine. (Image credit: Dr Rachel Druckenbrod, OD, VA Boston Healthcare System.)

sympathetic stimulation due to denervation hypersensitivity of alpha-1 receptors, and dilation of the Horner pupil occurs without effect (or with very minimal effect) on the normal pupil. This creates a reversal of anisocoria of at least 0.5 mm (typically 2 mm or more) which is diagnostic of Horner syndrome (**FIGURE 12.18**). Sensitivity of apraclonidine testing has been estimated to be greater than 90%.[69] It is important to note that the use of topical apraclonidine is contraindicated in pediatric patients due to risk for central nervous system (CNS) depression; in these patients, topical dilutions of 10% cocaine (the historical diagnostic drop for confirmation of Horner syndrome) is still used. Cocaine acts as an indirect sympathetic agonist by preventing reuptake of norepinephrine into the presynaptic terminal; since Horner syndrome features a paucity of norepinephrine due to deficient sympathetic signaling, topical cocaine has no effect on the Horner pupil but creates dilation of the normal pupil. Posttest anisocoria of at least 1 mm is diagnostic of Horner syndrome.[69]

Once Horner syndrome is suspected based on clinical findings and confirmed by in-office pharmacologic testing, additional workup is required. Full medical history, review of systems, and base neurological exam including full cranial nerve evaluation should be pursued in-office at first suspicion for Horner syndrome. The patient should be questioned about longevity of Horner symptoms, and attempts should be made to identify congenital cases (supported by long-standing presence and iris heterochromia) which do not require further workup. Patients should also be asked about recent neck or thoracic surgical procedures which can result in iatrogenic Horner syndrome. Acute cases which are concerning for potentially life-threatening lesions should be emergently sent for neuroimaging. These include (but are not necessarily limited to):

- cases of Horner syndrome accompanied by other neurological signs and symptoms
- cases suspicious for Pancoast syndrome (ipsilateral brachial plexopathy and Horner syndrome due to tumor at the lung)
- any Horner syndrome accompanied by neck or head pain
- patients reporting recent head or neck trauma
- patients with past medical history of cancer

Choice of imaging modality is usually guided by clinical suspicion for Horner's localization, though the entire sympathetic chain may be imaged using a combination of CT, MRI, CTA, and/or MRA. Treatment of Horner syndrome is focused on addressing the underlying etiology. Though not typically bothersome, patients who notice chronic ptosis may pursue surgical blepharoplasty or use topical phenylephrine or alpha agonist eye drops to temporarily lift the eyelid.[69]

NEOPLASM

Similar to those seen in hemorrhagic strokes, the ocular and visual sequelae of neoplasms depend primarily on the structures being affected due to direct invasion or secondary compression. The presenting symptoms can be identical to those described above, with the exception that they are generally more insidious in onset due to slow growth of the tumor; this phenomenon can also delay presentation, as patients can adapt to slow visual changes to some degree. It is important to recall that while brain neoplasia is far less common than stroke among the adult population, the opposite is true among children; the brain and CNS are the most common sites of pediatric solid cancers.[71] For all ages, meningioma is the most common type of nonmalignant brain tumor, while glioma is the most common malignant form. The occipital lobe is involved in less than 1% of cases of primary brain tumor.[71] Metastatic cancer to the brain is estimated 10 times more prevalent than primary brain tumors, and 20% to 40% of patients with cancer will develop brain metastases.[72] Common primary cancer sites which ultimately metastasize include lung, breast, skin (particularly melanoma), kidney, and the gastrointestinal tract. Large-cell lung cancer may be the most common type to metastasize to the occipital lobe.[73] All patients presenting to the optometrist with neurological manifestations (especially visual field loss) should be questioned about oncologic history. Cancers of the lung, breast, and colon are covered in Oncology (Chapter 8) and melanoma in Dermatology (Chapter 13).

Neoplastic Vision Loss

The prototypical visual field deficit secondary to neoplasm is the bitemporal hemianopia resulting from chiasmatic compression secondary to a sellar tumor such as pituitary adenoma or craniopharyngioma. This is covered in detail later in the chapter (with headache syndromes; also see Chapter 6 for pituitary). Like stroke, homonymous hemianopic or quadrantanopic field loss may result from intracranial neoplasm affecting the visual cortex, and visual-spatial or other perceptual disorders can similarly result from involvement of higher visual association areas. The features of neurological visual field loss detected on optometric examination cannot distinguish between stroke and neoplasm, and patients must undergo neuroimaging.

Tumors affecting the anterior (prechiasmal) visual pathway result most often in vision loss from direct involvement of the optic nerve(s) and/or the retina(e). Rather than homonymous visual field loss, these patients usually present with monocular vision loss associated with features of afferent visual dysfunction (such as dyschromatopsia and relative afferent pupillary defect) and structural abnormalities of the optic nerve and/or retina on physical examination of the globe. Examples of prechiasmal neoplasia include primary tumor formation of the optic nerve (eg, optic nerve glioma) or its sheath (eg, optic nerve meningioma); primary tumor formation of the retina (eg, retinoblastoma); and direct metastatic tumor invasion of the optic nerve or the retina. Primary or metastatic tumors of the orbit can also secondarily lead to vision loss from optic nerve compression, often with tell-tale features such as proptosis/globe displacement and restrictive ophthalmoplegia. Metastatic eye disease is covered further in Oncology (Chapter 8). Optic nerve glioma deserves special attention for its association with neurofibromatosis type 1 (NF1). Gliomas in NF1 can occur anywhere along the visual pathway and affect up to a quarter of patients with NF1, though only about half are symptomatic (Chapter 6).[16,74] These more commonly arise in childhood, for which reason children with NF1 are screened clinically for visual field deficits.[75] Bilateral optic nerve glioma is considered pathognomonic for NF1. Primary optic nerve glioma can also occur in isolation and may lead to monocular blindness despite multimodal treatment.[76]

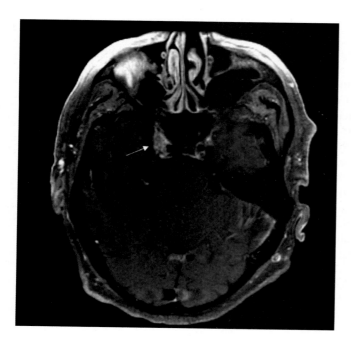

FIGURE 12.19 T1-weighted post-contrast image of a 73-year-old man with squamous cell carcinoma of the right cavernous sinus (arrow) from perineural spread of a forehead lesion. He presented with slowly progressive palsies of right cranial nerves III, V, and VI. (Image credit: Dr. Rachel Druckenbrod, OD, VA Boston Healthcare System.)

Neoplastic Ophthalmoplegia

Numerous types of cancer, both primary CNS and metastatic, can enter the cerebrospinal fluid (CSF) space and coat the inner meningeal layers in a process called *leptomeningeal carcinomatosis*. This generally causes visual symptoms via malignant cells infiltrating the cranial nerve roots as they exit the brainstem. Invasion of the optic nerves can also occur.[77] Symptoms generally begin with single cranial nerve palsy, which may involve ocular muscle paresis, but will progress to involve multiple cranial nerve roots. Leptomeningeal carcinomatosis can be the presenting symptom of cancer and should be considered in any patient with progressive eye movement abnormalities involving more than a single nerve. As mentioned previously, cancer involving the orbit can create a restrictive ophthalmoplegia, and cancer involving the cavernous sinus may also present with ophthalmoplegia from involvement of multiple cranial nerves (**FIGURE 12.19**).

HEADACHE SYNDROMES

The purpose of this section is to provide a relevant review of headache disorders that are important to the optometrist. The *International Classification of Headache Disorders, Third Edition (ICHD-3)*, has created standard criteria for more than 300 different headache types and may serve as an additional resource independent of this chapter. The onus is not on the optometrist to make a definitive headache syndrome diagnosis. However, it is critical to be aware of the ocular findings associated with certain headache types, as well as characteristics of secondary headaches, to ensure appropriate referral for further workup and management.

Primary Headache Syndromes

Primary headache disorders feature recurrent headaches that are not caused by a separate disease process, that is the headache is not a symptom of another disease, but a stand-alone diagnosis. Treatment of primary headaches is directed at the headache pain itself. Subtypes of primary headache include migraine, tension-type headache, cluster headache, and other defined primary headache syndromes (such as primary stabbing headache). Ninety percent of patients presenting with headache will have a primary headache disorder and a normal neurologic exam.[78] A thorough history, which includes location, quality, duration, time course, exacerbating factors, and associated symptoms, will help to distinguish primary from secondary headache syndromes (see below). The presence of associated symptoms such as visual disturbances, including scintillating scotomas, restricted peripheral visual fields, visual blurring, diplopia, and enlarged blind spots, may give a clue to the correct diagnosis. When examining a patient complaining of headache, the optometrist should pay special attention to vision, oculomotor function, the fundoscopic exam, and the presence of corneal injection and/or lacrimation, which all provide clues for headache classification.

The American Academy of Radiology recommends that most patients who present with nontraumatic, uncomplicated primary headache do not need neuroimaging.[79] However, those who present with concerning red flags based on history or physical examination should be considered for neuroimaging to exclude an underlying secondary cause (see below).[80]

Migraine

Migraine is a common primary headache disorder affecting millions of people worldwide. In the United States, the prevalence is estimated to affect about 17% of women and 6% of men.[81] Diagnosis is usually made under the age of 50, and there is a positive family history of migraine in a majority of cases. Among pediatric cases of migraine, motion sickness is a common feature (45%) and a useful minor diagnostic criterion in this age group.[82] Most migraine patients can identify one or more triggers, and avoidance is part of management. Triggers may include certain foods or odors, emotional stress, sleep disturbances, light, weather patterns, and hormonal changes associated with the menstrual cycle in women. Migraine has two major subtypes: migraine without aura and migraine with aura. These are sometimes referred to as "classic" and "common" migraine, respectively; however, these terms are nonspecific and their use is discouraged.

Migraine Without Aura

Migraine without aura is diagnosed after five attacks have occurred, with symptoms including two of the following four pain characteristics, and at least one associated other feature. Pain characteristics include:

- one-sided
- throbbing
- moderate to severe intensity
- aggravated by or causing avoidance of routine physical activities

Associated features include at least one of the following:

- light and/or sound sensitivity (photo- and/or phonophobia)
- nausea with or without vomiting

Attacks typically last 4 to 72 hours untreated, and patients characteristically prefer to rest in a dark and quiet place during at least part of the episode.[81]

Preceding the headache, a premonitory phase of nonpainful symptoms may occur with onset several hours or days prior to headache onset. Premonitory symptoms are categorized into fatigue and cognitive changes (including concentration difficulty, fatigue, memory impairment, depression, and irritability), homeostatic alterations (including food cravings, thirst, frequent urination, yawning, and sleep disturbance), and sensory sensitivities (including neck stiffness, photophobia, phonophobia, and nausea). The most commonly reported symptoms are tiredness, mood change, and yawning.[83]

The postdrome phase, which is relatively newly described, is the period between resolution of the throbbing headache and when the patient feels completely back to normal. During this phase, patients experience numerous nonheadache symptoms which are broadly grouped into neuropsychiatric, sensory, gastrointestinal, and general system symptoms. Neuropsychiatric symptoms include mood changes, concentration problems, and sleep disturbances. Sensory symptoms include head soreness, photo/phonophobia, and speech disturbances. Gastrointestinal symptoms including nausea, flatulence, constipation, vomiting, anorexia, food cravings, and abdominal pain. Systemic symptoms may include tiredness, urination, and fluid retention. The average duration of the postdrome reported varies from 18 to 25 hours.[84]

Migraine With Aura

Migraine aura is described in the *International Classification of Headache Disorders, Third Edition (ICHD-3)* as "recurrent attacks, lasting minutes, of unilateral fully reversible visual, sensory, or other central nervous system symptoms that usually develop gradually and are usually followed by headache and associated migraine symptoms."[85] The majority of migraine auras involve visual disturbances, followed by sensory, language, and motor symptoms. Visual aura symptoms are usually bilateral and symmetric, affecting one hemifield of both eyes.[81] Patients may or may not realize that both eyes are involved and may report monocular symptoms involving the eye on the same side as the involved hemifield. Simple visual auras are thought of as either *positive* or *negative* symptoms. Positive symptoms include small bright dots, flickering lights, white spots, colored dots, curved or circular jagged lines (**FIGURE 12.20**), and crescent or C-shaped forms, among others; negative symptoms can include scotoma, black spots, small black dots, hemianopia, tunnel vision, anopia, and disturbances of visual perception such as blurred/foggy vision. Disturbances of visual perception have been described by patients as looking through heat waves or water, deformed images, visual snow, fractured vision, oscillopsia, corona phenomena, and objects appearing closer or farther away than they actually are.[83] Additional less common visual symptoms include blurry vision, hallucinations, photopsia (perceived flashes of light), halos, obscurations, and micropsia (perceiving objects smaller than they are). Positive visual symptoms are far more common than negative ones,[88] though patients often experience more than one of the above disturbances in the same aura.[83] The aura usually starts at or near the center of fixation, gradually spreading laterally, and separate events may involve different sides of the visual field (ie, the

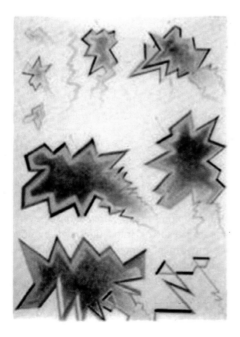

FIGURE 12.20 Illustrations of an aura of fortification spectra, at various stages of evolution, credited to Babinski (1890).[86,87] (Reprinted from Babinski J. De la migraine ophtalmique hystérique. *Arch Neurol.* 1890;20:305-335.)

aura is usually confined one side every time).[81] The prototypical description of migrainous "scintillating scotoma" involves a centrally located negative scotoma with an arc- or C-shaped peripheral leading edge of positive visual phenomena, sometimes with a feature of oscillatory motion-in-place ("shakiness"), which then gradually expands peripherally to one side before fading out of the visual field. Visual auras develop gradually over 5 to 20 minutes and typically last less than 4 hours.

It is important to recognize that visual auras may happen in the absence of a proceeding headache, a clinical phenomenon known as *acephalgic migraine*. Therefore, there is no obligate relationship between migraine aura and headache. However, clinicians should be vigilant to exclude other causes of new-onset transient visual phenomena in all patients with acephalgic migraine, most importantly ischemic events (ie, TIA) and occipital lobe mass lesion. Eliciting a detailed description of the patient's visual symptoms and understanding the typical features and demographic of acephalgic visual migraine is therefore critical. First, ischemic events do not generally cause the positive symptoms described above, nor do they typically spread slowly from a central focal point, building up over time (see discussions of visual field changes in cerebrovascular events and intracranial lesions). Transient monocular blindness is not typical of migraine, as symptoms should be binocular. Seizures involving the occipital lobe can cause positive visual phenomena similar to migraine; however, the duration of symptoms is generally considered to be brief (less than 5 minutes) and may be accompanied by other ictal features such as loss of consciousness or cognitive or emotional changes. Frequency of acephalgic migraine in the population is 0.7% with onset typically later in life (>age 50), and without a past or family history of migraine. Patients usually report numerous past episodes over the course of several years at the time of diagnosis, with stereotyped migrainous visual symptoms and no increased risk for stroke.[89] Acephalgic migraine in a younger person, or in an older person with acute onset or atypical description, is therefore immediately suspicious for alternative pathology. Since symptoms almost identical to migrainous visual aura have rarely been described due to occipital lobe mass lesions,[89] patients not fulfilling all typical features of acephalgic migraine and/or with acute onset of new symptoms should undergo neuroimaging. The optometrist should also perform an automated visual field exam, which can demonstrate shallow homonymous visual field loss not necessarily detectable by confrontation fields.

CLINICAL PEARLS
- Migraine-like visual aura symptoms can occur in the absence of headache, a diagnosis known as *acephalgic migraine*
- Acephalgic migraine symptoms are stereotypical, and other causes should be considered when the description is inconsistent
- TIA and occipital lobe mass lesions may produce symptoms that are similar to acephalgic migraine
- Features that should prompt neuroimaging in patients with acephalgic migraine-like symptoms include:
  - New-onset symptoms
  - Increase in frequency or acute-onset change in pattern of long-standing symptoms
  - Age <50
  - Age >50 with atypical descriptive features including:
    - Short duration of symptoms (seconds or <5 minutes)
    - Consistent localization of symptoms to one hemifield
  - Presence of detectable hemifield vision loss or subjective report of persistent hemifield scotoma
  - Suspicion for seizure activity

Although the pathophysiology of migraine aura is not fully understood, it is believed to be due to changes in activity in the visual cortex rather than primary disruption of ocular physiology. This phenomenon has been termed *cortical spreading depression* based on the pattern of changes seen in electrophysiologic and imaging studies.[90]

Retinal Migraine

Retinal migraine is a rare cause of TMVL.[91] It is defined by the *International Classification of Headache Disorders, Third Edition (ICHD-3)* as repeated attacks of monocular visual disturbance, including scintillations, scotoma, or blindness, associated with migraine headache. For the diagnosis, attacks must fulfill criteria for migraine with aura and criterion B which includes aura characterized by both of the following: fully reversible, monocular, positive, and/or negative visual phenomena (as described above) confirmed during an attack by way of clinical visual field exam and/or the patient's drawing of a monocular field defect. At least two of the following characteristics must also be present: spreading gradually over 5 or more minutes, symptoms lasting 5 to 60 minutes, and accompanied or followed within 60 minutes by a headache. Cases have been described with a prolonged monocular vision loss lasting from hours to week that fully resolved.[91]

Ophthalmologic evaluations are usually normal between attacks. If examined during an attack, it is important to distinguish between the loss of vision in one homonymous hemifield and the loss of vision in one eye. The patient should be instructed to alternately cover each eye; the description of hemifield loss with both eyes open is characteristic of a homonymous hemianopia rather than monocular blindness, and in this case should be present regardless of which eye is covered.[91] This should prompt investigation for postchiasmatic pathology. If, on the other hand, monocular blindness is identified, it should be vigilantly investigated to rule out other etiologies, as retinal migraine is very rare and is a diagnosis of exclusion (ICHD).

The differential diagnosis of retinal migraine includes amaurosis fugax (from various causes, including GCA), primary vascular disease of the central retinal artery or vein, hypercoagulable states such as macroglobulinemia, polycythemia, anticardiolipin antibody syndrome, and sickle cell disease (Chapter 8). Less common causes are orbital diseases including mass lesions, retinal detachment, and intermittent angle closure glaucoma. Interestingly, nearly half of patients with retinal migraines go on to develop permanent monocular vision loss, though the cause of this association is unclear.[91]

Trigeminal Autonomic Cephalalgias

Trigeminal autonomic cephalalgias (TACs) are a group of primary headache disorders that share similar clinical features but differ in timing, frequency, and treatment. The common features include severe headache associated with ipsilateral cranial autonomic features, some of which affect the eye. TACs include five distinct headache types—cluster headache, paroxysmal hemicrania, short-lasting unilateral neuralgiform headache attacks with conjunctival injection and tearing (SUNCT), short-lasting unilateral neuralgiform headache attacks with cranial autonomic symptoms (SUNA), and hemicrania continua. The most prevalent TAC is cluster headache; however, in the interest of a digestible framework they will be presented here in increasing order of typical duration.

Of note, a portion of TACs is secondary to pituitary tumors. Pituitary disease should be considered in all patients presenting with TAC. That said, only patients with atypical features or headaches refractory to standard treatment should undergo MRI and pituitary function testing.[92]

SUNCT and SUNA

SUNCT and SUNA are both rare primary headache disorders. They are characterized by very brief attacks of unilateral, severe stabbing or jabbing pain with associated cranial autonomic features.[93] SUNCT is defined by unilateral orbital or temporal pain that is stabbing or throbbing in quality and of moderate severity. There should be at least 20 attacks, lasting for 5 to 240 seconds, with ipsilateral conjunctival injection and lacrimation. In SUNA, there may be cranial autonomic symptoms other than conjunctival injection and lacrimation, or only one of those symptoms may be present.[85]

Neurologic examination is typically normal, although a small percentage (30%) of SUNCT and an even smaller percentage (11%) of SUNA patients may report ipsilateral sensory changes on the upper and middle face. MRI brain imaging may be normal with some incidental nonspecific findings, but in rare cases abnormal results may reveal vascular loops compressing on the trigeminal nerve and pituitary lesions.[93] Recommended workup includes MRI brain and arterial imaging of the head and neck. Treatment is lamotrigine, titrated up to a total daily dose between 100 and 200 mg. Second-line treatment includes topiramate and gabapentin.[94,95]

Cluster Headache

Cluster headache is defined by the ICHD-3 as attacks of severe, unilateral pain, which is orbital, supraorbital, temporal, or in any combination of these sites, lasting 15 to 180 minutes and occurring from once every other day to eight times per day. Headaches tend to occur in bouts or clusters lasting weeks to months, with intervening periods of more prolonged remission, sometimes lasting months to years. Headaches are associated with ipsilateral cranial autonomic features including conjunctival injection, lacrimation, miosis, ptosis and/or eyelid edema, nasal congestion, rhinorrhea, forehead and facial sweating, and/or with restlessness or agitation.[85] This last feature is particularly characteristic, and patients are often described as pacing the room and quite irritable. Cluster headaches are more common in men than women. There is often a delay to cluster headache diagnosis because of its cyclic nature and cranial autonomic features. With conjunctival injection and lacrimation being the most commonly associated symptoms, these patients may find their way to an optometry office before ever seeing a neurologist.[96]

Neurologic examination of a cluster headache patient may reveal mild ptosis and miosis on the side of the head pain, especially during or immediately following the attack. Impaired trigeminal sensation can sometimes be seen, which should trigger a search for an intracranial lesion. Other findings include ipsilateral tenderness of the carotid artery, periorbital swelling, and conjunctival injection. During a cluster period, a mild partial Horner syndrome ipsilateral to the pain is often present.[81] Cluster headaches are usually responsive to high-flow oxygen and triptans.

Secondary headaches mimicking cluster headache include acute-angle glaucoma, impacted molar tooth, maxillary sinusitis, Tolosa-Hunt syndrome (THS), temporal arteritis, trigeminal neuralgia, and paratrigeminal neuralgia. Carotid or vertebral artery dissections, cerebral arteriovenous malformations, stroke from moya moya disease, and subclavian steal syndrome may also present as similarly to cluster headache. As such, all patients with cluster headache should be evaluated with a brain MRI including dedicated views of the pituitary and cavernous sinus, and cerebrovascular imaging if dissection or other underlying vascular disease is suspected.[96] A neurologist can be enlisted to coordinate this workup.

Paroxysmal Hemicrania

Paroxysmal hemicrania is less common than cluster headache and is more common in women. It is defined as attacks of severe unilateral pain which is orbital, supraorbital, temporal, or in any combination of these sites. These attacks will last about 2 to 30 minutes and occurring several or many times a day. The mean attack frequency per day is 11, with a range of 2 to 50 per day.[97] Associated symptoms can include ipsilateral cranial autonomic features as have been described with other TACs.[85] Lacrimation is the most common associated autonomic feature during attacks, followed by conjunctival injection.[97]

Neurologic examination is typically normal between attacks. Differential diagnosis for paroxysmal hemicrania is similar to that of cluster headache, and again a brain MRI with MRA of the head and neck is recommended for workup.[94] Response to indomethacin is necessary for the diagnosis of paroxysmal hemicrania. Initial recommended dosing 150 mg daily, with increase to 225 mg daily if needed.[98] If indomethacin is ineffective, another diagnosis should be considered.

Hemicrania Continua

Hemicrania continua is similar to paroxysmal hemicrania in its response to indomethacin, but differs because it is continuous, often lasting greater than 3 months. The incidence and prevalence are unknown, but it is considered a very rare condition. It is characterized by unilateral frontal, orbital, or temporal pain that is sharp or throbbing.[92] A baseline persistent headache is always present with exacerbations of severe pain. During exacerbations, there is at least one ipsilateral cranial autonomic symptom, such as conjunctival injection, lacrimation, eyelid edema, ptosis, miosis, nasal congestion, rhinorrhea, and/or a sense of restlessness or agitation, or aggravation of the pain by movement.[85]

Neurologic examination is typically normal, although a portion (23%) of patients may report ipsilateral sensory changes in the face, and a slightly smaller and irregular pupil ipsilateral to the pain may be seen on exam.[92]

The differential diagnosis of long-lasting unilateral headache includes hemicrania continua, unilateral chronic migraine and new daily persistent headache, and other TACs, notably paroxysmal hemicrania. Hemicrania continua can be differentiated from chronic migraine and new daily persistent headache by the positive response to indomethacin. Hemicrania continua typically has fewer prominent cranial autonomic features than paroxysmal hemicrania. In addition, painful exacerbations in hemicrania continua are long lasting, usually several hours and less frequent, whereas those in paroxysmal hemicrania are short lasting (2-30 minutes) and occur many times per day.[92]

Once properly diagnosed, hemicrania continua is generally treatment responsive.[92] Response to indomethacin is necessary for the diagnosis. Dosing is the same as that used in paroxysmal hemicrania.[85]

Secondary Headache Syndromes

It is important to be able to distinguish primary headache syndromes from possibly devastating secondary headache syndromes that cannot be missed. The term secondary headache refers to headaches associated with underlying pathologies such as vascular disorders (ruptured aneurysm, venous sinus thrombosis, or arterial dissection), intracranial tumor, infection, or disorder of the eyes, ears, nose, sinuses, teeth, or mouth.[85] The term *referred headache pain* applies to pain originating from structures in and around the head, which is interpreted by the patient as a headache. As mentioned previously, a thorough history to help identify red flags will ensure that secondary causes of headache are not missed. One widely used mnemonic to ensure all important headache "red flags" are addressed is "2SNOOP4" (**TABLE 12.2**).

The best data exist to support sudden onset, onset after 50 years of age, and associated neurologic signs and symptoms as indicators of secondary headache. Of note, eye pain may be present in a primary headache disorder, secondary headache disorder, or primary ophthalmological condition.[99] This can be challenging to differentiate, but clinical cues can help to guide the differential diagnosis and appropriate treatment options.

Headache Secondary to Elevated Intracranial Pressure

Headache disorders related to high CSF pressure can be difficult to diagnose, mainly due to the overlap with features of primary headache disorders.[100] This section will cover two important clinical conditions with raised intracranial pressure and describe their clinical features, including important ophthalmoscopic findings.

TABLE 12.2 "2SNOOP4" Mnemonic for Evaluating Potential Secondary Causes of Headache

Exam/History Feature	Definition/Examples	Potential Secondary Etiology
Systemic signs/symptoms	• Fever, chills, night sweats • Myalgias • Weight loss	• Giant cell arteritis • CNS infection • Tumor
Secondary risk factors	• Immunocompromised state • History of cancer	• Opportunistic CNS infection • Metastatic cancer
Neurologic signs/symptoms	• Diplopia • Transient vision loss • Pulsatile tinnitus • Focal numbness or weakness	• Stroke, vasculitis, CVST • Tumor • Demyelinating disease • Leptomeningeal disease • Elevated intracranial pressure
Onset sudden	• Sudden onset or "thunderclap"	• Subarachnoid hemorrhage • RCVS
Onset age	• Age >50 when headache of *this character* began	• Tumor • Giant cell arteritis
Progressive	• No headache-free periods, which may be a change from prior episodic headache	• Elevated intracranial pressure • Headache when *standing* can indicate low intracranial pressure, usually due to CSF leak
Precipitated by Valsalva[a]	• Headache *begins* following Valsalva maneuver (most headaches are worse with Valsalva)	
Postural aggravation	• Worse when lying flat *or* standing up	
Papilledema		

CNS, central nervous system; CSF, cerebrospinal fluid; CVST, cerebral venous sinus thrombosis; RCVS, reversible cerebral vasoconstriction syndrome.

[a]Valsalva maneuver worsens most headaches, but rarely causes a headache to begin.

Adapted from Dodick DW. Pearls: headache. *Semin Neurol.* 2010;30(1):74-81. doi:10.1055/s-0029-1245000.

Pseudotumor Cerebri Syndrome

Pseudotumor cerebri syndrome is characterized by raised intracranial pressure and visual changes in the absence of an intracranial mass. Pseudotumor cerebri typically affects children and adults under the age of 50.[100] The typical patient is a woman of childbearing age with a body mass index in the obese range. Primary pseudotumor cerebri is also known as idiopathic intracranial hypertension (IIH), though the latter only applies when investigation has excluded other causes of elevated intracranial pressure (recognize that definitions vary; many clinicians use the terms pseudotumor cerebri and IIH synonymously, separating these entities from raised intracranial pressure from any identifiable cause, structural or otherwise).[100] The etiology of IIH is still not fully established. As obesity increases in the population, incidence of IIH is also rising. A recent study in the general US population showed an increase in the rate of IIH from 1.0 per 100,000 (years 1990-2001) to 2.4 per 100,000 (years 2002-2014).[101] Secondary causes of pseudotumor cerebri syndrome include cerebral venous abnormalities like venous thrombosis and jugular vein obstruction, decreased CSF absorption from previous intracranial infection or SAH, systemic venous hypertension, obstructive sleep apnea, and certain drugs such as vitamin A, retinoids, and corticosteroids. Hypoparathyroidism may be a rare but often underrecognized cause of raised intracranial pressure[102] (refer Chapter 6).

A definitive diagnosis of pseudotumor cerebri syndrome requires papilledema, normal neurologic examination (except for cranial nerve abnormalities, typically cranial nerve VI paresis), normal MRI brain, normal CSF composition, and an elevated lumbar puncture (LP) opening pressure greater than or equal to 250 mm CSF in adults and 280 mm CSF in children. Unilateral or bilateral abducens nerve palsy is supportive if papilledema is not present. If neither is present, at least three of the following neuroimaging criteria are required: empty sella, flattening of the posterior aspect of the globe, distention of the perioptic subarachnoid space with or without tortuous optic nerve, or transverse venous sinus stenosis.[103]

The earliest visual symptom of IIH is TVOs, which are episodes of visual blackout or dimming lasting seconds to minutes in one or both eyes. These episodes are generally precipitated by arising after bending over or from eye movements; vision returns to baseline after each episode, and episodes may occur many times daily. Increased intracranial pressure may produce diplopia, most frequently from a unilateral or bilateral abducens palsy. The resulting diplopia is constant, binocular, and horizontal and is worse at a distance. Other visual symptoms include visual acuity loss and visual field defects (in chronic disease), visual distortion, and photopsia. Nonvisual symptoms are common and can include headache, pulsatile tinnitus, low-frequency hearing loss, neck pain, dizziness, and back pain.[104]

Headache is the most common presenting symptom of IIH overall. The headache in IIH is typically severe and stabbing, constant or daily with daily pulsatile pain that gradually increases in intensity, may be accompanied by nausea, and is often associated with neck pain.[105] Migrainous symptoms such as photophobia, phonophobia, worsening with activity, nausea, and vomiting are highly prevalent and can confuse diagnosis.[106]

Papilledema refers to optic nerve swelling from increased intracranial pressure (**FIGURE 12.21**). The papilledema in pseudotumor cerebri is usually bilateral and symmetric. Visual acuity, color vision, and pupillary exam are normal in the acute phase, which help to distinguish papilledema from other causes of optic neuropathy which can appear similar (such as bilateral AION or bilateral anterior optic neuritis). Visual field examination is also acutely normal or shows characteristically enlarged blind spots (**FIGURE 12.21**).

The severity of papilledema is subjectively graded on live fundus examination or from fundus photodocumentation using the Frisen scale (**FIGURE 12.22**): grade I (minimal) characterized by a C-shaped halo; grade II (mild) with a circumferential halo; grade III (moderate) with obscuration of at least one segment of a major blood vessel leaving the optic disc; grade IV (marked) with total obscuration of a segment of a major blood vessel on the optic disc; and grade V (severe) with total obscuration of all blood vessels on and leaving the optic disc.[107] Though not always present, other ophthalmoscopic signs highly suggestive of raised intracranial pressure include loss of the spontaneous venous pulsation (SVP) at the optic disc and the presence of peripapillary retinal folds at the temporal disc margin (Paton folds) (**FIGURE 12.21**).[108,109] It is important to recognize that some people with normal intracranial pressure have no detectable SVP, so its absence is only suggestive of high intracranial pressure if SVP was previously known to be present.

It is helpful to document the disc and retinal appearance photographically with fundus photography for subsequent comparison over time. Optical coherence tomography (OCT), orbital ultrasound, and fluorescein angiography are other useful imaging modalities that can confirm the presence of bilateral optic nerve edema suspicious for raised intracranial pressure and exclude causes of pseudopapilledema, such as optic nerve head drusen.[103,110] OCT has the added advantages of quantifying retinal nerve fiber layer thickness for comparison over time and detecting macular fluid accumulation as a cause for vision loss (**FIGURE 12.23**).

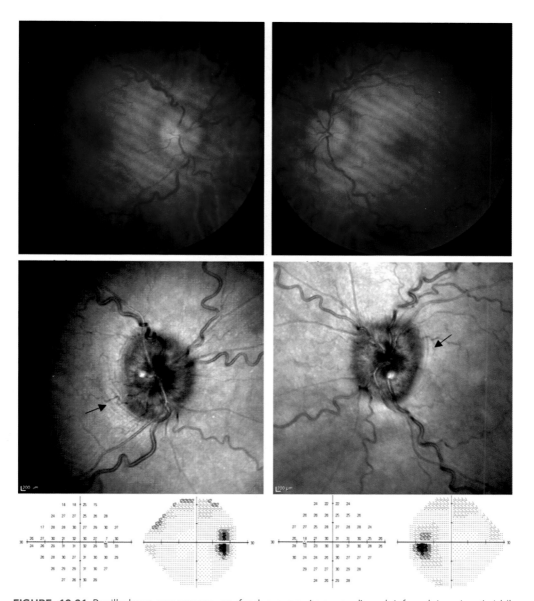

FIGURE 12.21 Papilledema appearance on fundus exam (top panel) and infrared imaging (middle panel). Paton folds are visible in both images, temporal to the discs (black arrows in the infrared images). Papilledema characteristically creates enlargement of the physiological blind spot on visual field testing (bottom panel), though not in all cases. (Image credit: Dr Rachel Druckenbrod, OD, VA Boston Healthcare System.)

Ultimately, LP with elevated opening pressure measurement ($\geq$250 mm H_2O in adults, $\geq$280 mm H_2O in children) is required to formally make a diagnosis of papilledema. LP should be performed only after confirming absence of a mass lesion with imaging, since LP in the presence of intracranial mass poses risk for brainstem herniation. MRI brain should include contrast administration to detect tumors and meningeal processes (Chapter 15). Brain magnetic resonance venography is also indicated to assess for venous sinus thrombosis and venous stenosis as causes of raised intracranial pressure.[100,104] As indicated above, neuroimaging signs suggestive of pseudotumor cerebri syndromes include empty

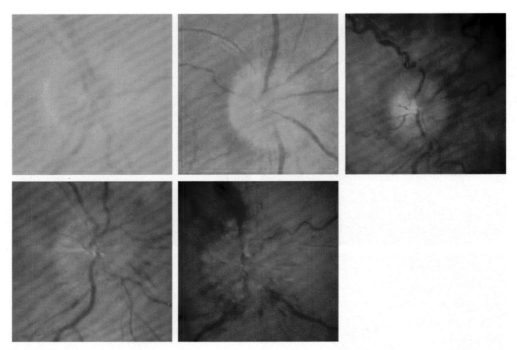

FIGURE 12.22 Varying severity of papilledema is graded subjectively using the Frisen scale. Top-left: Minimal papilledema (Frisen grade I). Top-middle: Mild papilledema (Frisen grade II). Top-right: Moderate papilledema (Frisen grade III). Bottom-left: Marked papilledema (Frisen grade IV). Bottom-right: Severe papilledema (Frisen grade V). (Image credit: Dr. Rachel Druckenbrod, OD, VA Boston Healthcare System.)

sella, flattening of the posterior aspect of the globe, and distention of the perioptic subarachnoid space with or without tortuous optic nerve (**FIGURE 12.24**). The LP is ideally performed in the standard lateral decubitus position and not the prone position (used when fluoroscopic guidance is needed) since the latter may falsely increase the opening pressure. False elevations or falsely normal readings can occur even with ideal technique, since the intracranial pressure demonstrates normal, constant fluctuation and can be elevated secondary to increased intra-abdominal or intra-thoracic pressure.[100]

Visual loss is the major morbidity in IIH. Historic hospital-based series reported bilateral blindness in up to 10%, which results from chronic optic nerve edema and subsequent permanent optic atrophy.[111] At a minimum, optometric examination in pseudotumor should include a measurement

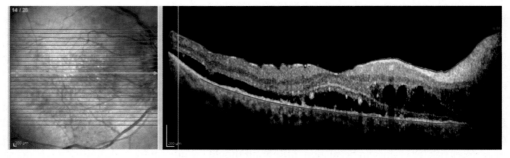

FIGURE 12.23 Spectral domain optical coherence tomography image depicting marked subretinal and intraretinal fluid in the right eye of a 70-year-old man with papilledema due to cerebral venous sinus thrombosis. Visual acuity measured 20/50, without optic atrophy. (Image credit: Dr. Rachel Druckenbrod, OD, VA Boston Healthcare System.)

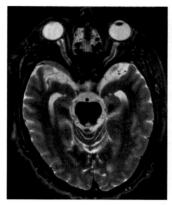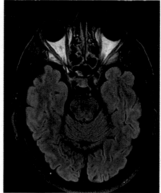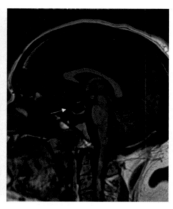

FIGURE 12.24 Magnetic resonance imaging findings in papilledema. Left: Tortuosity to the optic nerves with increased cerebrospinal fluid signal in the perioptic subarachnoid space. Middle: Flattening of the posterior sclerae. Right: "Empty" sella turcica; note the infundibulum of the pituitary gland appears to contact the floor of the sella turcica. (Image credit: Dr Rachel Druckenbrod, OD, VA Boston Healthcare System.)

of visual acuity in each eye, assessment of visual fields, pupil examination to look for afferent pupillary defect or poor pupillary reaction, and a fundoscopic exam.[104] Automated perimetry is very sensitive to detect visual field loss from early optic atrophy due to papilledema.[100] Visual field loss characteristically begins nasally and then extends superiorly and inferiorly to circumferential loss in advanced cases.

The Idiopathic Intracranial Hypertension Treatment Trial showed effectiveness of acetazolamide for improving visual fields, papilledema grade, and quality-of-life measures in patients with mild visual loss.[105,106] Acetazolamide is most effective for visual symptoms during the first month while the dose is being uptitrated. It is recommended to use the maximally tolerated dosage, up to 4 g daily, accompanied by a low-sodium, weight-reduction diet in patients with IIH with mild visual loss.[112] Patients with more extensive visual field loss may need more aggressive therapy including therapeutic LP, temporary lumbar drain, permanent lumbo-peritoneal shunt, optic nerve sheath fenestration, and venous sinus stenting, although there are no clear evidence-based guidelines for the utility of any of these treatments. Weight loss, even 10 to 15 lb, is critically important as it can be curative. Bariatric surgery can be considered for morbidly obese patients.[113]

Cerebral Venous Sinus Thrombosis

Cerebral venous sinus thrombosis (CVST) is a relatively uncommon but important cause of raised intracranial pressure and is due to occlusion of the cerebral veins by a blood clot. In addition to increased intracranial pressure, this can also result in SAH, stroke, or focal edema due to decreased venous outflow. It is more common in young adults and children, with about 75% of the adult patients being women. Risk factors include prothrombotic states (pregnancy, postpartum state, malignancy, and use of estrogen-containing hormonal contraceptives), direct injury to the sinuses or the jugular veins, and infections like otitis and mastoiditis. Headache is the presenting symptom in over 90% of adult cases.[114] Fundoscopic examination usually reveals papilledema. Definitive diagnosis is made by cerebral venous imaging.

The objective of treatment is to lower the intracranial pressure in order to prevent herniation or venous infarction, relieve headache, and reduce papilledema. Anticoagulation is the mainstay of treatment, though osmotic therapy to manage intracranial pressure may be necessary depending on extent of thrombus. Oral acetazolamide, dosed similarly to use in IIH, may also reduce the intracranial pressure. Often, this agent must be continued for weeks to months.[115]

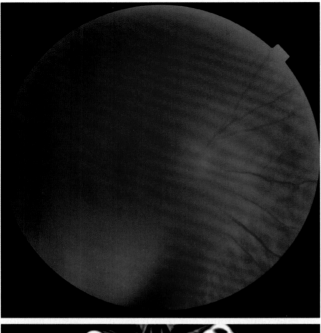

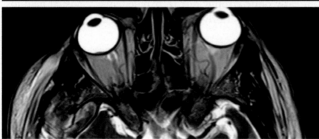

FIGURE 12.25 Terson syndrome in a 50-year-old man who suffered a fall and sustained a large subdural hematoma that required emergent craniotomy for evacuation. He was evaluated by optometry once medically stable, 3 months after his injury. Top panel: Large, non-clearing vitreous hemorrhage of the right eye. Visual acuity was 20/720. Note the vitreous hemorrhage is partially dehemoglobinized (white), due to chronicity. After successful vitrectomy, his visual acuity was 20/20. Bottom panel: MRI acquired 4 days after his fall, demonstrating right intraocular hyperintensity which likely represents accumulation of blood and distention of the subarachnoid space around the right optic nerve. (Image credit: Dr Rachel Druckenbrod, OD, VA Boston Healthcare System.)

Headache Secondary to Vascular Disorders

Headaches associated with ophthalmologic pathology can arise from many different vascular pathologies within the CNS. These include SAH, carotid artery dissection, and THS. Other causes addressed elsewhere in this chapter are ischemic stroke, hemorrhage stroke, and cortical venous sinus thrombosis.

Subarachnoid Hemorrhage and Terson Syndrome

SAH is an uncommon type of hemorrhagic stroke which leads to significant morbidity and mortality. Spontaneous rupture of an intracranial aneurysm is the underlying cause in most cases of nontraumatic SAH. Intracranial aneurysms occur in 2% to 6% of the population, but the vast majority of aneurysms are asymptomatic and will never lead to SAH. The occurrence of SAH peaks between age 50 and 60 years and is more common in women than in men.[116] Sudden onset of the "worst headache of life" or thunderclap headache, reaching maximum severity within 1 minute of onset, is the cardinal symptom of SAH. Headache is present in approximately 70% of patients; it is the only symptom in about 50% of cases, which may lead to a delayed diagnosis or misdiagnosis. Misdiagnosis is associated with increased risk of death and severe disability.

Noncontrast head CT is the diagnostic test of choice for SAH. If SAH is suspected and CT scan does not result in a definitive diagnosis, then additional testing by LP (which will demonstrate red

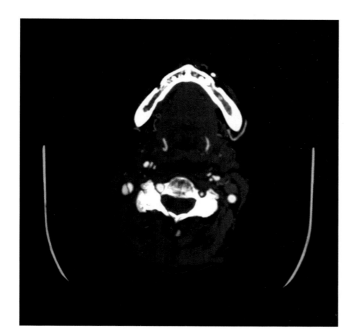

FIGURE 12.26 Dissection of the right internal carotid artery, with the false lumen visible adjacent to the artery. Compare to the round appearance of the normal left internal carotid artery. (Courtesy of Daniel Ginat, MD.)

blood cells and potentially products of blood degradation in the CSF) is recommended.[116] Normal imaging and LP results may occur if the headache has been present for more than 2 weeks, and a high suspicion should prompt further workup with a brain MRI and cerebrovascular imaging.

Approximately 10% of patients who survive SAH become legally blind. Ophthalmologic damage in SAH generally results from TS. TS is defined as any intraocular hemorrhage resulting from SAH, traumatic brain injury, or intracranial hemorrhage and has been reported to occur in 2% to 28% of SAH.[117] TS is hypothesized to occur due to rapid increases in intracranial pressure leading to venous congestion and upstream leakage of small blood vessels and/or forced efflux of blood and CSF into the eye via the optic nerve sheath. It is not frequently diagnosed in the acute hospital setting as it is often only noticed in the rehabilitation setting as consciousness and mobility improve.[117,118] TS is associated with increased Glasgow Coma Score (GCS) and increased risk for mortality.[119] Fundoscopic exam and OCT are considered the gold standards for diagnosis, though hemorrhages can be seen with ultrasound and CT or MRI scan (FIGURE 12.25). Controversy exists regarding the role of early surgical evacuation versus conservative therapy. Nonclearing vitreous hemorrhage may be addressed once the patient is medically stable with pars plana vitrectomy and internal limiting membrane peel, with good visual acuity outcomes.[120] Permanent visual acuity changes including blindness can result in some cases from prolonged exposure of the retina to blood products.[117,121]

Cervical Arterial Dissection

Arterial dissection (FIGURE 12.26) is defined as separation of and extravasation of blood into the normally adjoined layers of the artery. Carotid and, to a lesser extent, vertebral artery dissections are particularly relevant to the optometrist due to the potential for visual sequelae. Headache is frequently the earliest symptom of carotid artery dissection and is reportedly present in 60% to 95% of patients. The headache is usually sudden and severe at onset and can be similar to that associated with SAH. The headache is typically unilateral to the dissection with a constant steady ache. Direct or indirect trauma to the neck may cause internal carotid artery dissection, but the cause of most spontaneous dissections is not known.[122] Visual signs and symptoms can include ipsilateral Horner syndrome and transient or persistent monocular vision loss from RAO by thromboembolism. Preferred imaging techniques are CT angiography, MR angiography, and axial MRI scans with fat saturation, which demonstrates the lack of flow void, intramural blood, and mural expansion of the dissection.[123] Dissection of the vertebral arteries can also present with headache but is not generally associated with visual symptoms unless oculomotor brainstem nuclei or the occipital lobe are infarcted.

Tolosa-Hunt Syndrome

A rare idiopathic inflammatory disorder of the cavernous sinus and orbit, THS is characterized by severe and unilateral periorbital headache associated with painful and restricted eye movements, with attacks recurring every few months to years.[124] THS is a diagnosis of exclusion and must be differentiated from identifiable causes of orbital and cavernous sinus inflammation. It is included as one of the painful cranial neuropathies by the IHS in its headache classification. Diagnostic criteria require unilateral headache with presence of granulomatous inflammation of the cavernous sinus, superior orbital fissure or orbit as seen on MRI or biopsy, and palsies of one or more of the oculomotor nerves (cranial nerves III, IV, and/or VI) on the same side.[85] The annual incidence is estimated to be 1 case per million per year with an average age of 41 years at onset.

Pain is the most common presenting symptom and is described as sharp stabbing, and severe. It is generally periorbital but can be retro-orbital and radiate into the frontal and temporal areas. Ophthalmoplegia can lag up to 30 days, with the oculomotor nerve being most commonly affected (80%) followed by abducens nerve (70%), ophthalmic branch of trigeminal nerve (30%), and trochlear nerve (29%).[125] Treatment with corticosteroids produces a rapid improvement in the pain, with the ophthalmoparesis responding more slowly (weeks to months).[99]

Headache Secondary to Intracranial Mass Lesions

Brain tumors are an uncommon cause of headache[126] but are relevant to the optometrist as they can present with visual symptoms due to mass effect on the visual structures and pathways. It is thought that no more than 30% of patients diagnosed with a brain tumor report headache on presentation, and only 1% to 2% report headache as a lone clinical symptom.[127] The headache is described as dull, deep, and aching and may be associated with nausea and vomiting.[124] The pain is characteristically worsened by lying or bending down and is improved by rest. It is accentuated by exertion, coughing, sneezing, or vomiting. The headache is often generalized.[127]

In particular, pituitary tumors are commonly associated with disabling headache presumed secondary to dural tension or cavernous sinus invasion.[128] Pituitary macroadenoma (size > 1 cm) can cause visual field defects by compressing the optic chiasm or the optic nerve. Reported prevalence of visual deficits secondary to pituitary adenoma vary from 9% to 32%. Patients characteristically describe a bitemporal hemianopia (loss of vision in the lateral hemifield of each eye) due to compression of decussating fibers from the nasal retina at the optic chiasm (**FIGURE 12.27**). That said, any lesion affecting the chiasm can cause these deficits, so the pattern of visual loss is not pathognomonic. The tumor volume strongly correlates with the severity of the visual field effect.[129] Rapid-onset bilateral vision loss, bilateral ophthalmoplegia, and severe headache are highly suspicious for pituitary apoplexy, a medical emergency that results when a preexisting pituitary adenoma (diagnosed or undiagnosed) rapidly enlarges due to hemorrhage or infarction. These patients can rapidly progress to blindness if not treated and mortality can occur from hypopituitarism; thus, suspicion of pituitary tumor warrants urgent medical evaluation. The pituitary gland is covered in Chapter 6.

Headache Secondary to Disorders of the Eye

Patients with head or eye pain may be challenging to evaluate, as both primary and secondary headache disorders may produce symptoms referable to the trigeminal system, eye, and orbit.[123] Overall, primary ophthalmic pathology is an uncommon cause of headache pain; when present, diagnosis is apparent with thorough ocular examination. Headaches of ophthalmic etiology are usually due to asthenopia (eye strain), though structural causes may infrequently present with primary complaint

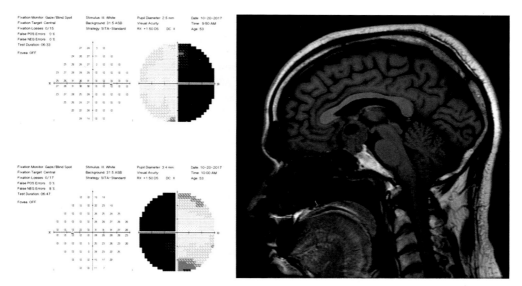

FIGURE 12.27 Bitemporal visual field loss in a 53-year-old man with pituitary macroadenoma. Left panels: Absolute temporal loss of visual field in the right (top) and left (bottom) eyes. Right panel: Cystic pituitary macroadenoma with suprasellar extension and chiasmal compression, measuring 2.5 × 2.5 × 3.3 cm. (Image credit: Dr Rachel Druckenbrod, OD, VA Boston Healthcare System.)

of headache, include anterior segment and orbital pathologies as well as prodromal pain from herpes zoster ophthalmicus (HZO; Chapter 9) or impending cranial mononeuropathy.

Asthenopia is the most common etiology of ophthalmic headache and is typically associated with one of more of the following[130]:

- Uncorrected refractive error
- Binocular vision abnormalities (especially convergence insufficiency)
- Accommodative dysfunction (including presbyopia)
- Glare from lighting
- Flickering light stimuli (eg, from computer screens)
- Compromised quality of viewing material (ie, poor contrast, poor legibility, small targets)

All of these situations place stress and strain on the accommodative and vergence systems, which are intimately linked; dysfunction in one or both systems may contribute to asthenopia. Sustained effort to maintain clear and single vision in the face of accommodative and/or vergence strain creates symptoms of eye and headache pain. Some component of corneal pain from dry eye/tear film insufficiency may simultaneously contribute, as blink rate decreases with increased effort and prolonged duration of visual focus. Headache associated with asthenopia is usually fronto-occipital or retro-orbital.

Structural etiologies of ophthalmic headache usually involve dry eye disease or intraocular inflammation, and less commonly orbital disease.[99,123,131,132] Stimulation of trigeminal nociorecep-tors within the cornea (in keratitis) or uvea (in uveitis and scleritis) creates referred pain which is interpreted by the patient as a periorbital headache. The accompanying conjunctival injection and photophobia/tearing in scleritis and uveitis may occasionally lead to misdiagnosis of TAC syndrome. Orbital inflammation (such as dacryoadenitis, idiopathic orbital inflammatory disease, and orbital cellulitis) may also occasionally present as a headache, especially when onset is more insidious. In the early stages of disease activity, clinical signs may be very subtle. Trochleitis is an uncommon inflammation of the superior oblique tendon as it passes through the trochlea that creates periorbital pain localizing to the superomedial orbit which worsens on abduction in upgaze. It may be idiopathic or associated with rheumatological disease (such as rheumatoid arthritis or systemic lupus erythematosus) and is akin to *tennis elbow of the eye*. Exam demonstrates localized tenderness and swelling in the vicinity of the superior oblique. Trochleitis is responsive to steroid injections. Structural ophthalmological causes of "headache" pain are typically rapidly responsive to appropriate ophthalmic management.

Acute primary angle closure, due to sudden obstruction of the anterior chamber angle, is an uncommon but important structural ophthalmologic cause of headache. Pain results from rapid elevation of eye pressure to symptomatic levels. Risk factors include advanced age, female gender, Asian race, and high hyperopia. In truth, only a small subset of patients with demographic risk factors or anatomical predisposition actually develop acute angle closure, so questions surrounding its pathophysiology remain.[133] Besides pain, ocular injection, corneal edema, and middilated pupil are also usually present.[123,134] Patients may complain of nausea, vomiting, and colored haloes around lights, a constellation of symptoms which can be misinterpreted as migraine with aura.[135] However, optometric examination with slit lamp biomicroscopy and measurement of intraocular pressure reveals the diagnosis.

Patients with optic neuritis frequently complain of eye or periorbital pain, worsened by eye movements. Optic neuritis is discussed in more detail below.

Though not quite primary ophthalmic causes, HZO and microvascular ocular motor cranial neuropathy are two conditions in the realm of optometric care which can create a prodromal periorbital pain which may be interpreted as headache.[123] Initially, examination may be entirely normal. Pain can precede the characteristic skin rash in HZO by several days, and rarely a rash never develops at all (*zoster sine herpete*). Pain in HZO is often described as a burning or shooting pain, is distributed unilaterally along the first division of the trigeminal nerve (V1), and can worsen when the affected area of skin is touched (allodynia). Prodromal pain may similarly occur with isolated third, fourth, or sixth nerve palsies of microvascular origin, preceding symptoms of diplopia by 5 to 10 days (though more commonly, when present pain is coincident with diplopia).[15] Patients complain of mild discomfort to severe pain of the ipsilateral brow or eye, and pain symptoms gradually improve over time, usually resolving well in advance of diplopia. A high index of suspicion is necessary to identify prodromal pain in HZO and cranial mononeuropathy and the diagnosis is confirmed in retrospect, once clinical signs of disease are manifest (Chapter 9).

OPTIC NEURITIS

Optic neuritis is inflammation of the optic nerve and presents as acute and painful vision loss. There are many causes of optic neuritis, including infectious, inflammatory, infiltrative, and paraneoplastic causes, though the most common cause is demyelinating disease, usually associated with multiple sclerosis (MS) as discussed below.[136,137] These patients are typically younger than 50 years and female, though optic neuritis can occur in any demographic. Most patients have abrupt central vision loss ranging from mild deficit to no-light-perception, though some may experience slowly progressive loss over days or weeks. In most adults the vision loss is unilateral, whereas it is generally bilateral in children or adults who are seropositive for myelin oligodendrocyte glycoprotein IgG (MOG-IgG) or anti-aquaporin-4 (AQP4) IgG antibodies.[136] These entities are increasingly recognized as distinct forms of demyelinating disease associated with optic neuritis and are collectively referred to as neuromyelitis optica spectrum disorders (NMOSDs). Some patients may also experience brief transient symptoms of positive visual phenomena, usually photopsias. There is associated eye pain in a vast majority of patients (>90%) which is often deep and retro-orbital, described as an aching sensation that worsens with eye movement and may precede the visual symptoms.

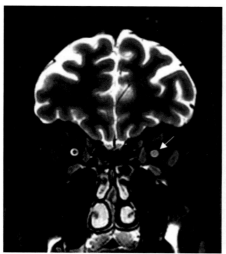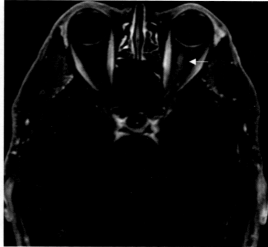

FIGURE 12.28 Fat-suppressed orbital MRI of patient with left optic neuritis. The affected nerve (white arrows) shows T2 hyperinensity (left, coronal scan) and enhancement following administration of gadolinium contrast (right, sagittal scan). (Image credit: Dr. Rachel Druckenbrod, OD, VA Boston Healthcare System.)[136]

Examination reveals clinical signs which are characteristic for optic neuropathy, including decreased visual acuity, decreased contrast sensitivity, dyschromatopsia, and a relative afferent pupillary defect. Various visual field defects are possible though central or paracentral scotoma is most common.[137] Unrelated to optic neuritis, patients with demyelinating brain or chiasmal lesions can show homonymous hemianopia/quadrantanopia or bitemporal visual field loss. The fundoscopic exam including appearance of the optic nerve head is generally normal in acute demyelinating optic neuritis associated with MS (ie, the neuritis involves only the retrobulbar optic nerve), although anterior disc swelling occurs in up to a third of these cases. Uncommonly, mild retinal vasculitis and a mild vitritis may be present.[137]

Diagnosis of demyelinating optic neuritis is usually clinical based on characteristic findings, though MRI is also sensitive for the diagnosis, and brain and spinal cord MRI will help to give valuable clue toward to the underlying etiology (typical brain findings in demyelinating disease are discussed below). MRI of the orbits with fat suppression and gadolinium is the most sensitive diagnostic test (95%) for optic neuritis (**FIGURE 12.28**); however, a normal orbital MRI scan does not exclude optic neuritis. The pattern of inflammation on MRI in combination with the clinical exam features may help differentiate between autoimmune, infectious, and granulomatous processes.[136] A brain MRI is standard to assess the prognosis for developing MS and prior to consideration of disease-modifying therapy for MS.[123] An abnormal MRI at symptom onset is the single most important predictor of the future risk of MS up to 15 years after the onset of optic neuritis[138] (Chapter 15). CSF studies in acute optic neuritis are typically notable for a mild CSF pleocytosis. Specific additional CSF and serological studies should be considered to evaluate other inflammatory, autoimmune, granulomatous, and infectious causes.[136]

High-dose corticosteroids are the standard treatment for acute optic neuritis, though most cases of demyelinating or idiopathic optic neuritis will resolve spontaneously with subsequent visual acuity of at least 20/40 in the absence of treatment. If infection is prominent in the differential diagnosis of a patient with optic neuritis, it is prudent to begin appropriate antibiotic therapy as soon as possible.[123] The Optic Neuritis Treatment Trial demonstrated that intravenous steroids (1000 mg/d for 3 days) followed by oral prednisone (1 mg/kg/d for 11 days) accelerated the recovery of vision, but after 1 month there was no significant difference in visual acuity, visual fields, color vision, or contrast sensitivity.[139] Nearly all patients began to recover at least one line of vision by 3 weeks.[140] In patients with abnormal MRI results, IV steroids at time of attack decreased the risk of subsequently developing MS when compared with oral dosing, though this effect has not been replicated.[141] Oral steroids in standard doses have no effect on the rapidity of recovery and were also associated with a higher recurrence rate and are now considered contraindicated in patients with acute optic neuritis.[139] Plasma exchange may be needed for patients with corticosteroid-refractory optic neuritis or that associated with NMOSD.

Optic Neuritis and Multiple Sclerosis

Optic neuritis occurs in approximately 70% of MS and can be the first symptom in 25% of these patients. The Optic Neuritis Treatment Trial has defined the clinical profile of patients with demyelinating optic neuritis, determined the value of corticosteroid treatment, and quantified the risk of developing MS. This trial has standardized the approach to the diagnosis, treatment, and subsequent follow-up in patients with demyelinating optic neuritis.[140]

MS is a chronic disease of inflammation and white matter demyelination within the CNS. Autoreactive lymphocytes infiltrate the CNS and create an inflammatory cascade resulting in demyelination and neuronal degeneration, with subsequent scarring.[142] Most patients diagnosed with MS are females between the ages of 35 and 64, with peak diagnosis in the third decade. There is a geographic association with Northern latitudes.[143] No pathogenic biomarker for MS has been identified, and the exact etiology of the disease remains unknown. There is likely an interplay between genetic predisposition and environmental factors. Patients with MS are more likely to have other autoimmune diseases (including autoimmune thyroid disease, psoriasis, and inflammatory bowel disease).[142]

Though many patients present with optic neuritis as described above, visual signs and symptoms of an acute attack can also include double vision due to palsy of extraocular muscles or internuclear ophthalmoplegia (in particular, bilateral internuclear ophthalmoplegia), impaired eye closure due to facial weakness, or nystagmus due to lesions in the brainstem or cerebellum. The disease usually starts with a relapsing-remitting course (so-called relapsing-remitting MS) followed by progressive deterioration of neurological function over time (secondary-progressive MS), though some patients exhibit a particularly-aggressive course with continued and steady progression from onset (primary progressive MS). Motor signs and symptoms occur as initial symptoms in up to 40% of cases and occur as part of the disease process in a majority; symptoms include asymmetric weakness of the lower and/or upper extremities, which can progress to spasm, clonus (sustained deep tendon reflexes), and/or paroxysmal dystonia. Exam shows a flaccid weakness with reduced deep tendon reflexes in the initial phase, which evolves to a spastic paresis or plegia with associated hyperreflexia. Sensory abnormalities are even more common and include symptoms of numbness, tingling, burning, tightness, or pain. L'Hermitte sign is described as an electric sensation radiating down the spine or extremities (often down the back of the neck with extension). Cerebellar signs such as ataxia and dysmetria develop over time in many patients, as do disturbances of speech, bowel and bladder dysfunction, fatigue, and neurocognitive dysfunction.[143] Sensory (including visual symptoms) and motor dysfunction may be worsened by hot temperatures as with showering and exercise, a phenomenon known as Uhthoff phenomenon. The diagnosis of MS is based on neurologic symptoms and signs, as well as dissemination of CNS lesions in space and time (see below). Brain MRI typically shows multiple T2-hyperintense white matter lesions in the subcortical, periventricular (abutting the lateral ventricles), juxtacortical (abutting the cortex), or infratentorial (brainstem, cerebellar peduncles, or cerebellum (**FIGURE 12.29**).[144] MRI of the spinal cord may show T2-hyperintense lesions extending one or two vertebral segments, most often in the cervical spinal cord. CSF

78. Dodick DW. Pearls: headache. *Semin Neurol.* 2010;30(1):74-81. doi:10.1055/s-0029-1245000.

79. Douglas AC, Wippold FJ, Broderick DF, et al. ACR appropriateness criteria headache. *J Am Coll Radiol.* 2014;11(7):657-667. doi:10.1016/j.jacr.2014.03.024.

80. Hadidchi S, Surento W, Lerner A, et al. Headache and brain tumor. *Neuroimaging Clin N Am.* 2019;29(2):291-300. doi:10.1016/j.nic.2019.01.008.

81. Martelletti P, Steiner TJ, eds. *Handbook of Headache.* New York, NY: Springer Science & Business Media; 2011.

82. Barabas G, Matthews WS, Ferrari M. Childhood migraine and motion sickness. *Pediatrics.* 1983;72(2):188-190.

83. Viana M, Sances G, Linde M, et al. Clinical features of migraine aura: results from a prospective diary-aided study. *Cephalalgia.* 2017;37(10):979-989. doi:10.1177/0333102416657147.

84. Bose P, Karsan N, Goadsby PJ. The migraine postdrome. *Continuum (Minneap Minn).* 2018;24(4, Headache):1023-1031. doi:10.1212/CON.0000000000000626.

85. Headache classification committee of the International Headache Society (IHS) the International Classification of Headache Disorders, 3rd edition. *Cephalalgia.* 2018;38(1):1-211. doi:10.1177/0333102417738202.

86. Babinski J. De la migraine ophthalmique hysté rique. *Arch Neurol.* 1890;20:305-335.

87. Schott GD. Exploring the visual hallucinations of migraine aura: the tacit contribution of illustration. *Brain.* 2007;130(6):1690-1703. doi:10.1093/brain/awl348.

88. Hansen JM, Goadsby PJ, Charles AC. Variability of clinical features in attacks of migraine with aura. *Cephalalgia.* 2015;36(3):216-224. doi:10.1177/0333102415584601.

89. Shams PN, Plant GT. Migraine-like visual aura due to focal cerebral lesions: case series and review. *Surv Ophthalmol.* 2011;56(2):135-161.

90. Charles A. The migraine aura. *Continuum (Minneap Minn).* 2018;24(4, Headache):1009-1022. doi:10.1212/CON.0000000000000627.

91. Grosberg BM, Solomon S, Friedman DI, Lipton RB. Retinal migraine reappraised. *Cephalalgia.* 2016;26(11):1275-1286. doi:10.1111/j.1468-2982.2006.01206.x.

92. Cittadini E, Goadsby PJ. Hemicrania continua: a clinical study of 39 patients with diagnostic implications. *Brain.* 2010;133(7):1973-1986. doi:10.1093/brain/awq137.

93. Cohen AS, Matharu MS, Goadsby PJ. Short-lasting unilateral neuralgiform headache attacks with conjunctival injection and tearing (SUNCT) or cranial autonomic features (SUNA) – A prospective clinical study of SUNCT and SUNA. *Brain.* 2006;129(10):2746-2760. doi:10.1093/brain/awl202.

94. Burish M. Cluster headache and other trigeminal autonomic cephalalgias. *Continuum (Minneap Minn).* 2018;24(4, Headache):1137-1156. doi:10.1212/CON.0000000000000625.

95. Newman LC. Trigeminal autonomic cephalalgias. *Continuum (Minneap Minn).* 2015;21(4):1041-1057. doi:10.1212/CON.0000000000000190.

96. Bahra A, Goadsby PJ. Diagnostic delays and mis-management in cluster headache. *Acta Neurol Scand.* 2004;109(3):175-179. doi:10.1046/j.1600-0404.2003.00237.x.

97. Cittadini E, Matharu MS, Goadsby PJ. Paroxysmal hemicrania: a prospective clinical study of 31 cases. *Brain.* 2008;131(4):1142-1155. doi:10.1093/brain/awn010.

98. Antonaci F, Sjaastad O. Hemicrania continua: towards a new classification? *J Headache Pain.* 2014;15(1):8. doi:10.1186/1129-2377-15-8.

99. Friedman DI. The eye and headache. *Continuum (Minneap Minn).* 2015;21(4):1109-1117. doi:10.1212/CON.0000000000000204.

100. Mriedman DI. Papilledema and idiopathic intracranial hypertension. *Continuum (Minneap Minn).* 2014;20(4):857-876. doi:10.1212/01.CON.0000453314.75261.66.

101. Kilgore KP, Lee MS, Leavitt JA, et al. Re-evaluating the incidence of idiopathic intracranial hypertension in an era of increasing obesity. *Ophthalmology.* 2017;124:697-700. doi:10.1016/j.ophtha.2017.01.006.

102. Sheldon RS1, Becker WJ, Hanley DA, Culver RL. Hypoparathyroidism and pseudotumor cerebri: an infrequent clinical association. *Can J Neurol Sci.* 1987;14(4):622-625.

103. Friedman DI, Liu GT, Digre KB. Revised diagnostic criteria for the pseudotumor cerebri syndrome in adults and children. *Neurology.* 2013;81(13):1159-1165. doi:10.1212/WNL.0b013e3182a55f17.

104. Thurtell MJ. Idiopathic intracranial hypertension. *Continuum (Minneap Minn).* 2019;25(5):1289-1309. doi:10.1212/CON.0000000000000770.

105. Wall M, Kupersmith MJ, Kieburtz KD, et al. The idiopathic intracranial hypertension treatment trial. *JAMA Neurol.* 2014;71(6):693-701. doi:10.1001/jamaneurol.2014.133.

106. Friedman DI, Quiros PA, Subramanian PS, et al. Headache in idiopathic intracranial hypertension: findings from the idiopathic intracranial hypertension treatment trial. *Headache*. 2017;57(8):1195-1205. doi:10.1111/head.13153.

107. Frisén L. Swelling of the optic nerve head: a staging scheme. *J Neurol Neurosurg Psychiatry*. 1982;45(1):13-18. doi:10.1136/jnnp.45.1.13.

108. Jacks AS, Miller NR. Spontaneous retinal venous pulsation: aetiology and significance. *J Neurol Neurosurg Psychiatry*. 2003;74(1):7-9.

109. Sibony PA, Kupersmith MJ; OCT Substudy Group of the NORDIC Idiopathic Intracranial Hypertension Treatment Trial. "Paton's folds" revisited: peripapillary wrinkles, folds, and creases in papilledema. *Ophthalmology*. 2016;123(6):1397-1399.

110. Kardon R. Optical coherence tomography in papilledema: what am I missing? *J Neuroophthalmol*. 2014;(34 suppl):S10-S17.

111. Mollan SP, Ali F, Hassan-Smith G, Botfield H, Friedman DI, Sinclair AJ. Evolving evidence in adult idiopathic intracranial hypertension: pathophysiology and management. *J Neurol Neurosurg Psychiatry*. 2016;87(9):982-992. doi:10.1136/jnnp-2015-311302.

112. Wall M. Update on idiopathic intracranial hypertension. *Neurol Clin*. 2017;35(1):45-57. doi:10.1016/j.ncl.2016.08.004.

113. Okoroafor F, Karim MA, Ali A. Idiopathic intracranial hypertension and bariatric surgery: a literature review and a presentation of two cases. *Br J Neurosurg*. 2019;33(1):112-114. doi:10.1080/02688697.2018.1427211.

114. Patil VC, Choraria K, Desai N, Agrawal S. Clinical profile and outcome of cerebral venous sinus thrombosis at tertiary care center. *J Neurosci Rural Pract*. 2014;5(3):218-224. doi:10.4103/0976-3147.133559.

115. Stam J. Current concepts: thrombosis of the cerebral veins and sinuses. *N Engl J Med*. 2005;352(17):1791-1798. doi:10.1056/NEJMra042354.

116. Macdonald RL, Schweizer TA. Spontaneous subarachnoid haemorrhage. *Lancet*. 2017;389(10069):655-666. doi:10.1016/S0140-6736(16)30668-7.

117. Ren Y, Wu Y, Guo G. Terson syndrome secondary to subarachnoid hemorrhage: a case report. *World Neurosurg*. 2019;124:25-28. doi:10.1016/j.wneu.2018.12.084.

118. Czorlich P, Skevas C, Knospe V, et al. Terson syndrome in subarachnoid hemorrhage, intracerebral hemorrhage, and traumatic brain injury. *Neurosurg Rev* 2015;38(1):129-136. doi:10.1007/s10143-014-0564-4.

119. McCarron MO, Alberts MJ, McCarron P. A systematic review of Terson's syndrome: frequency and prognosis after subarachnoid haemorrhage. *Neurol Neurosurg Psychiatry*. 2004;75:491-493.

120. Skevas C, Czorlich P, Knospe V, et al. Terson's syndrome – Rate and surgical approach in patients with subarachnoid hemorrhage: a prospective interdisciplinary study. *Ophthalmology*. 2014;121(8):1628-1633.

121. Reale C, Brigandì A, Gorgoglione N, Laganà A, Girlanda P. Terson's syndrome. *Pract Neurol*. 2020:20(2):163-164. doi:10.1136/practneurol-2019-002326.

122. Silbert PL, Mokri B, Schievink WI. Headache and neck pain in spontaneous internal carotid and vertebral artery dissections. *Neurology*. 1995;45(8):1517-1522. doi:10.1212/WNL.45.8.1517.

123. Friedman DI, Gordon LK, Quiros PA. Headache attributable to disorders of the eye. *Curr Pain Headache Rep*. 2010;14(1):62-72. doi:10.1007/s11916-009-0088-8.

124. Chou DE. Secondary headache syndromes. *Continuum (Minneap Minn)*. 2018;24(4, Headache):1179-1191. doi:10.1212/CON.0000000000000640.

125. Amrutkar C, Burton EV. *Tolosa-Hunt Syndrome*. In: StatPearls. Treasure Island, FL: StatPearls Publishing; 2019.

126. Taylor LP. Mechanism of brain tumor headache. *Headache*. 2014;54(4):772-775. doi:10.1111/head.12317.

127. Boiardi A, Salmaggi A, Eoli M, Lamperti E, Silvani A. Headache in brain tumours: a symptom to reappraise critically. *Neurol Sci*. 2004;25(suppl 3):S143-S147. doi:10.1007/s10072-004-0274-8.

128. Levy MJ, Jäger HR, Powell M, Matharu MS, Meeran K, Goadsby PJ. Pituitary volume and headache: size is not everything. *Arch Neurol*. 2004;61(5):721-725. doi:10.1001/archneur.61.5.721.

129. Lee JP, Park IW, Chung YS. The volume of tumor mass and visual field defect in patients with pituitary macroadenoma. *Korean J Ophthalmol*. 2011;25(1):37-41. doi:10.3341/kjo.2011.25.1.37.

130. Sheedy JE, Hayes JN, Engle J. Is all asthenopia the same? *Optom Vis Sci*. 2003;80(11):732-739.

131. Fasih U, Shaikh A, Shaikh N. Aetiology of headache in clinical ophthalmic practice at a tertiary care hospital of Karachi. *J Pak Med Assoc*. 2017;67(2):166-170.

132. Kaimbo DK, Missotten L. Headaches in ophthalmology. *J Fr Ophtalmol*. 2003;26(2):143-147.

133. Zhang X, Liu Y, Wang W, et al. Why does acute primary angle closure happen? Potential risk factors for acute primary angle closure. *Surv Ophthalmol*. 2017;62(5):635-647.

134. Vortmann M, Schneider JI. Acute monocular visual loss. *Emerg Med Clin N Am*. 2008;26(1):73-96. doi:10.1016/j. emc.2007.11.005.

135. Ringeisen AL, Harrison AR, Lee MS. Ocular and orbital pain for the headache specialist. *Curr Neurol Neurosci Rep*. 2010;11(2):156-163. doi:10.1007/s11910-010-0167-6.

136. Bennett JL. Optic neuritis. *Continuum (Minneap Minn)*. 2019;25(5):1236-1264. doi:10.1212/ CON.0000000000000768.

137. Smith CH. Optic neuritis. In: Miller NR, Newman NJ, eds. *Walsh & Hoyt's Clinical Neuro-Ophthalmology*. Philadelphia, PA: Lippincott William & Wilkins; 2005:293-347.

138. Optic Neuritis Study Group. Multiple sclerosis risk after optic neuritis: final optic neuritis treatment trial follow-up. *Arch Neurol*. 2008;65(6):727-732. doi:10.1001/archneur.65.6.727.

139. Beck RW, Cleary PA, Anderson MM, et al. A randomized, controlled trial of corticosteroids in the treatment of acute optic neuritis. The Optic Neuritis Study Group. *N Engl J Med*. 1992;326(9):581-588. doi:10.1056/ NEJM199202273260901.

140. Volpe NJ. The optic neuritis treatment trial: a definitive answer and profound impact with unexpected results. *Arch Ophthalmol*. 2008;126(7):996-999. doi:10.1001/archopht.126.7.996.

141. Beck RW, Gal RL. Treatment of acute optic neuritis: a summary of findings from the optic neuritis treatment trial. *Arch Ophthalmol*. 2008;126(7):994-995. doi:10.1001/archopht.126.7.994.

142. Nourbakhsh B, Mowry EM. Multiple sclerosis risk factors and pathogenesis. *Continuum (Minneap Minn)*. 2019;25(3):596-610. doi:10.1212/CON.0000000000000725.

143. Balcer LJ. Multiple sclerosis and related demyelinating diseases. In: Miller NR, Newman NJ, eds. *Walsh & Hoyt's Clinical Neuro-Ophthalmology*. Philadelphia, PA: Lippincott William & Wilkins; 2005:3429-3525.

144. Thompson AJ, Banwell BL, Barkhof F, et al. Diagnosis of multiple sclerosis: 2017 revisions of the McDonald criteria. *Lancet Neurol*. 2018;17(2):162-173. doi:10.1016/S1474-4422(17)30470-2.

145. Solomon AJ. Diagnosis, differential diagnosis, and misdiagnosis of multiple sclerosis. *Continuum (Minneap Minn)*. 2019;25(3):611-635. doi:10.1212/CON.0000000000000728.

The pathogenesis of acne involves the pilosebaceous follicles of the skin, and there is evidence that suggests an epidermal barrier dysfunction in acne skin.[38] The process includes

- Follicular hyperkeratinization (abnormally rapid shedding of skin cells)
- *Cutibacterium acnes* proliferation, an otherwise normal skin flora, which triggers inflammation[39]
- Increased sebum production inside the pilosebaceous follicle[40]
- Inflammatory process, which includes innate and acquired immunity[41]

Additionally, several other factors likely play a role in acne development and severity:

- Neuroendocrine stimulus: Androgen hormones stimulate sebum production[42]
- Genetic: Earlier and more severe acne occurs with a family history of acne[43]
- External substances: Cosmetic products, especially those with an oily or creamy texture (containing easily melting hydrocarbons), can produce an acne pomade or acne lesions in the areas in contact with the product
- Medications: Exogenous steroids, as an example

At this time, more evidence is needed to establish a relation between acne and dietary factors.[36,37,44,45] The classification of the acne can be based on the morphologic characteristics of the lesions such as

- Acne vulgaris, which can be noninflammatory (opened and closed comedones) or inflammatory (papules and pustules). This includes acne pomade, which consists of comedones and small papules.
- Acne nodular, formed by cysts
- Acne conglobate, composed of all the lesions mentioned above with bridged comedones and deforming scars

The acne classification can be also based on its severity as mild, moderate, and severe. This is related to the number and type of lesions, compromised areas (face, neck, chest, or back), and scarring[37,46] (**FIGURE 13.2**).

Currently, no universal grading or classification system can be recommended.[37]

The treatment of acne is based on its severity and includes topical or systemic antibiotics that reduce the inflammatory process, retinoids (vitamin A derivates), which regulate the keratinization process, as well as hormonal therapy that controls sebum production, and dermatologic procedures to improve esthetic outcomes.[37]

The first line of treatment, by severity, includes

- Mild acne: Topical therapy with benzoyl peroxide or a retinoid, or the combination of both; or benzoyl peroxide and antibiotic; or benzoyl peroxide, retinoid, and antibiotic.[37]
- Moderate acne: Topical combination therapy with benzoyl peroxide and antibiotic; or retinoid and benzoyl peroxide; or retinoid, benzoyl peroxide, and antibiotic; or oral antibiotic plus topical retinoid, benzoyl peroxide, and antibiotic.[37]
- Severe acne: Oral antibiotic plus topical therapy (any of the combination therapies); or oral isotretinoin.[47]

The duration of the oral antibiotic therapy should be the shortest possible, and there should be an evaluation every 3 to 4 months to consider discontinuation. Oral antibiotic therapy should always be prescribed in conjunction with topical therapy to reduce the risk of bacterial resistance. After completion of the systemic treatment, continued topical maintenance treatment with benzoyl peroxide or retinoid is recommended.[37,48]

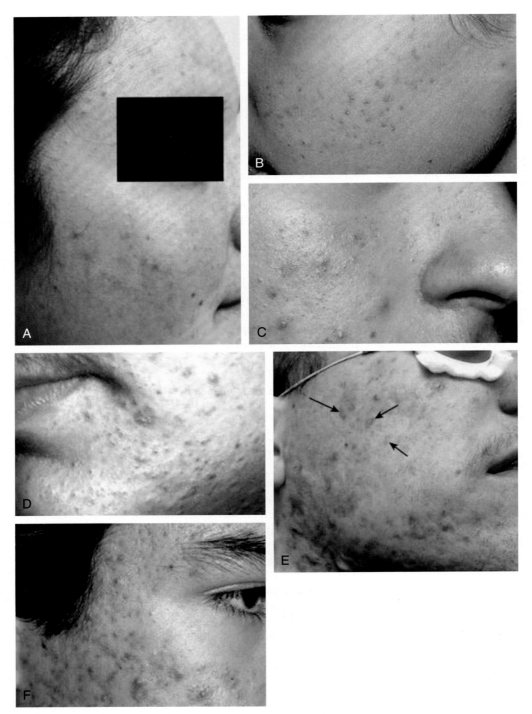

FIGURE 13.2 Acne. Mild acne examples (A and B); mostly blackheads and an occasional papule or pustule. C and D, Moderate acne examples. Seen here are multiple blackheads and whiteheads alongside pustules and papules. E and F, Severe recalcitrant acne examples. Note the nodules, cysts, and/or pits in both photos. (From Gonzales P. *The PA Rotation Exam Review*. Philadelphia, PA: Wolters Kluwer; 2018.)

Options for topical antibiotics include clindamycin, erythromycin, and azelaic acid. Benzoyl peroxide is recommended in patients on topical or systemic antibiotic therapy because it is effective in the prevention of bacterial resistance. Topical retinoid options are adapalene or tretinoin, which in conjunction with benzoyl peroxide, can be safely used in the management of preadolescent acne in children.[37] Systemic antibiotic therapy includes oral tetracyclines such as doxycycline and minocycline.[49,50] The use of oral erythromycin (restricted due to increased risk of bacterial resistance) and azithromycin is limited to patients who cannot use tetracyclines (pregnant women or children under 8 years of age).[37,51]

Oral isotretinoin is a retinoic acid derivate suitable for the treatment of severe nodular acne, recalcitrant moderate acne (treatment resistant), or for patients with scarring. This treatment decreases sebum production resulting in fewer acne lesions and less scarring.[37]

Low doses of isotretinoin between 0.5 and 1 mg/kg/d and a goal cumulative dose between 120 and 150 mg/kg is effective to treat acne while safely reducing the frequency and severity of its adverse effects.[37,52,53]

Routine monitoring of liver function and lipid profile is recommended at baseline and again when treatment response is achieved.[54] Two methods of contraception are necessary for women of childbearing age, as well as enrollment in the iPLEDGE risk management program to prevent isotretinoin exposure during pregnancy due to its teratogenic potential.[37,55-57]

It is recommended that elective procedures be delayed for 6 to 12 months after finishing treatment with isotretinoin to avoid the possible risk of delayed wound healing or keloid formation.[37,55]

Hormonal therapy with estrogen-containing combined oral contraceptives is effective as either adjuvant or monotherapy in the treatment of inflammatory acne in women. Premenstrual acne flares or excessive hair in a male distribution pattern (hirsutism), and the desire for contraception are indications for therapy.[58,59] The therapeutic effect is due to antiandrogenic properties, which decrease ovarian androgen production, increase hormone binding globulins (proteins that bind free testosterone, rendering it unavailable to produce the biological effect), and block androgen receptors.[37]

There are currently four combined oral contraceptives approved by the FDA for the treatment of acne. All of them include ethinyl estradiol combined with a progestin such as norgestimate, norethindrone acetate, drospirenone, or drospirenone/levomefolate.[37]

Treatment with oral contraceptives can be used in patients without a contraindication for use, including established pregnancy, antecedent thromboembolic event (Chapter 8), women breastfeeding less than 6 weeks postpartum, current breast cancer, smokers older than 35 years old, and women with liver disease.[37,58,60,61]

Acne complications include scarring, postinflammatory hyperpigmentation (dark spots that occur more frequently in darker skin tones), depression, and social withdrawal. Effective acne treatment can improve the emotional state of affected patients.[37] In 2013, it was estimated that the direct US healthcare cost of acne was $846 million.[62]

DERMATOLOGICAL MANIFESTATION OF DYSLIPIDEMIAS

Dyslipidemias are familial or acquired disorders of lipoprotein metabolism that manifest with one or more abnormalities in lipoprotein levels (elevated serum low-density lipoprotein cholesterol or triglycerides, decreased high-density lipoprotein cholesterol)[63] (Chapter 3).

Xanthomas are the skin manifestation of an underlying lipid abnormality. The pathogenesis of xanthomas is due to accumulation of lipid-laden macrophages (foam cells) in tissues. Xanthomas can be found in the skin, as well as in ligaments, tendons, fascia, or periosteum. Xanthomas are classified according to their presentation as planar, tuberous, tendinous, or eruptive. Eruptive xanthomas are the most common form of xanthomas and are associated with hypertriglyceridemia. Plane and tendon xanthomas are mostly associated with hypercholesterolemia, and tuberous xanthomas may be seen in both hypercholesterolemia and hypertriglyceridemia.[63,64]

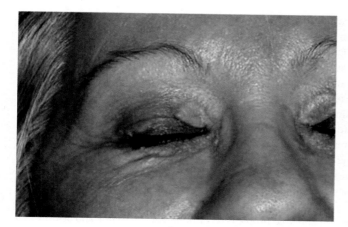

FIGURE 13.3 Xanthelasma. Yellowish plaque located on the upper eyelid toward the inner canthus is characteristic of this type of xanthoma. Patient reported a history of hyperlipidemia. (From DeLong L. *General and Oral Pathology for the Dental Hygienist*. 2nd ed. Philadelphia, PA: Wolters Kluwer; 2012.)

Plane xanthomas are slightly elevated lesions that can occur in any location, including flexural folds. They can be found as an individual lesion or as grouped lesions. Generalized plane xanthomas can involve large areas of the body. The most common presentation of plane xanthomas is yellowish plaques (elevated lesion) on the periorbital skin called xanthelasma[63-65] (FIGURE 13.3).

However, xanthelasmas can be seen in normolipidemic patients in up to 50% of cases.[64] Plane xanthoma on the palmar crease is known as xanthoma striatum palmar. Occurring less frequently, they are more strongly associated with hyperlipoproteinemia.[63]

Tuberous xanthomas are yellow nodules found more frequently over the surface of large joints or on the hands.[63-65] They tend to resolve within a few months of initiating systemic antihyperlipidemic treatment.[63,66]

Tendinous xanthomas are firm subcutaneous nodules found principally on the Achilles tendon or along the extensor finger tendons. Among all the types of xanthomas, these are the most recalcitrant to treat and may take years to resolve, and at times they persist indefinitely.[63-66]

Eruptive xanthomas are groups of yellow-orange papules with erythematous halos that appear suddenly. They principally occur on extensor surfaces of the extremities and buttocks. They typically resolve within weeks after reducing serum triglycerides level.[63-67]

The key issue in the management of xanthomas is treating the underlying lipid imbalance, other associated comorbidities, and discontinuing or lowering the dose of implicated medications. Approaches to lipid lowering includes lifestyle modification including exercise and a balanced diet and pharmacotherapy with lipid-lowering medications[63,68,69] (Chapter 3).

If there are functional or physical concerns related to the location of xanthomas, cryotherapy, ablative laser therapy, or surgical excision can be performed to improve symptoms.[70]

SKIN CANCER

Basal Cell Carcinoma

Basal cell carcinoma (BCC) is the most common cancer in humans and is included in the group of nonmelanoma skin cancers that affect more than 3.3 million persons annually in the United States.[71,72] BCC is a malignant keratinocyte epidermal tumor that predominantly affects the Caucasian population around the world.[73] It is a slow growing, locally invasive tumor with a low propensity to metastasize. The most significant clinical problem lies with its capacity for local tissue destruction.[73] The principal etiological factors are genetic predisposition and UV radiation exposure. The sun-exposed areas are the most commonly affected with a predilection for the head and neck[73] (FIGURE 13.4).

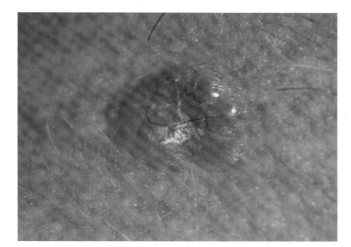

FIGURE 13.4 Enlarged nasal nodule in basal cell carcinoma. Note its depressed center and firm, elevated border. (From Edwards L. *Genital Dermatology Atlas.* 2nd ed. Philadelphia, PA: Wolters Kluwer; 2010.)

Other risk factors associated with the occurrence of BCC include fair skin (Fitzpatrick phototypes I and II), advanced age, male sex, immunosuppression, and arsenic exposure.[73,74]

The clinical and histopathological presentations of BCC are diverse, but it has to be suspected, especially in patients who present with a nonhealing skin lesion.

Clinical subtypes of BCC include the following:

- Nodular: The most common clinical presentation, occurring more frequently on the head and neck. Lesions typically appear as a translucent papule or nodule with telangiectasias and a rolled border. Sometimes larger lesions can have central necrosis and are referred as rodent ulcers.[75]
- Pigmented: These lesions are papules containing melanin, giving them a dark coloration.[75]
- Superficial: Occur most commonly on the trunk and appear as erythematous lesions that may be misdiagnosed as "eczema."[75]
- Morpheaform (sclerosing): An aggressive variant of BCC that may have an ivory-white appearance resembling a scar without antecedent trauma.[75]

The initial diagnostic impression of BCC is made clinically and can be supported with dermoscopy. Biopsy of the lesion is necessary to confirm the diagnosis.

The classification of BCC is based on the National Comprehensive Cancer Network Stratification of low- versus high-risk BCC, which includes clinical and pathological characteristics as follows[76]:

- Low risk: Lesion in area L* less than 20 mm, or in area M** less than 10 mm, well-defined borders, primary lesion, no association with immunosuppression or at a site of prior radiotherapy. Histological growth pattern of nodular or superficial without perineural invasion (PNI).
- High risk: Lesion in area L* equal or greater than 20 mm, or in area M** equal or greater than 10 mm, lesion in area H*** independent of the size, borders poorly defined, recurrent lesion after treatment, association with immunosuppression or on site of prior radiotherapy. Histological aggressive growth pattern like morpheaform and PNI.

---

*Area L includes the trunk and extremities excluding the hands, feet, pretibial area, and ankles.
**Area M includes the cheeks, forehead, scalp, neck, and pretibial area.
***Area H includes the central face, eyelids, eyebrows, periorbital skin, nose, lips, chin, mandible, pre- and postauricular area, temple, ear, genitalia, hands, and feet.

Although BCC does not commonly present periocularly, it comprises 80% to 95% of eyelid and medial canthus malignancies with a predilection for the lower eyelid. Infiltration of the orbit or globe itself occurs in less than 5% of patients, and it often occurs through the orbital periosteum when the tumor is located on the medial canthus. Extension to surrounding nerves, extraocular muscles, lacrimal sac, ethmoid sinus, or the cribriform plate is possible. BCC can also invade the superior orbital fissure via PNI and spread to the cavernous sinus or cerebral tissue.[77,78]

The mean duration from initial diagnosis of periorbital BCC to orbital invasion is 8.5 years, and it is more likely in high-risk periorbital carcinomas that include extensive lesions, infiltrative histopathological patterns, morpheaform type, tumors that recur after excision, and those localized on the medial canthus.[77,78]

Patients with orbital invasion can be asymptomatic or present with invasion of the bulbar conjunctiva, displacement of the globe, or immobility of the eye. For this reason, in high-risk BCC, complementary imaging studies should be done to exclude locally invasive disease to the eye.[77,78]

The treatment of BCC is performed based on the tumor risk stratification and considering risk of recurrence, preservation of the function, patient expectations, and potential complications.[74] Surgery remains the therapeutic standard when it is possible to be performed.

In low-risk primary BCC, curettage and electrodessication may be considered in nonterminal hair locations.[74,75] Surgical excision with 4 mm of margins and histological assessment is the recommended treatment.[74]

In high-risk BCC, Mohs micrographic surgery is recommended.[72,73] With this surgical technique it is possible to preserve tissue and ensure clean histopathological margins.

When surgical treatment is not feasible or preferred, cryosurgery, imiquimod, 5-fluorouracil, photodynamic therapy, or radiotherapy can be considered in low-risk BCC (understanding that the cure rate may be lower[72,73]).

Treatment for locally advanced or metastatic BCC requires multidisciplinary management. Surgery and radiotherapy are recommended for locally advanced diseases. For persistent tumors after treatment, cases where surgery and radiotherapy are contraindicated, and for metastatic disease, systemic treatment with smoothened inhibitor drugs should be considered. In cases of metastatic disease when therapy with smoothened inhibitors is not feasible, platinum-based chemotherapy should be considered or supportive care can be offered.[72]

Treatment options for patients with BCC metastatic to the eye are based on extent of the eye invasion, visual function, and comorbidities. It includes Mohs micrographic surgery with or without radiotherapy, exenteration with or without radiotherapy, smoothened inhibitors, or radiotherapy as monotherapy.[77-79]

Cutaneous Squamous Cell Carcinoma

Cutaneous squamous cell carcinoma (cSCC) is a keratinocyte tumor that is the second most common skin cancer after BCC. In the United States, the lifetime risk for its development is estimated at 9% to 14% for men and 4% to 9% for women.[80,81] There are between 200,000 and 400,000 new cases per year in the United States, and there are more than 3000 disease-related death cases.[81,82]

Risk factors for the development of cSCC include cumulative sun exposure, history of sun burns in childhood and youth, fair skin, chronic exposure to ionizing radiation, immunosuppression, infection with papilloma virus types 16 and 18 (especially for tumors arising in the genital area), and exposure to arsenic. Some genodermatosis such as albinism, xeroderma pigmentosum, and injured or chronically diseased skin such as long-standing ulcers, areas of chronic osteomyelitis, burns or scars, and areas of radiation dermatitis are more prone to develop cSCC.[80,81]

Sun-exposed areas including the head, neck, dorsum of the arms, and hands are common sites of presentation.[80,81] Periocular cSCC comprises 5% to 10% of eyelid tumors[77] (**FIGURE 13.5**).

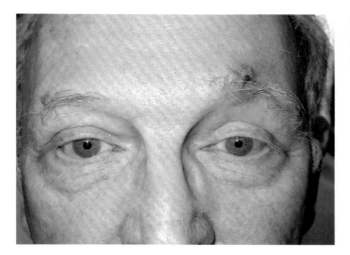

FIGURE 13.5 Squamous cell cancer on a chronic sun-exposed site. (From Hall BJ. *Sauer's Manual of Skin Diseases*. 11th ed. Philadelphia, PA: Wolters Kluwer; 2017.)

The precursor lesion of cSCC is actinic keratosis, which is a scaly lesion usually between 2 and 6 mm in diameter. Coloration may be similar to normal skin, reddish or brown. These lesions are more easily palpated than seen.[75,80] They are considered in situ squamous cell tumors. It is estimated that the annual rate of progression per lesion from an in situ cSCC to an invasive cSCC ranges from 0.025% to 20%.[80,83]

Persons with multiple actinic keratoses possibly have a 6% to 10% cumulative lifetime risk of having at least one invasive cSCC. This risk depends on the number of lesions and their evolution over time.[80,84]

Other forms of in situ cSCC include Bowen disease that manifests with sharply demarcated, erythematous, velvety, or scaly plaques in sun-exposed areas. Erythroplasia of Queyrat appears as red, smooth plaques on the glans penis, but this presentation is less frequent. The lower lip is also affected by cSCC and it presents as roughened, erythematous, or whitish scaly papules or plaques that may progress to a nodular lesion.[75,80]

In situ cSCC may progress to an invasive disease if not treated adequately.[80]

Invasive cSCC manifests as firm papules and plaques, flesh-colored or erythematous, with a smooth or hyperkeratotic surface (thickened outer skin layer). Some tumors can be pigmented, and ulceration may be present.[75,80]

Invasive cSCC has the potential to recur and metastasize. The 5-year recurrence and metastasis rates of primary cSCC are approximately 8% and 4%, respectively.[80,85] Among the main risk factors for recurrence and metastasis are the location (such as lesions on the eyelids, ears, and lips); size of more than 2 cm in diameter; deep invasion into the tissue; and perineural extension.[80] The risk of metastases may be two to three times higher in immunosuppressed patients.[81,86]

Patients can be asymptomatic or experience itching, pain, and altered sensation. The latter symptoms may raise the suspicion for PNI. Also, lesions may present with scales, crusts, small fissuring, or cutaneous horns and may be nonhealing with easy bleeding.[75,80]

The lower eyelid is the most common site of presentation in the periocular area, but cSCC can also be seen on the upper eyelid or medial canthus. Eyelid tumors usually present as a painless, flesh-colored, or erythematous plaque, with scaling or as a nodular lesion that can present with fissuring or ulceration. A less common presentation is as a verruciform lesion.[77,87] Among the in situ periocular tumors, 3% to 5% may progress to an invasive carcinoma presenting with PNI leading to orbital, periorbital, or intracranial invasion. Like BCC, cSCC may invade the cavernous sinus leading to cranial neuropathy.[88] The supraorbital nerve is most often affected by PNI.[77,89] PNI manifests with tenderness of the lesion, altered cutaneous sensation in the perilesional skin, palpebral ptosis, globe displacement (proptosis), or impacts on vision. Between 10% and 25% of these invasive tumors metastasize to regional lymph nodes, including parotid, preauricular, submandibular, or submental nodes, especially those recurrent lesions larger than 2 cm.[77,89]

The diagnosis of cSCC is made clinically and is confirmed with histopathological study of the biopsy specimen. A clinical examination of regional lymph nodes is always mandatory.[81]

A useful classification of the cSCC that orients the treatment was made by the current National Comprehensive Cancer Network (NCCN) and is based on the classification of the tumor as low or high risk as follows[90]:

- Low risk: Area L* less than 20 mm, or area M** less than 10 mm, well-defined borders, primary lesion, no immunosuppression, location is not on the site of previous radiotherapy or chronic inflammation, no rapidly growing tumor, and without neurologic symptoms. Histopathological findings include well to moderately differentiated tumor, no high-risk subtype, depth less than 2 mm, no perineural, vascular, or lymphatic invasion.
- High risk: Area L* equal or greater than 20 mm, area M** equal or greater than 10 mm, area H***, borders poorly differentiated, recurrent lesion, presence of immunosuppression, or on area of previous radiotherapy or chronic inflammation, rapidly growing tumor, and presence of neurologic symptoms. Histopathological findings include poorly differentiated tumor, high-risk subtype, depth equal or greater than 2 mm, perineural, vascular, or lymphatic invasion.

Staging imaging studies in high-risk tumors area recommended to evaluate the presence of deep structural involvement with extensive localized disease, nodal, or distant metastases.[81] In these cases, a sentinel nodal biopsy should be considered.[81,91] For periocular tumors, imaging studies help with surgical planning and may evaluate the presence of PNI which appears as an ocular adnexal pseudocyst.[89]

The treatment options for actinic keratoses include cryosurgery, electrodesiccation, curettage, topical fluorouracil, dermabrasion, or laser resurfacing.[80]

The treatment of cSCC is based on the tumor risk stratification and considering the risk of recurrence, preservation of function, patient expectations, and potential complications.[81] Surgery remains the therapeutic standard when it is possible to be performed.

In low-risk cSCC, curettage and electrodessication may be considered in nonterminal hair areas. Surgical excision with 4 to 6 mm margins to a depth of midsubcutaneous adipose tissue with histological margin evaluation is recommended.[81] If surgical therapy is not feasible or preferred, radiotherapy or cryosurgery may be considered in low-risk tumors with the understanding that the cure rate may be lower.[81] In high-risk cSCC, Mohs micrographic surgery is recommended.[81] The treatment of choice for eyelid tumors is Mohs surgery and the defect frequently requires oculoplastic reconstruction. Total or subtotal supraorbital nerve exenteration may be required if the tumor extends into the orbit.[77,89]

The management of locally advanced or metastatic disease should include a multidisciplinary group. Surgical resection is typically recommended with or without radiotherapy and possible systemic therapy for regional lymph node metastatic disease.[81] Chemotherapy and radiotherapy combined should be considered for inoperable disease.[81] For distant metastatic disease, chemotherapy with epidermal growth factor inhibitors and Cisplatin as a single agent or in combination therapy are recommended.[81]

General recommendations: After a diagnosis of a first nonmelanoma skin cancer, screening for new tumors should be performed at least annually. The patients should be counseled on skin self-examination and sun protection.[72]

---

*Area L includes the trunk and extremities excluding the hands, feet, pretibial area, and ankles.
**Area M includes the cheeks, forehead, scalp, neck, and pretibial area.
***Area H includes the central face, eyelids, eyebrows, periorbital skin, nose, lips, chin, mandible, pre- and postauricular area, temple, ear, genitalia, hands, and feet.

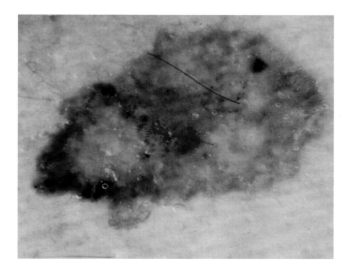

FIGURE 13.6 Superficial spreading melanoma. (From Johnson J. *Bailey's Head and Neck Surgery*. 5th ed. Philadelphia, PA: Wolters Kluwer; 2013.)

Melanoma

Cutaneous melanoma (CM) is a tumor originating from the melanocyte cells of the epidermis, leading to skin pigmentation. CM is potentially the most dangerous type of skin cancer, causing 90% of skin cancer–related mortality.[92] In the United States, 1 in 36 men and 1 in 52 women develop melanoma, with a higher prevalence in the Caucasian population.[93] The World Health Organization estimates that there are 132,000 new melanoma cases worldwide per year.[77]

Risk factors for development of melanoma include intermittent intense sun exposure, sun burns (especially in childhood), fair skinned individuals, persons with freckles, red or blond hair, an increased number of nevi, and family history of melanoma[94,95] (**FIGURES 13.6-13.8**).

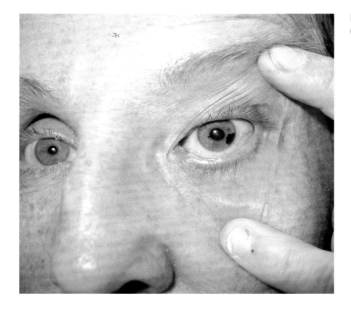

FIGURE 13.7 Ocular melanoma. (Image provided by Stedman's.)

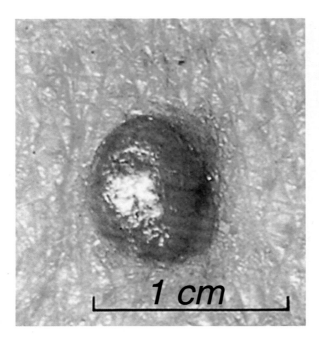

FIGURE 13.8 Nodular melanoma. (From Kronenberger J. *Lippincott Williams & Wilkins' Comprehensive Medical Assisting.* 5th ed. Philadelphia, PA: Wolters Kluwer; 2015.)

Clinical subtypes of melanoma include the following:

- Superficial spreading melanoma (SSM) is the most common subtype, accounting for approximately 70% of all CMs. However, it has a slow rate of progression. It appears more commonly on intermittently sun-exposed areas such as the lower extremities of women and the upper back of men. It frequently appears as a lesion with irregular borders and pigmentation. This includes shades of dark brown to black, bluish, pink, reddish, and grayish white. SSM is the most common subtype associated with preexisting nevi and may present as a focal area of darker pigmentation within the nevus.[96]
- Nodular melanoma (NM) is the second-most common subtype of melanoma and accounts for approximately 15% to 30% of all melanomas. NM appears more frequently as a de novo lesion as opposed to one arising from a preexisting nevus. The trunk is the most common location. Its appearance is most commonly a uniformly dark brown-blue or bluish-red raised nodular lesion. However, 5% are amelanotic (pink-reddish lesions without dark pigment). NM can have a rapid evolution to a vertical growth pattern invading deep into the skin which may confer a bad prognosis.[96]
- Lentigo maligna (LM) and lentigo maligna melanoma (LMM) are related lesions. The former is a subtype of melanoma in situ with a prolonged radial (horizontal) growth phase that may progress to an invasive (through the epidermis to involve the dermis) LMM subtype, which has a vertical growth. LMM constitutes 10% to 15% of all CM. LM and LMM are diagnosed more commonly in the seventh to eight decades of life, in contrast to the other subtypes which can be diagnosed at earlier stages of life. LM appears more frequently as a de novo lesion and just 3% of cases are associated with nevi. The most common site of presentation is on areas chronically exposed to the sun such as the face. This is especially true for the cheeks, nose, neck, scalp, and ears. It is frequently associated with photodamage. Its presentation is a flat lesion with irregular borders and shape. It may have different shades of brown, and it slowly progresses to a nodular lesion with a vertical growth pattern that confers a more aggressive behavior.[96]

- Acral lentiginous melanoma (ALM) prevalence differs among ethnic groups. For example, it constitutes only 2% to 8% of melanomas in Caucasians but represents the most common subtype in darker-pigmented individuals. ALM is diagnosed more often in older persons with a median age of onset of 65 years old. The most common site of presentation is on the sole of the foot, but it can also be seen on the palm and subungual (beneath the nail) locations. It presents as a lesion with irregular borders and pigmentation that can be brown, black, red, or a combination of colors. However, the most common color is brown-black. When ALM is located on the subungual area, it usually affects the great toe or thumb and appears as a brown to black discoloration or growth in the nail bed. Usually, the diagnosis of ALM is made late in life both due to the location and because it is often misdiagnosed. This late diagnosis usually leads to poor outcomes. This subtype of CM is not believed to be associated with sun exposure.[96]

Primary intraocular melanoma is rare, affecting 3000 North Americans each year.[97] The Collaborative Ocular Melanoma Study by the National Eye Institute determined that choroidal melanoma (a form of uveal melanoma) is the most common primary tumor of the eye.[98] Uveal melanoma may less commonly involve the iris (4%) or ciliary body (6%). Much less common than uveal melanoma are melanomas involving the conjunctiva (5%) and other sites (10%) such as the eyelid and lacrimal gland.[99] The symptoms of ocular melanoma include flashes and floaters, diplopia, decreased vision, redness, and eye pain.[77] Patients with cutaneous nevi (especially dysplastic cutaneous nevi) and freckles, iris nevi, and choroidal nevi are at increased risk for ocular melanoma.[99] High-risk features of choroidal nevi transformation to melanoma are shown in **TABLE 13.1** and can be remembered by the mnemonic "To Find Small Ocular Melanoma Use Helpful Hints."[100] Patients with one to two of these risk factors should be monitored at least every 6 months, and those with more than two risk factors should be referred to an ocular oncologist or retinal specialist for evaluation and consideration of treatment.

Factors that raise suspicion for malignancy in pigmented cutaneous lesions include the following[94]:

- A long-standing mole or a new mole including pigmented lesions on the nails, scalp, or mucous membranes which change in shape, color, or size
- Any mole which has three or more colors or has lost its symmetry
- A mole which is itching or bleeding

TABLE 13.1   High-Risk Features for Choroidal Nevus Transformation Into Choroidal Melanoma[100]

Feature	Hazard Ratio for Tumor Growth	P-Value
Thickness >2 mm	2.09	<.001
Fluid	3.16	.002
Symptoms	2.34	.002
Orange pigment	2.75	<.001
Margin ≤3 mm to the disc	1.82	.001
Ultrasonographic hollowness	2.92	<.001
Halo absence	6.48	.009

The diagnosis of CM is initially clinical, and dermoscopy can improve diagnostic accuracy. It is useful to implement the ABCDE algorithm for clinical CM detecting as illustrated[101]:

A (asymmetry): When the lesion is divided into two, the parts are not equal in shape.
B (border): Presence of irregular, poorly defined borders.
C (color): Color variegation. The presence of more than one color in the lesion.
D (diameter): Greater than 6 mm.
E (evolving): Changing of the lesion over time.

Other emerging noninvasive diagnostic techniques that can be considered are reflectance confocal microscopy, electrical impedance spectroscopy, optical coherence tomography, and gene expression analysis.[102] Adequate pictures of the lesion should be obtained and examination of the rest of the skin should take place to look for other lesions. An excisional (complete) biopsy with a margin of 1 to 3 mm around the lesion is recommended. The pathologic report should include Breslow, indicating the thickness of the tumor, presence of ulceration, and mitotic rate (cell proliferation). These are all important predictors of outcomes.[103]

The pathologic staging of CM known as "TNM" is defined by the eighth edition of the American Joint Committee on Cancer. It is based on tumor size (T), nodal involvement (N), and the presence of local or distant metastases (M). This determination of tumor stage directs patient management.[104]

For treatment of melanoma, surgery remains the first line of treatment for primary CM in situ or of any thickness.[103,105] Surgical excision should be performed with margins, depending on tumor thickness, and confirmation of histologically clear margins is recommended.[103]

For example, for CM in situ, excisions should be with margin between 0.5 and 1 cm and a depth to underlying adipose tissue. For invasive tumors, the margin should be between 1 and 2 cm and depth to muscular fascia. Performance of a sentinel lymph node biopsy (SLNB) in tumors with thickness equal or greater than 1 cm is also recommended. SLNB should also be considered in tumors with thickness between 0.8 mm and 1 cm or less than 0.8 mm with presence of other adverse features such as ulceration or lymphovascular invasion.[103] Sentinel lymph node state (positive or negative) has been regarded as the most important prognostic factor.[103,106]

In the event of positive sentinel lymph node, interdisciplinary evaluation is recommended for further management of the patient with consideration of complete lymph node dissection versus regional nodal surveillance.[103]

Patients who have been diagnosed with invasive CM should have a through history to identify symptoms and signs of disseminated disease. Examination should include total body skin including the biopsy site to detect new lesions and lymph node evaluation looking for visible or palpable metastases. The history and examination will direct the need for additionally laboratory and imaging studies.[103]

Although ocular metastatic melanoma is rare, patients with advanced (metastatic) CM must be monitored for the development of metastatic intraocular disease. Symptoms are the same as primary ocular melanoma, but the behavior is more aggressive.[98,107] The most common locations for ocular metastasis are the choroid, retina, vitreous, and ciliary body. Tumor metastases can be bilateral, diffuse, or multifocal.[107,108] The average time interval between the diagnosis of primary CM and metastatic ocular melanoma is 3 years.[107] The treatment for primary or metastatic ocular melanoma includes tumor resection and radiotherapy. Enucleation of the eye should be considered in patients with diffuse ocular disease or extraocular extension.[98,107,109]

The management of advanced CM (presence of nodal or distant metastases) should be performed by an interdisciplinary group. In these cases, improved survival has been demonstrated with drugs targeting the mitogen-activated protein kinase pathway (BRAF and MEK inhibitors) and immune checkpoint blockage to activated T lymphocytes (ie, monoclonal antibodies against cytotoxic T lymphocyte antigen 4 [CTLA-4], programmed death 1 [PD-1], and its programmed death ligand

107. Rosenberg C, Finger PT. Cutaneous malignant melanoma metastatic to the eye, lids, and orbit. *Surv Ophthalmol.* 2008;53:187-202.

108. Solomon JD, Shields CL, Shields JA, Eagle RC Jr. Posterior capsule opacity as initial manifestation of metastatic cutaneous melanoma. *Graefes Arch Clin Exp Ophthalmol.* 2011;249:127-131.

109. Singh P, Singh A. Choroidal melanoma. *Oman J Ophthalmol.* 2012;5:3-9.

110. Ugurel S, Rohmel J, Ascierto PA, et al. Survival of patients with advanced metastatic melanoma: the impact of novel therapies-update 2017. *Eur J Cancer.* 2017;83:247-257.

111. Andtbacka RH, Kaufman HL, Collichio F, et al. Talimogene laherparepvec improves durable response rate in patients with advanced melanoma. *J Clin Oncol.* 2015;33:2780-2788.

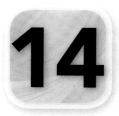

Pulmonary

Tanya Weinstock, Arti Tewari, and Gene Muise

OBJECTIVES

The lungs are a critical organ considering their role in oxygenation, and the importance of respiration is reflected as a key vital sign. In addition, the lungs aid in serum acid/base balance through CO_2 exchange and maintenance of normal arterial perfusion with angiotensin converting enzyme (ACE). Impaired lung function can result from obstructive or restrictive diseases. Obstructive diseases impair airflow and include asthma, chronic obstructive pulmonary disease (COPD), and cystic fibrosis (CF). Restrictive lung diseases result from poor lung compliance with impaired expansion during inhalation and include infections such as pneumonia (Chapter 9) and lung tissue damage with diseases such as sarcoid (Chapter 12). Lung diseases cause a range of symptoms with diffuse impacts in other organ systems. Relevant links to the eye include pharmacologic considerations such as drug adverse effects and drug interactions.

KEY CONCEPTS

Asthma and allergic disease
COPD

Drug therapy for asthma and COPD
Cystic fibrosis

SECTION 1: ASTHMA AND ALLERGIC DISEASE

Asthma is a heterogeneous disease that is usually characterized by airway inflammation and mucus production. It is typically defined by a history of respiratory symptoms such as wheeze, shortness of breath, chest tightness, and cough that vary over time in intensity with variable expiratory flow limitation. Respiratory symptoms typically occur following an exposure to a trigger such as allergens, exercise, environmental pollutants (eg, tobacco smoke), or respiratory viral infection.[1] In approximately 75% of cases, asthma is diagnosed before the age of 7. The population prevalence of asthma in the United States is 7.9%, with a higher incidence in children at 8.4% as is typical for this disease.[2]

The classic symptoms of asthma include wheezing, cough that is often worse at night, and shortness of breath. Symptoms are episodic and vary in severity with the time course of hours to days and may resolve spontaneously with removal of stimulating triggers. A mainstay of treatment is identifying and eliminating the allergens and other environmental exposures that are common causes of asthma exacerbations. Many patients with asthma have a strong family history of asthma or other atopic diseases, though a minority of asthma is considered nonallergic asthma, seen more often in adults.

Asthma is a heterogeneous clinical entity with presentations that can be considered allergic and nonallergic. The majority of asthma is allergic, especially in children. In allergic diseases, IgE is produced by plasma cells and responds to environmental triggers. Interactions between IgE and mast cells result in the release of histamine, leukotrienes, and other mediators, which results in a range of symptoms from asthma to atopic skin disease. Pulmonary symptoms also result from airway abnormalities including hypertrophy and hyperresponsiveness. The typical cascade of asthma thus begins with exposure to one or more triggers that results in airway inflammation and mucus secretion, airway narrowing, and the typical respiratory symptoms.

Diffuse wheezing is a typical physical exam finding during an asthma exacerbation. Wheezes are typically expiratory and have multiple pitches owing to involvement of airways of different sizes. In very severe exacerbations, wheezes may no longer be audible as air movement is extremely limited due to airway narrowing. Patients with severe airflow obstruction will exhibit tachypnea, tachycardia, and a prolonged inspiratory:expiratory (I:E) ratio. The I:E ratio refers to the proportion of the respiratory cycle spent inhaling versus exhaling; a normal ratio is 1:2; however, with symptomatic asthma, airway narrowing requires more time spent exhaling. Many patients with a low I:E ratio will exhibit tripod breathing; when seated, they use extended arms rested on the thighs to support the upper chest. There are certain extrapulmonary manifestations that can be seen in allergic asthma, including edema in the nasal cavities, nasal polyps, atopic dermatitis with lichenified plaques in a flexural distribution, and digital clubbing. Ocular findings include Dennie-Morgan lines and Hertoghe sign, in which there is loss of the lateral third of the brow (as also occurs in hypothyroidism) (**FIGURE 14.1**).

The diagnosis of asthma is confirmed with spirometry, where a maximal inhalation is followed by a forceful exhalation, leading to a measurement of forced expiratory volume in 1 second (FEV1) and forced vital capacity (FVC). This ratio is reduced in asthma, indicating an obstructive pattern characteristic of the disease. Once an obstructive physiology (versus restrictive) has been identified, the severity of airflow obstruction is categorized by the degree to which FEV1 is reduced below normal. Most importantly, asthma is characterized by reversibility of obstruction with the use of bronchodilators. Acute reversibility is tested by giving a dose (usually 2 puffs) of a bronchodilator and repeating spirometry after 15 minutes. An increase in FEV1 by more than 12% and greater than 200 mL confirms bronchodilator responsiveness.

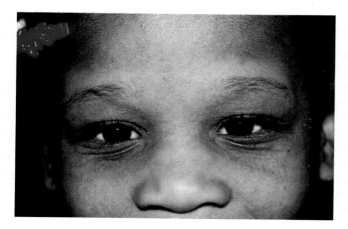

FIGURE 14.1 Eyelid atopic dermatitis. Note lichenification and the characteristic double fold (Dennie-Morgan line) that extends from the inner to the outer canthus of the lower eyelid and the "allergic shiners," the darkening color of the periorbital areas. (From Goodheart HP. *Goodheart's Photoguide of Common Skin Disorders.* 2nd ed. Philadelphia, PA: Lippincott Williams & Wilkins; 2003.)

> **BOX 14.1**   Key Components of an Asthma Action Plan
>
> **Green Zone:** Peak flow 80% to 100% of normal. Continue current treatment plan.
>
> **Yellow Zone:** Peak flow 50% to 80% of normal. Augment treatment; get help if not improving.
>
> **Red Zone:** Peak flow <50% of normal. Take an emergency treatment and get help.

Peak flow is often used to monitor patients with moderate or severe asthma. By adding an objective measure (the peak flow) to a patient's subjective symptoms, the disease can be monitored and managed over time through periods of exacerbation and remission. Peak flow can be measured by the patient in a community setting (eg, at home, in school) and consists of a single measurement made during a forceful exhalation. Bronchodilators are given to improve peak flow. An improvement of approximately 20% after bronchodilator administration is seen in asthma.

Asthma management focuses on addressing the symptoms of asthma (cough, chest tightness, wheeze, or shortness of breath), reducing the need for inhaled bronchodilators (short-acting beta-agonists [SABA]), reducing nighttime awakenings, and maintaining a normal level of activity. All of these goals reduce the risk of exacerbations and limit the need for urgent evaluations and hospitalization (**BOX 14.1**).

Asthma treatment has three major components:

- Environmental controls
- Reliever drug (bronchodilator)
- Controller drugs

Asthma action plans have come into practice to allow patients to manage their individual asthma therapy based on the severity of their symptoms. The patient's normal peak expiratory flow rate is used to construct a personalized asthma action plan with colored zones defined by percent change from the normal peak flow obtained while asymptomatic. Plans are implemented based on a patient's symptom diary and home measurement of peak flow day to day. The action plan includes specific instructions on treatments such as the dose and frequency of controller medications, use of reliever medication as needed or before exercise, and managing triggers to prevent an exacerbation. The plan also provides an indication of when disease severity requires assistance.

The standard stepwise approach to pharmacotherapy is based on increasing medications until asthma is controlled, while remaining cognizant of possible side effects.[3] When determining appropriate therapy for patients who are not already on a controller medication, the first step is classifying the severity of the patient's symptoms. Asthma severity is determined by considering symptoms over the past 2 to 4 weeks, current level of lung function (peak flow or FEV1/FVC values), and the number of exacerbations in the past year.

Mild *intermittent asthma* symptoms can be managed with a SABA bronchodilator alone when use is infrequent. When the SABA is required more than a few times per week for symptom relief (excluding use in prevention of exercise-induced asthma), daily controller medications are recommended. First-line options for controller therapies in so-called *persistent asthma* include two groups of medications: inhaled corticosteroids (ICS) or glucocorticoids and leukotriene receptor antagonists (LTRA). For more severe disease and frequent exacerbations, higher doses of glucocorticoid and the combined use of both of these drug classes are recommended. Long-acting beta-agonists (LABA) are also added to regimens used to treat more severe disease, although some LABA agents (namely formoterol) can be used as a reliever therapy as well. Patients with severe allergic asthma may also be candidates for biological therapies aimed at reducing the burden of IgE (such as omalizumab). Common pulmonary medications used in asthma as well as COPD are discussed later in the chapter (Section 3).

SEASONAL ALLERGIES

Seasonal allergies lead to allergic symptoms including rhinitis, sinusitis, and conjunctivitis occurring at a particular time of the year. There are a number of identified risk factors, including a family history of atopy, male sex, maternal smoking exposure in the first year of life, and a serum IgE level >100 U/mL before age 6. Presenting symptoms are typically sneezing paroxysms, rhinorrhea, and fatigue. Patients who also have seasonal allergic conjunctivitis (SAC) present with symptoms including ocular injection, itching, tearing, or burning. Allergic conjunctivitis is discussed further below. Allergy is classified both by temporal patterns and severity.

- Intermittent allergic rhinitis: symptoms are present less than 4 days a week or for less than 4 weeks.
- Persistent allergic rhinitis: symptoms are present more than 4 days a week and for more than 4 weeks.

Moderate to severe allergic rhinitis includes sleep disturbances, impairment of work performance, or impairment of daily activities.

Seasonal allergies are mostly caused by pollen from trees, grasses, and weeds. Pollination periods depend on the geographic area. Symptoms are therefore predictable and reproducible from year to year. Persistent nasal mucosal inflammation develops with repeat exposure, which leads to a more significant response to a smaller exposure as time passes.

Physical exam findings often include orbital edema or "allergic shiners" (**FIGURE 14.2**), accentuated transverse folds beneath the eyelids (Dennie-Morgan lines), and/or a transverse nasal crease caused by repeated rubbing. Labs are generally normal, including serum IgE. Allergy skin testing can confirm that the patient is sensitized, but is not necessary for diagnosis, which can be made clinically. In patients with poorly controlled symptoms or coexisting systemic manifestations of allergy such as asthma, atopic dermatitis, or recurrent sinusitis, testing for allergens may be more helpful as seasonal allergies can also overlap with sinusitis, asthma, and atopic dermatitis.

SAC or "hay fever conjunctivitis" is the most common form of allergic conjunctivitis and specifically occurs during allergy season, due to outdoor environmental exposures. It is clinically distinguished from the other most common forms of allergic conjunctivitis: acute allergic conjunctivitis

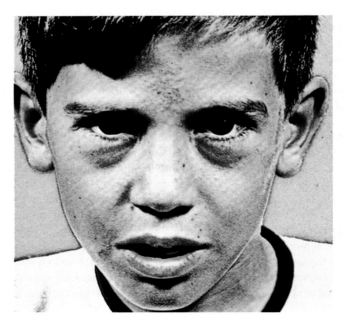

FIGURE 14.2 Perennial allergic rhinitis. The child suffering from perennial allergic rhinitis has an open mouth (cannot breathe through the nose) and edema and discoloration of the lower orbitopalpebral grooves ("allergic shiners"). (From Bickley LS. *Bates' Guide to Physical Examination and History Taking.* 8th ed. Philadelphia, PA: Wolters Kluwer; 2002.)

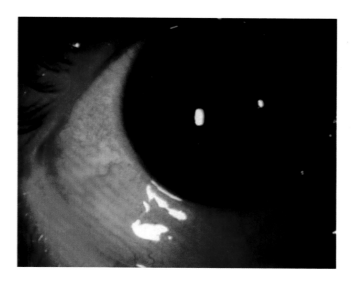

FIGURE 14.3 Diffuse hyperemia and bulbar chemosis are typical of seasonal allergic conjunctivitis. (From Gerstenblith AT. *Wills Eye Manual.* 6th ed. Philadelphia, PA: Wolters Kluwer; 2012.)

(sudden-onset due to acute allergen exposure) and perennial allergic conjunctivitis (a more chronic conjunctivitis related to year-round indoor allergen exposures, such as dust mites and mold). Diagnosis of SAC normally occurs first in childhood. Clinical history of atopy and/or other seasonal allergy symptoms, in particular allergic rhinitis, are often present. Hallmark symptoms are redness and itching, while burning, photophobia, tearing, and watery or mild mucoid discharge may also be present. Examination shows diffuse conjunctival hyperemia and chemosis (**FIGURE 14.3**) with a mild papillary reaction of the inferior palpebral conjunctiva. Upper tarsal papillary reaction is not typically prominent in SAC as in other more chronic and severe forms of allergic conjunctivitis. Ancillary testing to confirm the diagnosis is typically not necessary when history and examination findings are consistent. SAC is most commonly treated with topical antihistamines, mast cell stabilizers, or combination drops which include both of these drugs. Mild topical steroids (eg, loteprednol, etabonate) and topical lubrication agents also have a role. While some oral antihistamine-decongestant medications may prove useful in treating the conjunctivitis associated with seasonal allergies, isolated eye disease should be treated topically since oral agents carry risk for ocular side effects (see "Clinical Pearls") and systemic symptoms such as drowsiness.[4]

Seasonal allergy treatment starts with steps to avoid specific allergens. In some cases, particularly in children, remarkable improvement can be seen by simply having parents wash the child's hair nightly before bed. This ensures that pollen is not transferred to the pillowcase and inhaled all night. When allergens cannot be avoided, therapy can be initiated, often by patients using over-the-counter products without medical supervision.

Over-the-counter antihistamines, nasal glucocorticoids, and decongestants are readily available and typically used first-line. They all offer some degree of effectiveness for mild to moderate symptoms. Despite the easy availability of these medications, there are important precautions that are specific to each individual agent. First-generation antihistamines (such as diphenhydramine) are sedating and even nighttime dosing may impair next-day motor performance.[5] Stimulant effects of oral decongestants (phenylephrine, pseudoephedrine) can increase blood pressure and heart rate; they should be avoided in the setting of hypertension and some arrhythmias. In addition, some over-the-counter allergy relief medications contain a combination of drugs, which may include an analgesic such as acetaminophen or an NSAID, along with diphenhydramine and phenylephrine. The combinations are confusing for patients who are not familiar with the ingredients, which results in a heightened risk of drug-disease and drug-drug interactions as well as inadvertent overdoses (often in the analgesic component) when used together with other over-the-counter remedies.

SECTION 2: CHRONIC OBSTRUCTIVE PULMONARY DISEASE

COPD is a common, chronic pulmonary disease characterized by progressive fixed airflow obstruction. The reported prevalence of COPD diagnosed in the United States is 6.4%; however, the true rate is likely higher as people with mild airflow restriction are typically asymptomatic and unaware of their condition.[6] COPD is the third leading cause of death in the United States.[7] By far, the most common risk factor for the development of COPD is cigarette smoking. Other environmental factors such as air pollutants can influence COPD risk and are seen disproportionately in developing countries. Lower socioeconomic status is a risk factor for COPD. Advancing age and a history of asthma are also risk factors.

COPD is characterized by poorly reversible airway obstruction, which is confirmed by spirometry, and includes obstruction of the small airways and emphysema. Small airway obstruction leads to impaired gas exchange, air trapping, and shortness of breath, specifically in response to physical exertion. The mechanism of disease in COPD is not entirely understood, but there are associations with chronic inflammation, accelerated aging of the lung, and breakdown of the repair mechanism, leading to oxidative stress. Impaired gas exchange leads to hypercapnia (high CO_2 levels) and hypoxemia (low oxygen levels). Acute exacerbations are generally triggered by infection or environmental exposures, and frequent exacerbations are linked to overall poor prognosis.

One challenge with making an early diagnosis is that symptoms may be underreported in patients who minimally engage in physical activity. Presenting symptoms for COPD are typically a constellation of exertional dyspnea, cough, sputum production, chest tightness, or fatigue. Spirometry is the reference standard for the initial diagnosis and assessment of the severity of COPD which is reflected by a reduced FEV1 and FEV1:FVC ratio. If obstruction is present on spirometry, a short-acting bronchodilator can be administered with repeat spirometry to establish the diagnosis based upon incompletely reversible obstruction. Spirometry is also used to monitor for disease progression.

On physical exam, auscultation of prolonged airflow at the trachea during maximal forced effort can be useful in early diagnosis of obstruction. Breath sounds such as expiratory wheezing and rhonchi are rarely present in stable patients but can indicate an acute exacerbation.

In 1998, the Global Initiative for Chronic Obstructive Lung Disease (GOLD) was established. The purpose of this initiative was to focus on management and prevention of COPD. Guidelines were established, and the first consensus report for treatment of COPD was published in 2001. Currently, the global initiative for COPD promotes the "ABCD" assessment of COPD patients based on symptom severity and risk of exacerbation.[8]

- GOLD group A includes patients with low symptom severity and low risk of exacerbation.
- GOLD group B includes patients with high symptom severity and lower exacerbation risk.
- GOLD group C includes patients with low symptom severity but high exacerbation risk.
- GOLD group D includes patients with high symptom severity and high exacerbation risk.

When evaluating prognosis for patients with COPD, an assessment of risk for future acute exacerbations and death is of primary importance. A patient's history of COPD exacerbations, especially in the past year, has been shown to have a statistically significant relationship with increased risk for future exacerbations and death.[9]

Treatment at any level of disease severity should always include smoking cessation counseling including pharmacologic management when necessary. Appropriate immunizations against respiratory pathogens with seasonal influenza vaccine and pneumococcal vaccine (Chapter 9) are also an important part of treatment (TABLE 14.1).

Currently, the mainstay of pharmacotherapy for symptoms is with bronchodilators in the muscarinic antagonist class or β-agonist class. Muscarinic antagonists block M1 and M3 muscarinic

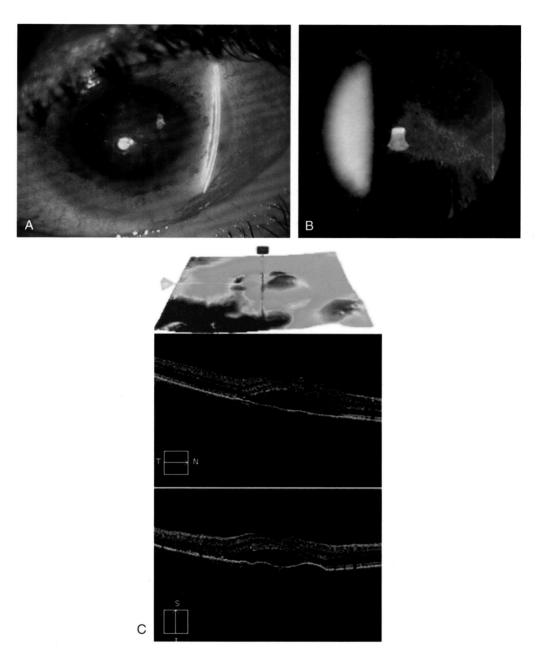

FIGURE 14.4 Systemic drugs used in allergy, asthma, and chronic obstructive pulmonary disease may demonstrate adverse ophthalmic effects. A, Acute angle closure may result from mydriasis caused by systemic anticholinergics and antihistamines. Note the shallow anterior chamber and mid-dilated pupil. B, Posterior subcapsular cataract is a well-known side effect of systemic corticosteroids. C, Central serous chorioretinopathy (as demonstrated by optical coherence tomography imaging) may flare or be exacerbated with the chronic use of systemic corticosteroids. (A, From Gerstenblith AT. *Wills Eye Manual.* 6th ed. Philadelphia, PA: Wolters Kluwer; 2012. B, Courtesy of Julia Monsonego, CRA. C, From Alfaro DV. *Age-Related Macular Degeneration.* 2nd ed. Philadelphia, PA: Wolters Kluwer; 2014.)

CF in adults leads to both acute and recurrent pancreatitis due to defective secretion of pancreatic acinar cells. Pancreatic dysfunction and insufficiency often lead to exocrine gland dysfunction and glucose intolerance, inducing CF-related diabetes. CF patients with diabetes should have regular monitoring for diabetic retinopathy with an optometrist. Focal biliary cirrhosis can also be due to inspissated bile causing elevations of serum alkaline phosphatase and lobular hepatomegaly. Some of these patients progress to periportal fibrosis, cirrhosis, and variceal bleeding.

CLINICAL PEARLS
Potential ocular involvement in CF includes:

- Dry eye syndrome
- Nyctalopia, xerophthalmia, and pigmented retinopathy from vitamin A deficiency
- Diabetic retinopathy in cases of CF-related pancreatic insufficiency

In adult male patients, infertility is common. More than 95% of men with CF are infertile due to defective sperm transport. Many also have absent vas deferens in the setting of disrupted organogenesis due to a defective CFTR. In females with CF, infertility is more common than the general population but not as common as in men with CF; this is thought to be due to abnormal production of cervical mucus.

Typical respiratory manifestations of CF include a persistent, productive cough, lung hyperinflation, and obstruction identified on pulmonary function tests. Over time, bronchiectasis develops with symptoms including a new cough, new increased sputum production, decreased exercise tolerance, increased fatigue, decreased appetite, and increased nasal congestion. FEV1 is typically the first change seen in pulmonary function assessment. The specific diagnosis is made from a change from baseline, not by specific parameters. As the disease progresses, patients are more likely to develop chronic bronchitis with typical organisms. In children, respiratory infections are most commonly caused by *Staphylococcus aureus* and *Haemophilus influenza* species. In adulthood, *Pseudomonas aeruginosa* infections are unfortunately more common, likely due to impaired clearance induced by a defective CFTR. Recurrent infection leads to bronchial wall destruction, loss of cartilaginous support, and eventually bronchiectasis.

The Cystic Fibrosis Foundation reported that roughly 35% of patients have at least one pulmonary exacerbation severe enough to require IV antibiotics in their lifetime. Roughly 20% of these patients fail to recover from these exacerbations. The leading cause of morbidity and mortality in patients is pulmonary disease, primarily due to acute infection. Medication therapy is focused on promoting secretion clearance and antibiosis.

Antibiotics are indicated in all consensus guidelines[19] for management of acute pulmonary exacerbations. When initiating empiric antibiotics (Chapter 9), the inclusion of double antibiotic coverage for *Pseudomonas* species has been shown to improve pulmonary function and reduce sputum bacterial density. Refining therapy is based on growth of cultures from expectorated sputum. Many patients grow multiple organisms, and in these cases, a combination of antibiotics that cover all isolates is crucial, but may result in long-term administration of broad-spectrum antibiotics. Pseudomonal infections are treated typically with piperacillin-tazobactam or carbapenems plus a fluoroquinolone or amikacin. A similar regimen is used for concomitant methicillin-sensitive *S. aureus*. For methicillin-resistant *S. aureus*, vancomycin or linezolid would be added to typical pseudomonal coverage. The duration of antibiotics is based on symptom resolution, so the course of therapy can be anywhere from 10 days to several weeks.

Medications to clear respiratory secretions include inhaled DNase, hypertonic saline, and mannitol. DNase is an endonuclease that cleaves strands of denatured DNA that are released during the inflammatory state by degrading neutrophils. This action decreases the viscosity of typically purulent sputum. Hypertonic saline is typically used in conjunction with DNase. The high osmolality of hypertonic saline draws water from the airway to re-establish the surface area that is usually infiltrated by sputum in patients with CF. Inhaled mannitol is primarily used as a second-line option for patients who fail DNase and hypertonic saline.

New therapies recently FDA approved in the last 8 years include oral CFTR modulator therapy, which functions to amplify or correct protein function and can treat 90% of gene mutations in CF. These therapies have been shown to markedly improve respiratory symptoms, FEV1, incidence of exacerbation and infection, and quality of life. Noncongenital cataracts in children taking the CFTR modulator ivacaftor have been reported, and monitoring is recommended.

Other therapies include chest physiotherapy and anti-inflammatory medications, such as azithromycin and glucocorticoids. Glucocorticoids are typically used in patients exhibiting asthma-like symptoms, including wheeze or chest tightness. Chronic azithromycin is often added for its anti-inflammatory purposes. Optimization of nutritional status and supervised exercise will also help patients' overall health and well-being.

REFERENCES

1. Dharmage SC, Perret JL, Custovic A. Epidemiology of asthma in children and adults. *Front Pediatr.* 2019;7:246. doi:10.3389/fped.2019.00246.

2. *2017 National Health Interview Survey (NHIS).* Accessed February 28, 2020. https://www.cdc.gov/asthma/most_recent_national_asthma_data.htm.

3. Global Initiative For Asthma (GINA). *Global Strategy for Asthma Management and Prevention.* 2019. https://ginasthma.org.

4. O'Brien TB. Allergic conjunctivitis: an update on diagnosis and management. *Curr Opin Allergy Clin Immunol.* 2013;13(5):543-549.

5. Zhang D, Tashiro M, Shibuya K, et al. Next-day residual sedative effect after nighttime administration of an over-the-counter antihistamine sleep aid, diphenhydramine, measured by positron emission tomography. *J Clin Psychopharmacol.* 2010;30(6):694-701.

6. Wheaton AG, Cunningham TJ, Ford ES, Croft JB; Centers for Disease Control and Prevention (CDC). Employment and activity limitations among adults with chronic obstructive pulmonary disease – United States, 2013. *MMWR Morb Mortal Wkly Rep.* 2015;64(11):290-295.

7. National Center for Health Statistics. *Health, United States 2015 With Special Feature on Racial and Ethnic Health Disparities.* Hyattsville, MD: US Dept Health and Human Services; 2016.

8. The Global Initiative for Chronic Obstructive Lung Disease. *Global Strategy for the Diagnosis, Management and Prevention of Chronic Obstructive Pulmonary Disease* :2020 Report. http://www.goldcopd.org.

9. Cardoso J, Coelho R, Rocha C, Coelho C, Semedo L, Bugalho Almeida A. Prediction of severe exacerbations and mortality in COPD: the role of exacerbation history and inspiratory capacity/total lung capacity ratio. *Int J Chron Obstruct Pulmon Dis.* 2018;13:1105-1113. doi:10.2147/COPD.S155848.

10. Garbe E, LeLorier J, Boivin J, Suissa S. Inhaled and nasal glucocorticoids and the risks of ocular hypertension or open-angle glaucoma. *J Am Med Assoc.* 1997;277(9):722-727. doi:10.1001/jama.1997.03540330044033.

11. Salpeter SR, Buckley NS, Ormiston TM, Salpeter EE. Meta-analysis: effect of long-acting beta-agonists on severe asthma exacerbations and asthma-related deaths. *Ann Intern Med.* 2006;144(12):904-912.

12. Bartlett JD, Jaanus SD. Ocular adverse drug reactions to systemic medications. In: Bartlett JD, Jaanus SD, eds. *Clinical Ocular Pharmacology.* 5th ed. St. Louis, Missouri: Butterworth-Heinemann; 2008:701-59

13. Lachkar Y, Bouassida W. Drug-induced acute angle closure glaucoma. *Curr Opin Ophthalmol.* 2007;18(2):129-133

14. Haimovici R, Gragoudas ES, Duker JS, Sjaarda RN, Elliott D. Central serous retinopathy associated with inhaled or intranasal corticosteroids. *Ophtahlmology.* 1997;104(10):1653-1660

15. Fardin B, Weissgold DJ. Central serous chorioretinopathy after inhaled steroid use for post-mycoplasmal broncho-spasm. *Br J Ophthalmol.* 2002;86(9):1065-1066

16. Roddy MF, Greally P, Clancy G, Leen G, Feehan S, Elnazir B. Night blindness in a teenager with cystic fibrosis. *Nutr Clin Pract.* 2011;26(6):718-721.

17. Joshi D, Dhawan A, Baker AJ, Heneghan MA. An atypical presentation of cystic fibrosis: a case report. *J Med Case Reports.* 2008;2:201.

18. Morkeberg JC, Edmund C, Prause JU, Lanng S, Koch C, Michaelsen KF. Ocular findings in cystic fibrosis patients receiving vitamin A supplementation. *Graefes Arch Clin Exp Ophthalmol.* 1995;233(11):709-713.

19. Mogayzel PJ Jr, Naureckas ET, Robinson KA, et al. Cystic fibrosis pulmonary guidelines. Chronic medications for maintenance of lung health. *Am J Respir Crit Care Med.* 2013;187(7):680-689.

15 Neuroimaging: Diagnostic Imaging of the Orbit and Visual Pathway

Daniel T. Ginat and Emily R. Humphreys

LEARNING OBJECTIVES

This chapter reviews diagnostic imaging of the orbit and visual pathway as it pertains to optometry. In particular, relevant anatomy and lesions depicted on CT and MRI are reviewed. Neuroimaging modalities can be used to help confirm, classify, and localize suspected orbital or neurological pathology detected during an optometric examination.

KEY CONCEPTS

- Neuroradiology modalities and basic principles
- Basic imaging anatomy

- Examples of abnormal pathology on imaging

IMAGING MODALITIES AND BASIC PRINCIPLES

Certain orbital and neurological signs and symptoms discovered during optometric examination warrant neuroimaging, primarily with computed tomography (CT) and magnetic resonance imaging (MRI). Clinical findings that warrant neuroimaging include:

- noncongenital ptosis
- proptosis
- ophthalmoplegia
- optic nerve edema
- optic neuropathies
- visual field defects
- pupillary defects
- vision loss without a specific ocular cause

Image modality choice is dependent on the underlying suspected pathology and is guided by patient characteristics and the clinical exam findings. In clinical practice, it is appropriate to defer to the expertise of the radiologist for guidance. CT and MRI each have advantages and disadvantages, as indicated in **TABLE 15.1**. In addition, the reader may also reference the American College of Radiology Appropriateness Criteria for further guidance regarding the selection of pertinent imaging.

TABLE 15.1 **Comparison of Computed Tomography (CT) and Magnetic Resonance Imaging (MRI) for Neuroimaging**

Modality	Advantages	Disadvantages
CT	• Excellent delineation of bone • Better suited for trauma cases • Short scan time	• Ionizing radiation exposure • Can be limited by metal artifacts
MRI	• Superior soft-tissue delineation, particularly of the optic nerve • Better suited for characterizing different types of tumors	• Relatively long scan time • Can induce claustrophobia • Often loud • Can be limited by metal artifacts

Computed Tomography

CT scans are acquired using x-rays transmitted through the patient at a variety of angles, producing images based on the differences in x-ray attenuation (or reduction of intensity) through the body. Different tissues attenuate x-rays to varying degrees, and this can be quantified using Hounsfield Units (HU), as depicted in **TABLE 15.2**. In addition, CT images can be viewed in different anatomic levels and "window" settings, such as "bone window," which normalizes the grayscale to a range that better highlights bone, and "soft-tissue window," which does the same for soft tissue.

Magnetic Resonance Imaging

Magnetic resonance imaging (MRI) uses a magnetic field to align water protons in the body with the direction of the scanner magnetic field. In the body's natural state, proton spins are randomly oriented. Once protons are aligned, radio waves are pulsed—exciting the protons to a higher energy level. When the radio waves are turned off, the protons return to their baseline state. This process releases a radio-frequency signal, which is detected by coils and converted into an image using a computer. Different tissues will produce different signals based on their innate physical characteristics, with corresponding differing intensities on the final image.

MRI exams comprise various "sequences" that provide different views of the anatomy based on differing characteristics of tissue signal. Different sequences have different patterns of proton excitation and relaxation. Utilizing multiple sequences during one MRI scan improves diagnostic capability. There are many MRI sequences available, of which a few of the most common are discussed below and summarized in **TABLE 15.3**:

- *T1-weighted images (T1W)*: T1 (longitudinal relaxation time)-weighted sequences are considered "fat-weighted," in which fat appears bright and cerebrospinal fluid (CSF) is dark. Gadolinium-based contrast is also bright (see section on contrast), and therefore is administered with T1W sequences.
- *T2-weighted images (T2W)*: T2 (transverse relaxation time)-weighted sequences are considered "water-weighted," where CSF is bright and fat is dark. T2W images are useful for inflammatory optic neuropathies, as the pathologic nerve will appear brighter than the normal nerve or other white matter.
- *Fluid attenuation inversion recovery (FLAIR)*: FLAIR sequences suppress CSF signal in T2W images of the brain, making certain lesions more conspicuous (eg, white matter lesions in multiple sclerosis located next to the ventricles, which may be masked by the bright CSF without FLAIR). This sequence is not routinely performed to evaluate the orbital contents.

TABLE 15.2 Attenuation Values of Different Materials on CT		
Tissue	**CT**	**Attenuation (HU)**
Air		−1000
Fluid (CSF, vitreous)		0-15
Brain		20-45
Fat		−200 to −50
Bone		200-1000

CSF, cerebrospinal fluid; CT, computed tomography; HU, Hounsfield units.
Image credit: Dr Daniel T. Ginat, MD.

TABLE 15.3 Comparison of Tissue Appearance on Various Magnetic Resonance Imaging (MRI) Sequences

Tissue	T1-Weighted (T1W)	T2-Weighted (T2W)	T2-Weighted (T2W) FLAIR
Fluid (CSF, vitreous)			
White matter			
Gray matter			
Fat			

CSF, cerebrospinal fluid; FLAIR, fluid-attenuated inversion recovery; T1, longitudinal relaxation time; T2, transverse relaxation time.

Image credit: Dr Daniel T. Ginat, MD.

- *Diffusion-weighted images (DWI)*: Diffusion-weighted sequences are used to detect acute infarct. This sequence is sensitive to the movement of protons. Restricted diffusion, such as in the case of acute ischemia, confines the protons within the intracellular and extracellular spaces, resulting in less dissipation of signal.
- *Fat-suppressed images*: Since fat is bright on T1 and T2 sequences, eliminating signal from fat helps make some lesions more conspicuous. This is especially useful when assessing orbital pathology, given the large volume of intraorbital fat.

Imaging Planes

Both CT and MRI can produce cross-sectional images in different planes: axial, coronal, and sagittal (**FIGURE 15.1**). Viewing pathology in more than one plane can be helpful to analyze areas of interest. For example, coronal views are good for looking at the orbital contents, sinuses, and the relationship of the pituitary to the chiasm. Axial scans are beneficial for viewing the brainstem, globe, cavernous sinus, and occipital lobe. Viewing the pituitary gland and brainstem with sagittal scans are also helpful. Images are oriented with the right side of the body on the left, and vice versa, as if one was standing at the patient's feet and looking toward the head as they lie on the imaging table.

Contrast Agents

Intravenous contrast can be administered with CT and MRI. When contrast is used, blood within vessels, blood leaking out of vessels, highly vascularized soft tissue (eg, tumors, inflammation), and demyelination will appear brighter ("enhance") on the selected images. Pre- and postcontrast images can be compared and are especially useful in cases of inflammation, as postcontrast images will show significant enhancement in comparison to precontrast images. For example, the optic nerve will usually be relatively bright on T2W images compared with the brain due to any kind of optic neuropathy (eg, glaucoma, optic neuritis, ischemic optic neuropathy), but it will only enhance with contrast due to inflammatory pathologies like optic neuritis (Chapter 12).

CT uses iodine-based contrast, whereas MRI uses gadolinium-based contrast. Allergies can be a problem with contrast agents, most commonly the iodine-based contrast agents. Typically, contrast is avoided altogether if the patient has a history of severe allergic reaction. Contrast is a relative contraindication for minor allergic reactions; some patients may receive an antihistamine and steroids prior to administration of the contrast to help reduce risk.

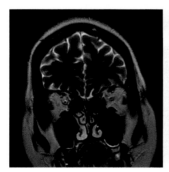 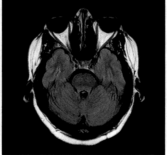 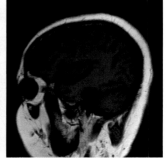

FIGURE 15.1 Coronal (T2-weighted), axial (T2-weighted FLAIR [fluid-attenuated inversion recovery]), and sagittal (T1-weighted) sequences of a normal brain. (Image credit: Dr Daniel T. Ginat, MD.)

An additional contraindication for contrast administration is poor kidney function. Typically serum creatinine and glomerular filtration rate are checked prior to the administration of contrast. The iodine-based x-ray contrast carries a higher risk of acute kidney injury. Newer gadolinium agents are likely less toxic than once believed, and it is up to the radiologist whether kidney function is ordered prior to contrast administration for MRI. The newer gadolinium agents are also less likely to cause a rare but serious complication known as nephrogenic systemic fibrosis. This toxic reaction results from gadolinium remaining in body tissues for an extended period, typically due to poor kidney function.

BASIC IMAGING ANATOMY

The normal imaging anatomy of the orbit and visual pathway is illustrated in **TABLES 15.4** and **15.5**. Associated abnormalities are described and depicted in the following sections.

TABLE 15.4   **Imaging Anatomy of the Orbit**

Structure	CT (Soft-Tissue Window)		T2W MRI		T1W MRI	
	R	L	R	L	R	L
Anterior chamber (a) Lens (b) Posterior chamber (c) Posterior globe wall (d), including sclera and uvea						
Optic nerve (a) Optic nerve sheath (b)						
Superior rectus (a) Superior oblique (b) Medial rectus (c) Inferior rectus (d) Lateral rectus (e)						

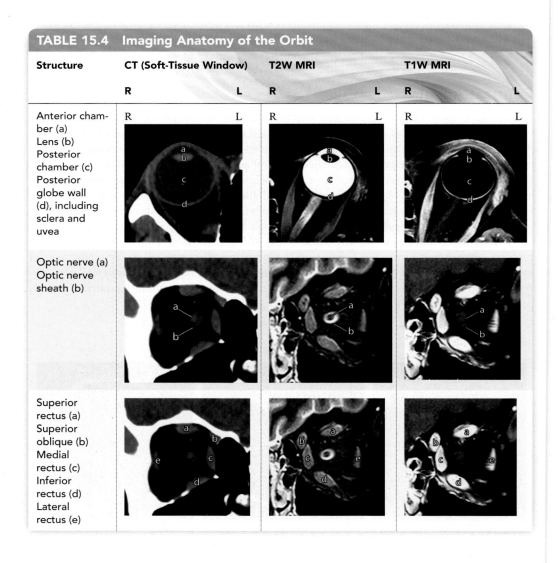

TABLE 15.4   Imaging Anatomy of the Orbit   (Continued)

Structure	CT (Soft-Tissue Window)		T2W MRI		T1W MRI	
	R	L	R	L	R	L
Lacrimal gland (a) Nasolacrimal duct (b)	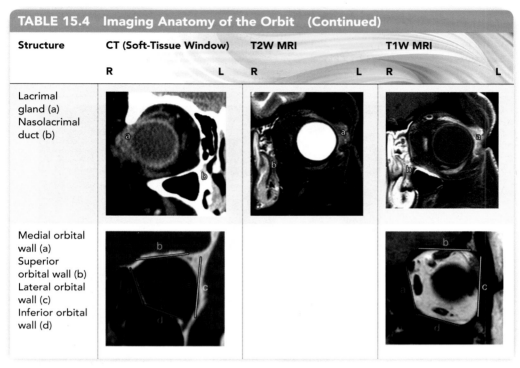					
Medial orbital wall (a) Superior orbital wall (b) Lateral orbital wall (c) Inferior orbital wall (d)						

CT, computed tomography; T1W, T1-weighted; T2W, T2-weighted.
Image credit: Dr Daniel T. Ginat, MD.

TABLE 15.5   Imaging Anatomy of the Visual Pathway

Visual Pathway Structure	T1-Weighted MRI Coronal Plane		T1-Weighted MRI Axial Plane	
	R	L	R	L
Optic nerve	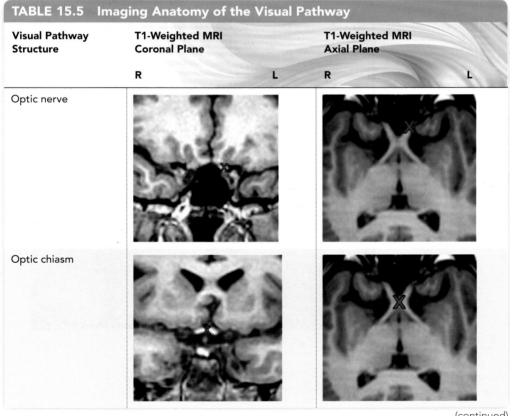			
Optic chiasm				

(continued)

TABLE 15.5 Imaging Anatomy of the Visual Pathway (Continued)

Visual Pathway Structure	T1-Weighted MRI Coronal Plane		T1-Weighted MRI Axial Plane	
	R	L	R	L

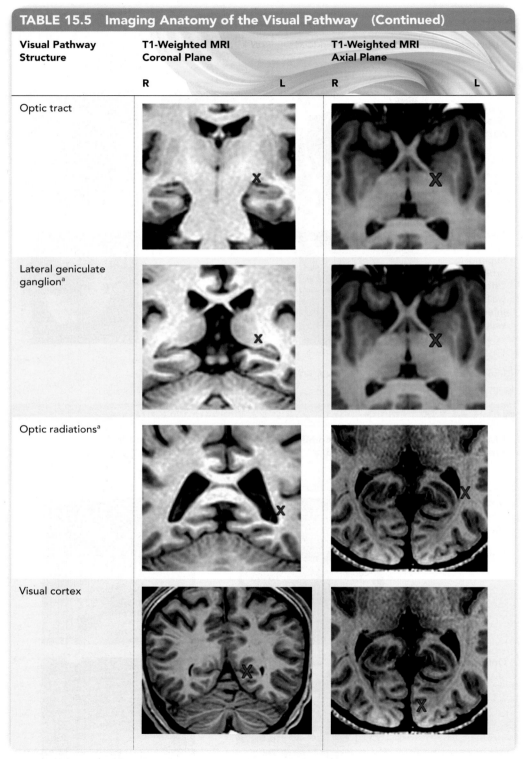

Optic tract

Lateral geniculate ganglion[a]

Optic radiations[a]

Visual cortex

MRI, magnetic resonance imaging.

[a]Approximate location.

Image credit: Dr Daniel T. Ginat, MD.

IMAGING OF ORBITAL ABNORMALITIES

Developmental globe abnormality: The globe normally measures approximately 22 to 25 mm in diameter beyond 1 year of age. Deformity of the globe can be caused by staphylomas or colobomas. Enlargement of the globe, known as buphthalmos, is most frequently seen in congenital glaucoma. In contrast, microphthalmos is a globe measuring less than 16.5 mm and is often associated with congenital anomalies (**FIGURE 15.2**).

Retinal and choroidal pathology: Although CT and MRI are not necessarily performed to identify retinal and choroidal detachment, these imaging modalities can sometimes delineate these pathologies and discover associated lesions (**FIGURE 15.3**). In addition, for cases of retinoblastoma, MRI can be used to evaluate for episcleral tumor extension (**FIGURE 15.4**) and the possibility of intracranial "trilateral" retinoblastoma.

Orbital trauma: Eye exams may be difficult to perform in cases of orbital trauma due to periorbital edema and/or patient discomfort. Thus, CT is the gold standard for orbital assessment. Orbital wall fractures are common following trauma, particularly fractures of the orbital floor and medial wall. When there is outward displacement of the orbital wall fragments, these are referred to as blowout fractures. Clinical hallmarks of a blowout fracture include facial swelling, gaze-evoked diplopia (typically worse in upgaze), pain on eye movement, and enophthalmos >2 mm. There can also be hypoesthesia of cranial nerve V2 due to injury to the infraorbital canal. Orbital fractures may require surgical intervention, especially if there is entrapment of the extraocular muscles in the setting of gaze restriction (**FIGURE 15.5**). Inferior rectus entrapment due to orbital floor fracture is the most common. Besides fracture, hemorrhage and globe injury can also be depicted on CT (**FIGURE 15.6**). Penetrating orbital trauma may be accompanied by emphysema or retained foreign bodies (**FIGURES 15.7** and **15.8**).

Sinusitis and preseptal versus *orbital cellulitis* (Chapter 9): The orbital septum acts as an anterior barrier to the orbit. The septum extends from the orbital rims and through the eyelids. Any infection anterior to the septum is considered preseptal cellulitis, whereas infection behind the septum is considered orbital cellulitis, a much more concerning diagnosis due to the possibilities of vision

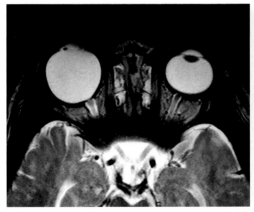 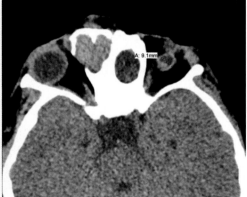

FIGURE 15.2 (Left) Axial T2-weighted MRI shows marked enlargement of the right globe (buphthalmos) related to severely increased intraocular pressure. (Right) Microphthalmia of the left globe in a patient with Bosma arhinia microphthalmia syndrome, a congenital syndrome characterized by nose and eye abnormalities. (Image credit: Dr Daniel T. Ginat, MD.)

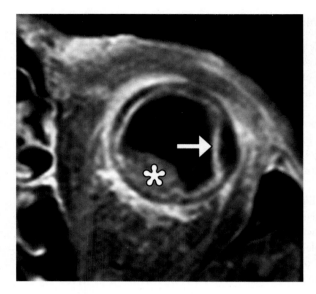

FIGURE 15.3 Axial postcontrast T1-weighted MRI shows choroidal detachment (arrow) and an intraocular metastasis (*) in a patient with head and neck cancer. (Image credit: Dr Daniel T. Ginat, MD.)

loss from optic nerve compression and retro-orbital, intracranial extension of the infection. In cases of periorbital cellulitis, imaging is useful to assess whether the infection is confined preseptally or if there is also postseptal involvement, as well as to identify a potential source of the infection, such as sinusitis. CT is particularly suitable for evaluating the sinonasal cavities, in which acute sinusitis can manifest as mucosal thickening and fluid. CT is useful to look for abscess formation in cases of orbital cellulitis (**FIGURE 15.9**), which should be surgically drained as part of management. Otherwise, MRI is suitable for evaluating intracranial and intraorbital extension of infection from invasive fungal sinusitis, in which the inflammatory changes can be subtle (**FIGURE 15.10**). As always, a clinical

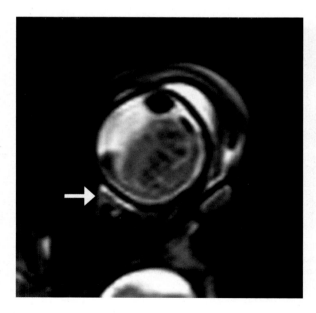

FIGURE 15.4 Axial fat-suppressed T2-weighted MRI shows a large intraocular retinoblastoma with extrascleral extension (arrow). (Image credit: Dr Daniel T. Ginat, MD.)

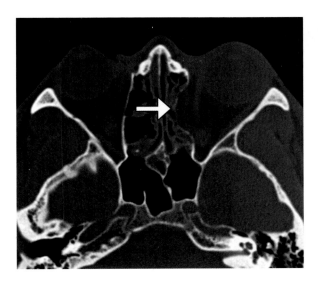

FIGURE 15.5 Axial CT image shows a chronic left medial orbital wall blowout fracture (arrow) with associated enophthalmos. (Image credit: Dr Daniel T. Ginat, MD.)

ophthalmological exam should be correlated with imaging findings, looking for clinical evidence that differentiates preseptal from orbital cellulitis.

Lesions of the lacrimal glands and drainage system: The lacrimal gland is situated in the superotemporal aspect of the orbit and normally measures up to 20 mm in length and 5 mm in width in adults. Enlargement of the lacrimal gland can be focal or diffuse and caused by neoplasm, infection, or inflammatory conditions (**FIGURE 15.11**). CT scan is primarily for screening and visualization of the lacrimal gland, whereas MRI is particularly useful for distinguishing the fluid-filled lacrimal duct from neoplasm (**FIGURE 15.12**).

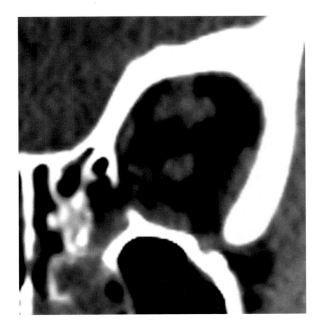

FIGURE 15.6 Coronal CT image shows a left medial orbital wall blowout fracture with medial rectus entrapment. This patient would have difficulty in adduction and potentially upgaze, as well as pain on eye movement. (Image credit: Dr Daniel T. Ginat, MD.)

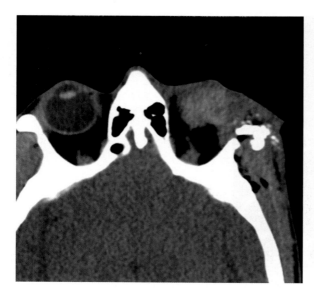

FIGURE 15.7 Axial CT image of left orbital trauma with left periorbital swelling, left lateral orbital wall fracture, intraocular hemorrhage, and globe rupture. (Image credit: Dr Daniel T. Ginat, MD.)

Thyroid eye disease versus *orbital inflammation* (Chapter 6): The extraocular muscles normally range in size from 2 to 5 mm in cross-sectional width. Enlargement of the extraocular muscles can result from neoplasm, inflammation, traumatic edema or hemorrhage, or thyroid eye disease. In thyroid eye disease specifically, there is a predilection for the inferior, medial, and superior rectus muscles, respectively, often with hypoattenuation of the enlarged muscle belly, and sparing of the muscle tendons on CT (**FIGURE 15.13**). In contrast, the extraocular muscles in cases of rheumatic orbitopathy and orbital pseudotumor (also known as idiopathic orbital inflammatory syndrome) tend to be associated with diffuse muscle thickening and surrounding orbital inflammation (**FIGURE 15.14**).

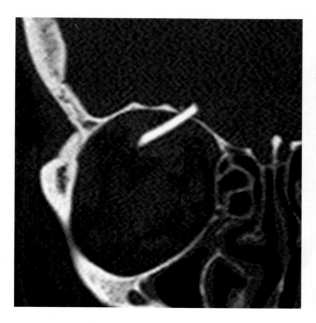

FIGURE 15.8 Coronal CT image shows a foreign body in the right upper orbit with intracranial extension through the superior orbital wall. (Image credit: Dr Daniel T. Ginat, MD.)

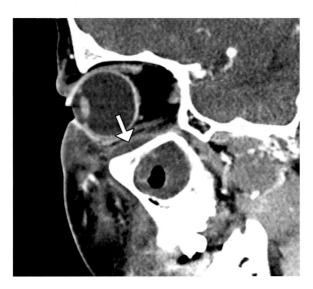

FIGURE 15.9 Sagittal CT image shows inferior periorbital cellulitis, an inferior orbital subperiosteal abscess (arrow), and maxillary sinusitis. Given the abscess posterior to the septum, this represents orbital cellulitis, likely originating from sinusitis. (Image credit: Dr Daniel T. Ginat, MD.)

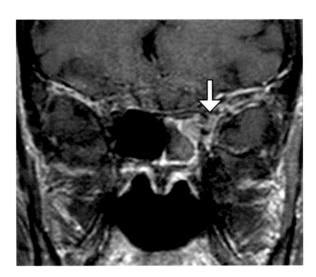

FIGURE 15.10 The patient has a history of diabetes mellitus and recent left eye surgery, and presents with headache and visual disturbance from orbital apex syndrome in the setting of invasive fungal sinusitis. Coronal fat-suppressed postcontrast T1-weighted MRI shows enhancement in the left orbital apex (arrow) and adjacent sphenoid sinus. (Image credit: Dr Daniel T. Ginat, MD.)

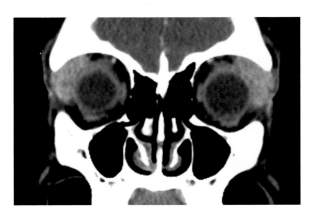

FIGURE 15.11 Coronal CT image shows diffuse enlargement of the bilateral lacrimal glands in a patient with sarcoidosis. (Image credit: Dr Daniel T. Ginat, MD.)

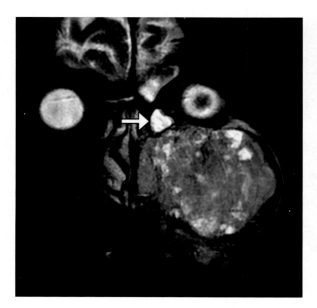

FIGURE 15.12 Coronal T2-weighted MRI shows a large left sinonasal tumor that obstructs the left nasolacrimal duct with dilatation of the left lacrimal sac (arrow). (Image credit: Dr Daniel T. Ginat, MD.)

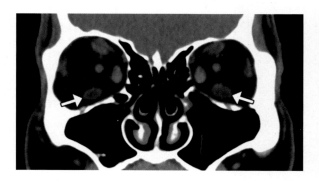

FIGURE 15.13 Coronal CT image depicts swelling of the bilateral inferior rectus muscles with hypoattenuation (arrows) in a patient with thyroid eye disease. There is also relatively mild swelling of the medial and superior rectus muscles. (Image credit: Dr Daniel T. Ginat, MD.)

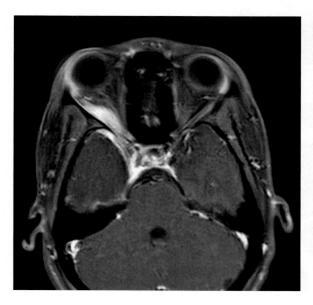

FIGURE 15.14 Axial CT image portrays right lateral rectus muscle swelling from idiopathic orbital pseudotumor with involvement of the right cavernous sinus (Tolosa-Hunt syndrome) in a patient with right cranial nerve III palsy and right peri-orbital and temporal pain. (Image credit: Dr Daniel T. Ginat, MD.)

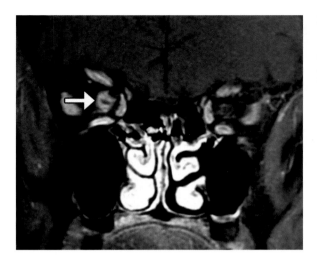

FIGURE 15.15 Coronal fat-suppressed postcontrast T1-weighted MRI shows an enhancing mass surrounding the right optic nerve (arrow), which corresponds to a meningioma. (Image credit: Dr Daniel T. Ginat, MD.)

The tendons are often inflamed in these cases, differentiating them from thyroid eye disease, and other orbital contents, such as the lacrimal gland, may also show signs of inflammation.

Optic nerve and nerve sheath lesions (Chapter 11 and 12): MRI can be useful for localizing tumors of the optic nerve sheath versus optic nerve, such as meningiomas and gliomas, respectively (**FIGURES 15.15** and **15.16**). Otherwise, MRI can assess for abnormality of the optic nerve in the setting of optic neuritis, which can be caused by multiple sclerosis, neuromyelitis optica (Devic disease), toxic substance exposure, systemic lupus erythematosus, and sarcoidosis, for example. MRI typically demonstrates contrast enhancement of the affected optic nerves and can reveal accompanying lesions in the brain, such as demyelinating plaques in the white matter (**FIGURE 15.17**). MRI imaging is not often used to evaluate cases of other noninflammatory optic neuropathies, such as glaucoma or ischemic optic neuropathy, in which only mild thinning of nerve size and mildly

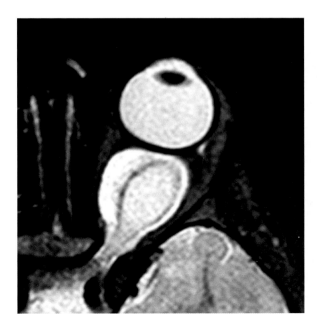

FIGURE 15.16 Axial T2-weighted MRI shows enlargement and high T2 of the left optic nerve that corresponds to an optic nerve glioma in a patient with neurofibromatosis type 2. (Image credit: Dr Daniel T. Ginat, MD.)

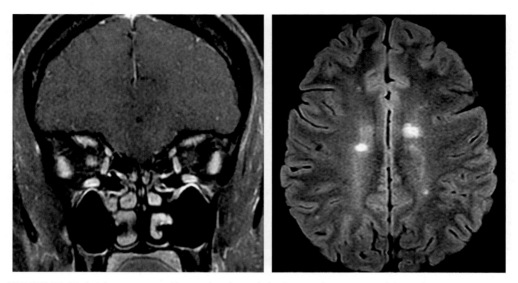

FIGURE 15.17 Axial postcontrast T1-weighted MRI (left) shows enhancement of the right optic nerve, and the axial T2-weighted FLAIR (fluid-attenuated inversion recovery) (right) shows demyelinating white matter lesions in the brain in a patient with multiple sclerosis. (Image credit: Dr Daniel T. Ginat, MD.)

increased T2W signal might be apparent (**FIGURE 15.18**). Nevertheless, imaging can be helpful in cases of unclear clinical diagnosis to help differentiate inflammatory from noninflammatory optic neuropathy. Neuroimaging is also useful for evaluating patients with papilledema. While the orbital imaging can demonstrate optic nerve bulging and optic nerve sheath dilatation, imaging is primarily indicated to help identify underlying intracranial causes, such as cerebral venous sinus thrombosis, intracranial tumors, or pseudotumor cerebri (**FIGURES 15.19** and **15.20**). These can be accompanied by secondary signs of elevated intracranial pressure such as hydrocephalus, a partially empty

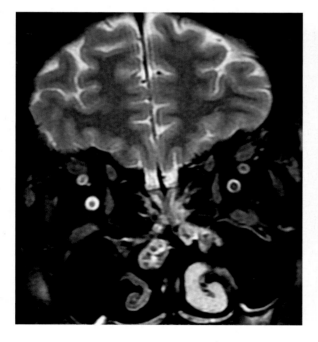

FIGURE 15.18 Coronal T2-weighted MRI shows atrophy and mild T2 hyperintensity of the right optic nerve associated with glaucoma, but normal left optic nerve. (Image credit: Dr Daniel T. Ginat, MD.)

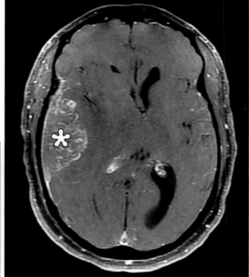

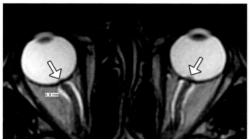

FIGURE 15.19 Axial T2-weighted MRI (left) shows dilatation of the bilateral optic nerve sheaths and edema of the optic nerves (arrows). Axial postcontrast T1-weighted MRI (right) shows a large right cerebral convexity meningioma (*) with associated midline shift and entrapment of the left lateral ventricle, indicating increased intracranial pressure. (Image credit: Dr Daniel T. Ginat, MD.)

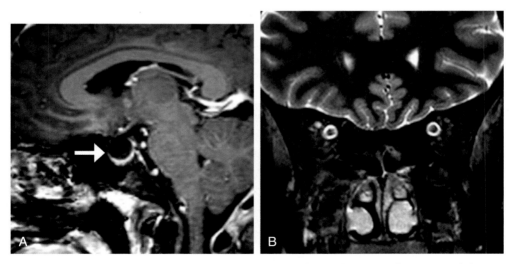

FIGURE 15.20 Sagittal T1-weighted MRI (A) shows an enlarged partially empty sella (arrow) and the coronal T2-weighted MRI of the orbits (B) shows dilatation of the optic nerve sheaths in a patient with pseudotumor cerebri. (Image credit: Dr Daniel T. Ginat, MD.)

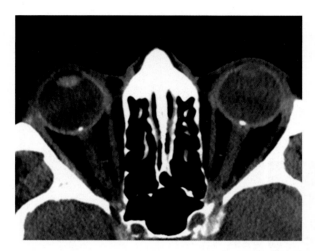

FIGURE 15.21 Axial CT image shows punctate calcifications at the bilateral optic nerve heads related to drusen. (Image credit: Dr Daniel T. Ginat, MD.)

sella turcica ("empty sella sign"), and narrowing of the transverse venous sinuses. Otherwise, in cases of pseudopapilledema in the setting of optic disc drusen, CT can reveal corresponding punctate calcifications (**FIGURE 15.21**).

IMAGING OF SELLAR, SUPRASELLAR, AND CAVERNOUS SINUS ABNORMALITIES

Pituitary tumors (Chapter 6): Large pituitary tumors can impinge upon the optic chiasm, leading to bitemporal hemianopsia. Since the average distance between the optic chiasm and the pituitary gland is 10 mm, pituitary macroadenomas are defined as lesions greater than 10 mm in size and are more likely to impact vision. Lesions <10 mm in size are considered microadenomas and are less likely to impact vision. High-resolution coronal T2-weighted MRI images are useful for delineating the relationship of the tumors with respect to the optic chiasm and nerves (**FIGURE 15.22**). While pituitary macroadenomas are more common in adults, craniopharyngiomas should be considered as a possibility for sellar and suprasellar tumors with a mixture of cystic and solid components, particularly in children (**FIGURE 15.23**).

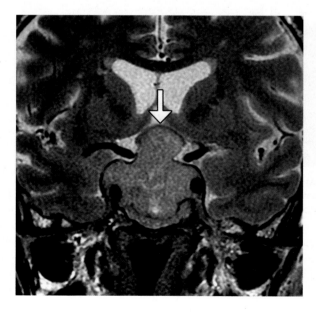

FIGURE 15.22 Coronal T2-weighted MRI shows a pituitary macroadenoma with suprasellar extension compressing the optic chiasm (arrow). Note the homogenous solid characteristics. (Image credit: Dr Daniel T. Ginat, MD.)

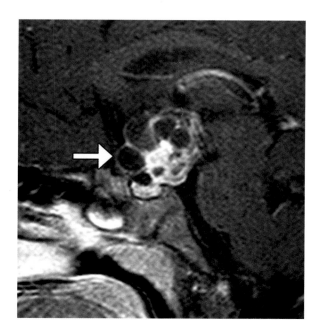

FIGURE 15.23 Sagittal postcontrast T1-weighted MRI of a large suprasellar cra-niopharyngioma with solid and cystic components (arrow) in a child with gradual vision loss. (Image credit: Dr Daniel T. Ginat, MD.)

Cavernous Sinus lesions

The cavernous sinus contains a venous plexus, internal carotid artery, and cranial nerves III, IV, V1, V2, and VI. A variety of abnormalities can occur within the cavernous sinuses, including infectious, granulomatous, and inflammatory conditions, neoplasms, and vascular lesions. MRI is particularly useful for depicting cavernous lesions in the setting of esotropia (**FIGURE 15.24**). Otherwise, vascular imaging is more appropriate for evaluating patients with suspected carotid cavernous fistulas (**FIGURE 15.25**).

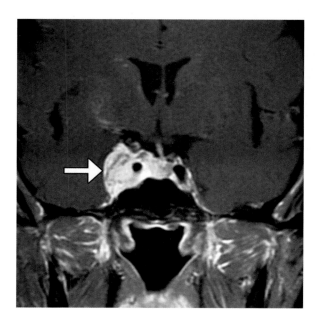

FIGURE 15.24 Coronal T1-weighted MRI shows a right cavernous sinus meningioma (arrow). (Image credit: Dr Daniel T. Ginat, MD.)

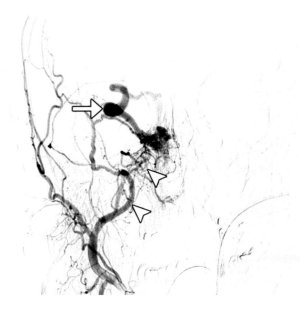

FIGURE 15.25 Frontal digital subtraction angiogram shows fistulous connection between the external carotid artery and cavernous sinus (arrowheads) with early opacification and dilatation of the right superior ophthalmic vein (arrow). (Image credit: Dr Daniel T. Ginat, MD.)

BRAIN ABNORMALITIES

Ischemic cerebral or brainstem infarction (Chapter 12): MRI is the gold standard for identifying cerebrovascular infarction, which can be associated with visual field loss when the occipital lobes are involved or with diplopia from oculomotor abnormalities when the brainstem is involved (**FIGURES 15.26** and **15.27**). Acute infarcts display restricted diffusion on DWI, while chronic infarcts appear as encephalomalacia.

    Intracranial hemorrhage (Chapter 12): CT imaging without contrast is the modality of choice for evaluating suspected acute intracranial hemorrhage (**FIGURE 15.28**). Acute hemorrhage is typically hyperattenuating on CT, and the attenuation normally decreases over time.

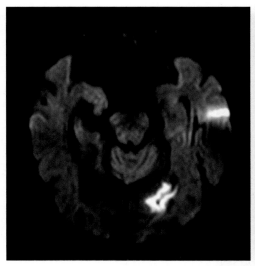
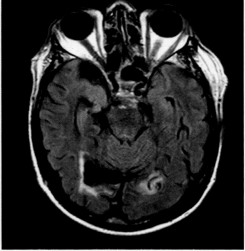

FIGURE 15.26 Axial diffusion-weighted image (DWI) (left) and T2-weighted FLAIR (fluid-attenuated inversion recovery) (right) MRI show an acute infarct in the left occipital lobe and a chronic infarct in the right occipital lobe in a patient with cortical blindness. (Image credit: Dr Daniel T. Ginat, MD.)

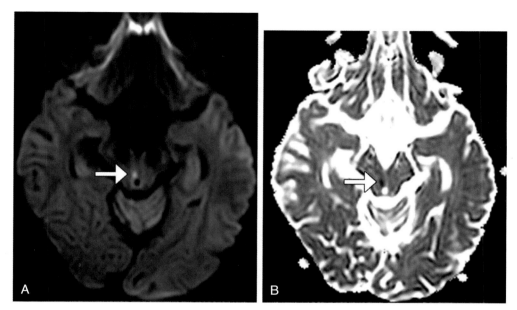

FIGURE 15.27 Axial diffusion-weighted images (DWI) (A) and ADC (apparent diffusion coefficient) map (B) show a punctate acute infarct (arrows) in a patient with internuclear ophthalmoplegia (INO). (Image credit: Dr Daniel T. Ginat, MD.)

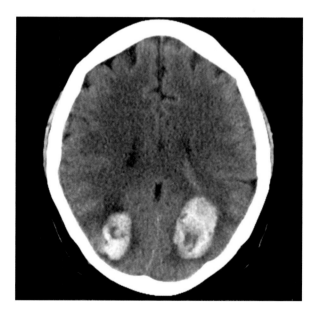

FIGURE 15.28 Axial CT image shows acute hemorrhage of occipital lobe metastases bilaterally. (Image credit: Dr Daniel T. Ginat, MD.)

BIBLIOGRAPHY

1. Expert Panel on Neurologic Imaging. ACR appropriateness Criteria* orbits vision and visual loss. *J Am Coll Radiol.* 2018;15(5S):S116-S131. http://www.mrisafety.com/.

2. Weber AL, Sabates NR. Survey of CT and MR imaging of the orbit.*Eur J Radiol.* 1996;22(1):42-52. doi:10.1016/0720-048x(96)00737-1.

3. Szatmáry G. Imaging of the orbit. *Neurol Clin.* 2009;27(1):251-284. doi:10.1016/j.ncl.2008.09.008.

4. Hesselink JR, Karampekios S. Normal computed tomography and magnetic resonance imaging anatomy of the globe, orbit, and visual pathways. *Neuroimaging Clin N Am*. 1996;6(1):15-27.

5. Kubal WS. Imaging of orbital trauma. *Radiographics*. 2008;28(6):1729-1739. doi:10.1148/rg.286085523.

6. Nguyen VD, Singh AK, Altmeyer WB, Tantiwongkosi B. Demystifying orbital emergencies: a pictorial review. *Radiographics*. 2017;37(3):947-962. doi:10.1148/rg.2017160119.

7. Kruger JM, Cestari DM, Cunnane MB. Systematic approaches for reviewing neuro-imaging scans in ophthalmology. *Digit J Ophthalmol*. 2017;23(3):50-59. doi:10.5693/djo.03.2016.05.001.

8. Learned KO, Nasseri F, Mohan S. Imaging of the postoperative orbit. *Neuroimaging Clin N Am*. 2015;25(3):457-476. doi:10.1016/j.nic.2015.05.008.

9. Toosy AT, Mason DF, Miller DH. Optic neuritis. *Lancet Neurol*. 2014;13(1):83-99. doi:10.1016/S1474-4422(13)70259-X.

10. Nadarajah J, Madhusudhan KS, Yadav AK, Chandrashekhara SH, Kumar A, Gupta AK. MR imaging of cavernous sinus lesions: pictorial review. *J Neuroradiol*. 2015;42(6):305-319.

Index